The Fevered Fight

The Fevered Fight

A Medical History of the American Revolution

1775–1783

Martin R. Howard

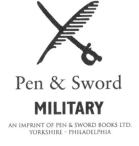

Pen & Sword

MILITARY

AN IMPRINT OF PEN & SWORD BOOKS LTD.
YORKSHIRE - PHILADELPHIA

First published in Great Britain in 2023 by
Pen & Sword Military
An imprint of
Pen & Sword Books Ltd
Yorkshire - Philadelphia

ISBN 978 1 39908 482 6

Typeset in INDIA By IMPEC eSolutions
Printed and bound in England
By CPI UK Ltd.

Pen & Sword Books Ltd. incorporates the Imprints of Pen & Sword Archaeology,
Atlas, Aviation, Battleground, Discovery, Family History, History, Maritime,
Military, Naval, Politics, Railways, Select, Transport, True Crime, Fiction,
Frontline Books, Leo Cooper, Praetorian Press, Seaforth Publishing,
Wharncliffe and White Owl.

For a complete list of Pen & Sword titles please contact

PEN & SWORD BOOKS LIMITED
47 Church Street, Barnsley, South Yorkshire, S70 2AS, England
E-mail: enquiries@pen-and-sword.co.uk
Website: www.pen-and-sword.co.uk

or

PEN AND SWORD BOOKS
1950 Lawrence Rd, Havertown, PA 19083, USA
E-mail: uspen-and-sword@casematepublishers.com
Website: www.penandswordbooks.com

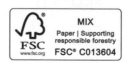

Contents

Acknowledgements

I am very grateful to Matthew Spring who generously provided me with a copy of Thompson Forster's journal. The expert staff at The National Archives and National Army Museum in London have provided valuable assistance in the search for archival material. The National Anthropological Archives at the Smithsonian Institute and the Guilford Courthouse National Military Park have given kind permission for the use of illustrations. Thanks to Rupert Harding and Amy Jordan at Pen & Sword.

List of Colour Illustrations

List of Black and White Illustrations

List of Maps

Major Events of the American Revolutionary War 1775–1783

1775

April 19	First shots at Lexington and Concord
April	Start of siege of Boston
May 10	Rebels capture Fort Ticonderoga
June 16	Washington appointed commander-in-chief of Continental Army
June 17	Battle of Bunker Hill
September	American invasion of Canada
December 9	Battle of Great Bridge
December 31	Failed American assault on Quebec

1776

March 4	British evacuation of Boston
May (–July)	American retreat from Quebec
June 28	Battle of Sullivan's Island (Charleston)
July 4	Declaration of Independence
August 27	Battle of Long Island
September 16	Battle of Harlem Heights
October 11	Battle of Valcour Island
October 29	Battle of White Plains
November 16	British capture Fort Washington
December 26	First Battle of Trenton

1777

January 2	Second Battle of Trenton
January 3	Battle of Princeton
July 7	Battle of Hubbardton
July 8	Battle of Skenesborough
August 6	Battle of Oriskany
August 16	Battle of Bennington
September 11	Battle of Brandywine
September 19	Battle of Freeman's Farm
September 20	Battle of Paoli
September 26	British occupation of Philadelphia
October 4	Battle of Germantown
October 7	Battle of Bemis Heights
October 17	Burgoyne's surrender at Saratoga

1778

February	France signs friendship treaty with rebels
June	British evacuation of Philadelphia
June 28	Battle of Monmouth
August 29	American/French attack on Newport (Rhode Island)
December 29	British capture of Savannah

1779

16 July	Battle of Stony Point
July 24 (–August)	Penobscot Expedition
August (–Sept.)	Sullivan Expedition
October 18	American/French attack on Savannah

1780

March 29 (–May)	Siege of Charleston
May 29	Battle of Waxhaws
July	Rochambeau and troops arrive at Rhode Island
August 16	Battle of Camden
October 7	Battle of King's Mountain

1781

January 17	Battle of Cowpens
March 15	Battle of Guilford Courthouse
April 25	Battle of Hobkirk's Hill
May	Washington and Rochambeau meet at Wethersfield
September 5	Battle of the Virginia Capes (Chesapeake)
September 8	Battle of Eutaw Springs
September 28	Start of siege of Yorktown
October 19	Cornwallis's surrender at Yorktown

1782

November	Preliminary articles of peace in Paris

1783

April	Cessation of hostilities agreed
September	Treaty of Paris
November	Final British evacuation of New York

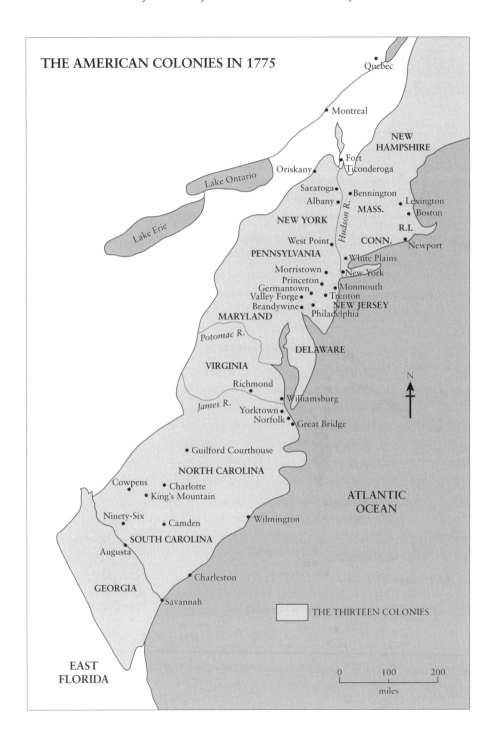

THE AMERICAN COLONIES IN 1775

Quebec

Montreal

NEW HAMPSHIRE

Lake Ontario

Fort Ticonderoga

Oriskany

Saratoga • Bennington • Lexington
Albany • MASS. • Boston

NEW YORK

Hudson R.

R.I.

West Point CONN. • Newport

PENNSYLVANIA White Plains

Morristown • New York
Princeton •
Germantown • Monmouth
Valley Forge • Trenton
Brandywine • NEW JERSEY
Philadelphia

Lake Erie

MARYLAND

Potomac R.

DELAWARE

VIRGINIA

Richmond

James R. Williamsburg
Yorktown •
Norfolk • Great Bridge

• Guilford Courthouse

NORTH CAROLINA

Cowpens • Charlotte
• King's Mountain

Ninety-Six
• Camden

Wilmington

ATLANTIC OCEAN

SOUTH CAROLINA

Augusta

• Charleston

GEORGIA

Savannah

THE THIRTEEN COLONIES

EAST FLORIDA

N

0   100   200
miles

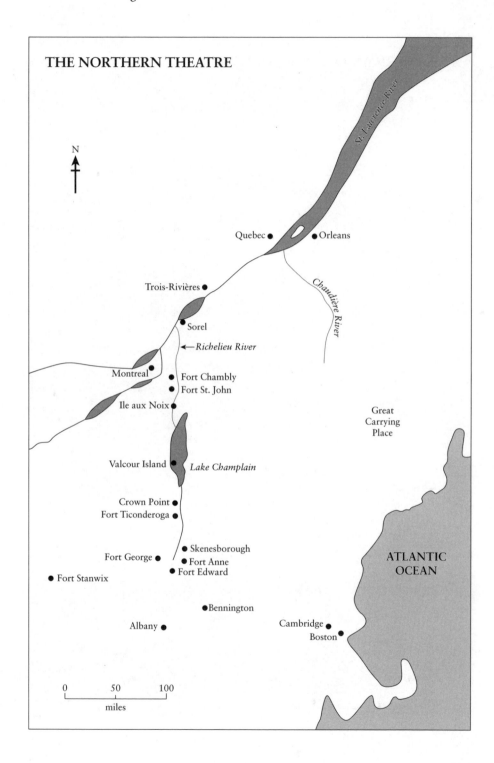

THE NORTHERN THEATRE

N

St. Laurence River

Quebec ● ● Orleans

Chaudière River

Trois-Rivières ●

● Sorel

← *Richelieu River*

Montreal ●
● Fort Chambly
● Fort St. John

Ile aux Noix ●

Great
Carrying
Place

Valcour Island ● *Lake Champlain*

Crown Point ●
Fort Ticonderoga ●

● Skenesborough
Fort George ● ● Fort Anne
● Fort Edward

● Fort Stanwix

ATLANTIC
OCEAN

●Bennington

Cambridge ●
Albany ● Boston ●

0   50   100

miles

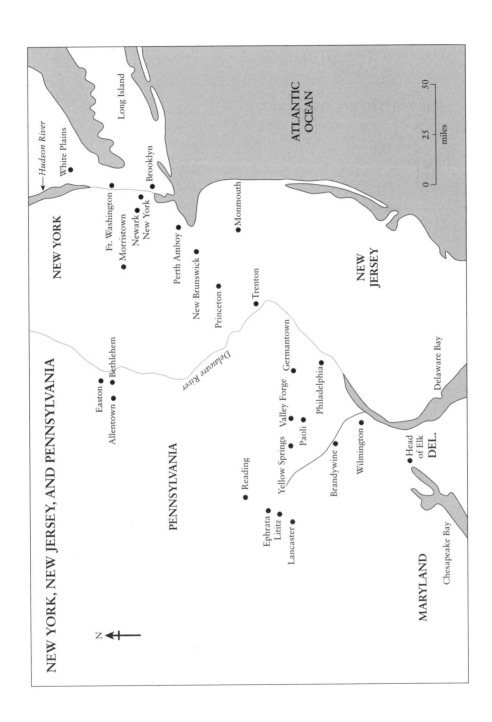

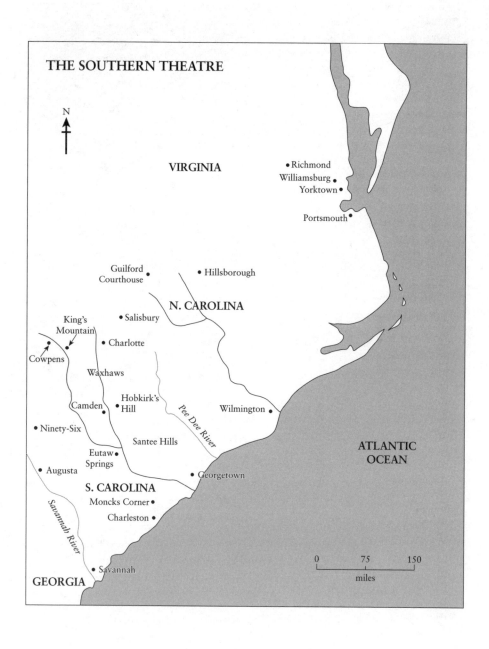

THE SOUTHERN THEATRE

N

VIRGINIA

• Richmond
Williamsburg •
Yorktown •

Portsmouth •

Guilford •
Courthouse

• Hillsborough

N. CAROLINA

King's
Mountain

• Salisbury

Cowpens

• Charlotte

Waxhaws

Hobkirk's
Camden • Hill

Wilmington •

• Ninety-Six

Santee Hills

Pee Dee River

• Augusta

Eutaw •
Springs

• Georgetown

ATLANTIC
OCEAN

S. CAROLINA

Moncks Corner •

Charleston •

Savannah River

0   75   150

miles

• Savannah

GEORGIA

Medicine and War

Chapter 1

Civilian and Military Medicine on the Eve of the Revolution

On mules and dogs the infection first began,
And last the baneful arrows fixed in Man.
Homer, The Iliad, Book One

When Cotton Mather of Massachusetts died in 1728, he was survived by only two of his fifteen children.[1] This was not exceptional. More than 85 percent of babies in early South Carolina died before reaching the age of two.[2] By the 1780s in Philadelphia, it was still the case that 50 per cent of all deaths occurred under the age of ten years. The most dangerous decades were the first, the third and the fourth. A typical Massachusetts man aged twenty years could expect to live another thirty-four years.[3] This was better than his cousin in the slums of London who, at the outset of the American Revolution, could expect five years less.[4] Due to the risks of pregnancy and the complications of childbirth women often only lived into their forties. The wealthy of all societies, with their access to better nutrition and medical care, might live longer, but they were not spared life's fragility. Martha Washington knew from personal experience that 'sickness is to be expected'.[5]

In Britain, the medical profession was divided into three parts — the physicians, surgeons, and apothecaries. Physicians were the elite, usually having a university degree and often limiting their practice to the upper classes. Surgeons were trained by apprenticeship. Their role was mainly to administer first aid for emergencies and their status was low. The apothecaries were also regarded as inferior to the physicians, their apprenticeship enabling them to sell and prescribe drugs and to act as general practitioners to the wider population.[6]

Within London and a few miles around, some regulatory control was exerted by the College of Physicians, the Corporation of Surgeons, and the Society of Apothecaries. The provinces were a different world, with many 'medical practitioners' having no legal title to practise either medicine or surgery. At the time of the American Revolution there were more than 4,000 medical men resident in England and Wales. These included 149 physicians, 274 surgeons, and 351 apothecaries in London.[7] When George III was crowned in 1760, there were seven general hospitals, two asylums and six special hospitals in the capital and seventeen institutions in the provinces.[8] Conditions on the wards were usually atrocious with mortality rates between 6 and 13 per cent.[9]

Unsurprisingly, colonial medicine had much in common with the British system. The earliest American doctors to arrive from Europe were probably a small number of English physicians who came to the first settlements. In Virginia, there were likely only three or four such men prior to 1700 and over the next century only one in nine Virginia practitioners received any formal training.[10] The British occupational distinction in the hierarchy of physicians, surgeons and apothecaries was blurred, with physicians also performing surgery and dispensing drugs.[11] Philip Cash describes five classes of medical men, the vast majority receiving their training under the apprenticeship system. This education was often extremely limited, with many failing to master the most basic skills.[12] An observer in 1750 complained that '[q]uacks abound [here] like locusts in Egypt'.[13]

There was, however, an emerging expertise in American medicine on the eve of the war with Britain. Of the 3,500 legitimate medical practitioners in the thirteen colonies in 1775, no fewer than 400 had medical degrees. At home, these were conferred by King's College in New York and the College of Philadelphia. Some had travelled to prestigious European medical schools, especially Edinburgh, where 200 Americans had attended by the end of the eighteenth century. The most fortunate were able to walk the wards of the Pennsylvania Hospital. This was founded in 1751 and was the first institution in the country recognisable as a modern hospital. A similar facility opened in New York in 1771.[14] Although they provided valuable training opportunities and undermined local quacks, these first American hospitals were no better than their equivalents in London. A visitor to Philadelphia in 1777 saw, 'a dreadful Scene of human Wretchedness. The Weakness and Languor, the Distress and Misery, of these Objects is a truly Woeful Sight'.[15] Between 1753 and 1777 about 12 per cent of the patients died despite the exclusion of those with terminal disease or infection.[16]

Thus, American medicine at the outset of the Revolution was not static. Some improvements were being made in education, regulation and the cross-fertilisation of ideas. More courses were on offer, there was easier access to European books and journals, and more autopsies were being performed.[17] The War provided the catalyst for further medical professionalization, but it is also true that many American doctors carried the torch of revolution. Twenty-one physicians were members of the First Provincial Congress of Massachusetts and 1,400 doctors volunteered for the army and navy.[18] Some served as officers of all ranks up to major-general.[19] Benjamin Rush, arguably the most distinguished American physician of the eighteenth century, captured the mood after Lexington; 'The first gun that was fired at an American cut the cord that had tied the two countries together'.[20]

The term 'fever' was central to the classification of diseases in the eighteenth century. James Lind defined it as 'an indisposition of the body attended commonly with an increase of its heat'.[21] This is recognisable today, but at the time of the Revolution fever was regarded as a disease rather than a symptom. It has been estimated that it caused 80 per cent of all deaths and the medical fight against it might be compared with the ongoing battle against cancer.[22] It was classified according to its periodicity. There were 'intermittent fevers' characterised by paroxysms and complete remissions. In 'remittent fevers' the remissions were less complete and in 'continuous fevers' there was no respite.[23] These broad terms were widely applied but there were variations and other factors were considered including season and location. Sir John Pringle, the great authority on army diseases of the period, divided fevers into inflammatory, bilious and putrid types. He also emphasised that different disorders tended to occur during the summer or the winter or in camp or garrison.[24] It is often possible to identify modern disease entities from this contemporary nomenclature. Intermittent (or intermitting) and remittent (remitting) fevers were commonly malaria, while continuous fevers associated with a specific location (e.g. hospital) were likely to be typhus or perhaps typhoid.

The British population was afflicted by a litany of potentially life-shortening diseases including respiratory infections, typhus, cholera, smallpox, malaria, tuberculosis and dysentery. In civilian America the greatest fear was of epidemics of yellow fever, smallpox and diphtheria but colonial health was most affected by diseases which occurred relentlessly year after year such as dysentery, malaria, and respiratory infections. Typhus was mainly limited to the port cities and typhoid to the northern settlements. Measles, whooping cough and mumps were all present but not a great cause of mortality. American Indian communities were especially susceptible to smallpox and influenza.[25]

The cause of these disorders was little understood but there were two fundamental theories, both of which attracted supporters. Many believed that diseases were caused by 'miasma' or 'miasmata', invisible poisons which were exuded from rotting organic material, the soil and standing water.[26] In his account of the diseases afflicting the British Army in Germany in the decade prior to the Revolution, Donald Monro attributed an outbreak of dysentery to the troops 'being often exposed to the putrid Steams of dead Horses, of the Privies, and other corrupted Animal and Vegetable substances after their juices had been highly exalted by the Heat of Summer'.[27] Robert Jackson, a British army doctor in the American Revolutionary War, explained that malaria was caused by the exhalations from the swamps and moist ground of the southern colonies; 'Daily experience still proves it'.[28]

Others were less convinced. Although there was no concept of bacterial or viral infections or the roles of insects and rodents as disease vectors, the contagion theory was gaining ground. Benjamin Franklin wrote to Benjamin Rush in 1773 expressing the view that influenza 'may possibly spread by Contagion as well by a particular Quality of Air'. He had seen that the disease was passed from person to person in enclosed spaces.[29] Three years later in Canada, Thomas Dickson Reide, surgeon's mate to the 29th Regiment, had no hesitation in blaming contagion alone as the source of intermittent fever.[30]

As neither theory explained all circumstances, even the most intelligent medical men resorted to fanciful speculation. Jackson asserted that the number of sick soldiers in his care doubled in the period approaching a new or full moon.[31] Conversely, doctors in civilian and military life recognised real associations between demographic factors and disease. Benjamin Rush, reflecting on the causes of disease in the American Continental Army, commented that it was always healthier on the move than when in camp, that young men under twenty years old were most vulnerable to camp diseases, and that the recruits from the American south were more sickly than their northern and eastern compatriots. Black soldiers were also unhealthier than the men of European origin in the ranks. He noted that fevers could be spread by clothes and blankets.[32]

Unfortunately, the treatment of disease was led more by the archaic medical theories of antiquity than by more enlightened considerations. In the mid-eighteenth century it was still widely believed that the state of disease was a disturbance in the balance of the body's humours (phlegm, blood, black bile, yellow bile). This perceived disequilibrium provided the rationale for the 'anti-inflammatory' or 'antiphlogistic' regimes which were ubiquitous. The combination of bleeding by the lancet or other means, drenching in cold water, blistering, and the administration of drugs such as purgatives (designed to induce diarrhoea), emetics (to induce nausea and vomiting), and agents producing profound sweating and salivation formed the mainstay of treatment.[33] Changes in diet and vegetable drugs were probably mostly harmless but this cannot be said of the minerals (e.g. mercury, antimony) which were also advocated. The 'biologicals' such as insect parts and excreta were presumably judged to be potent due to their repulsiveness.[34] All these agents were listed in contemporary formularies, the *Lititz Pharmacopoeia* of 1778 being the first published in America.[35]

Such therapies were only likely to make the patient more miserable and even shorten life, but they were widely accepted in civilian and military practice. Forward-thinking Americans such as George Washington, Abigail Adams and Franklin all recommended bleeding and blistering for their sick family members.[36] Rush supported the use of emetics, laxatives and blisters.[37] Many memoirists of the Revolutionary War testify to the restorative effects of a 'puke' or the passage of copious stools. Any perceived benefit was probably a placebo effect or a spontaneous recovery, but the multiplicity of interventions meant that even when the patient's symptoms improved it was difficult to know which part of the therapy had been active. Thomas Dickson Reide admitted that 'no two [medical] authors agree in the same opinion, or mode of treatment; yet almost every one points out what he terms a *successful method of cure*, and recommends it with enthusiasm'.[38] That this scepticism was shared by some soldiers is obvious from the following guidance to army doctors taken from the satirical *Advice to the Officers of the British Army* published in 1782.

> 'Whenever you are ignorant of a soldier's complaint, you should first take a little blood from him, and then give him an emetic and a cathartic — to which you will add a blister. This will serve, at least, to diminish the number of your patients.'[39]

While a true understanding of the causation of disease and its effective treatment was held back by the entrenched views of antiquity, there were preventive

advances in ~~preventative~~ measures. French and British authors observed that the greatest loss of life occurred among the children of the poor. Improvements in infant hygiene led to a gradual fall in mortality in the years after 1750.[40] As we will see, there was increasing emphasis on the importance of hygiene in armies. Beyond this, there were the more specific interventions of quarantine and inoculation.

Quarantine was used in the British Army both routinely to prevent the spread of diseases from military transports and to counter the dissemination of particular disorders such as smallpox.[41] The author of the *Military Guide* of 1781 makes this explicit.

> 'When any man is taken ill of the smallpox, or any other pestilential disorder, he should immediately, upon the discovery of this disease, be sent to a private and remote lodgings as can be had; and all soldiers prevented from visiting him, lest the visitors catch such distempers, and communicate the infection.'[42]

Americans used quarantine to fight smallpox outbreaks. Sufferers might be sent to 'lonely house[s] in the middle of the woods' or even offshore.[43] Johann Conrad Dohla, a Hessian soldier in British service, was on Rhode Island in 1778. He noted that a small island below Newport was called Pest or Smallpox Island (now Coasters Harbor Island); 'The people and children who have smallpox are sent there, because this is considered a contagious and most dirty disease'.[44]

Vaccination for smallpox using cowpox was not given before the end of the eighteenth century but inoculation was already well known in Europe. It was probably first employed in the American colonies in Boston in 1721 when puritan minister Cotton Mather convinced Zabdiel Boylston to try the operation. The live *Variola* virus was deliberately introduced into an incision on the patient's arm or hand. The actual procedure was usually preceded by an unpleasant dietary regimen. After an incubation period, smallpox resulted but this was generally in a much milder form than the naturally contracted disease and lifelong immunity was conferred. Inoculation was not risk-free, but fatality rates were much lower than those encountered in severe epidemics. During the Boston 1721 outbreak, only 2 per cent of the inoculated citizens died.[45] The gruelling and mysterious nature of inoculation made it controversial and there was resistance. The colony of Virginia outlawed it during the Revolution, leading to a robust response from one of the procedure's greatest advocates, George Washington.

> 'Surely the daily instances which present themselves of the amazing benefits of inoculation must make converts of the most rigid opposers and bring repeal of the most impolitic law which restrains it.'[46]

American troops were especially vulnerable to smallpox, many having no previous exposure. Large-scale inoculation of the Continental Army carried real risks, not least that the British might seize the moment to attack. After much deliberation, Washington ordered a mass inoculation in early 1777.[47] Inoculation was also used successfully by the British Army. This might be voluntary or involuntary. General William Howe at the siege of Boston recommended the procedure in those not previously afflicted but he gave his men a choice, whereas General Guy Carleton in Canada made inoculation obligatory in all who had not had smallpox.[48]

The British surgeon Benjamin Gooch, in his surgical textbook of 1767, outlines the reasonable expectations of the patient. The surgeon, according to Gooch, should:

> 'pronounce whether the patient wou'd recover or not; whether the cure would be easy or difficult; if it would prove a short or tedious work; if it would be a perfect or imperfect cure; in which condition he [the patient] might be afterwards.'[49]

From accounts of civilian surgery of the period it seems that such standards were exceptional. The absence of anaesthesia, antisepsis, blood transfusion and antibiotics meant that most civilian surgeons limited themselves to more minor interventions such as the treatment of cuts, abscesses, burns, dislocated joints, and simple fractures. Antiphlogistic measures such as bleeding and purging might be resorted to.[50]

Surgical skill was a rarity, but a few better trained surgeons did attempt more invasive operations. These included trephination (trepanning), amputation, the management of hernias and hydroceles, and lithotomy (the removal of bladder and kidney stones). This level of expertise often emanated from Europe. John Jones was born in Long Island in 1729 and received his medical degree from

Rheims in France. His surgical prowess allowed him to perform lithotomy in only slightly more than a minute. Jones's work, *Plain Concise Practical Remarks in the Treatment of Wounds and Fractures*, was reprinted in 1776 and proved to be of great value to the surgeons of the Continental Army.[51]

On the cusp of the Revolution, experience of military medicine in America was very limited. In eighteenth-century Europe, the speciality was in evolution, with the administration of military medicine increasingly becoming the responsibility of government. This approach acknowledged the special challenges faced by army physicians and surgeons.[52]

The most obvious distinction between civilian and military surgery was the frequency and nature of trauma. At the Battle of Great Bridge in December 1775, a Virginian soldier 'saw the horrors of war in perfection, worse that can be imagin'd; 10 and 12 bullets thro' many; limbs broke in 2 or 3 places; brains turned out. Good God, what a sight!'[53] These wounds were the predictable result of the weaponry used by the armies of the period. The lead musket ball was round, often jagged, and about three quarters of an inch in diameter. When fired at longer ranges, over 200 yards, it might cause a minor injury or be deflected by pieces of equipment or objects in pockets. At medium range, the soft ball tended to flatten on impact, resulting in a large conical-shaped wound. At short range, less than 50 yards, it was capable of breaking limb bones and dislocating joints. John Hunter, the most scientific and original British army surgeon of the eighteenth century, gained his experience as a staff surgeon in the Belle Isle Expedition and in Portugal during the 1760s. He noted that a musket ball at slow velocity was quite likely to change direction in the body. A ball of greater velocity cut through the tissues more like a sharp instrument.[54] Thrusts with sword or bayonet led to penetrating injuries, whereas slashing with a sword caused lacerations.[55]

Artillery most commonly fired roundshot which was likely to kill immediately or cause devastating injuries.[56] At the Battle of White Plains in 1776, Corporal Thomas Sullivan and his comrades were on the receiving end of a British cannonade; 'one [rebel] with his head shot off and between his feet, and the other with the head and half his breast shot off'.[57] British army surgeon John Ranby, whose 1744 text on wound surgery was highly influential, noted that cannon balls caused 'great lacerations of the parts endued with an exquisite sensation. These are ever attended with an excruciating pain'.[58]

There were attempts at classification and prognostication. Jones divided wounds into four types: the incised, the punctured, the lacerated and the contused. He observed that when there was healing, this usually occurred in nine stages culminating in a dry scar.[59] Gooch emphasised the importance of identifying 'mortal' wounds; those which would be fatal in the absence of treatment.[60] Some injuries were mysterious, the most well described being the 'wind-of-ball' phenomenon. American surgeon James Thacher was on the battlefield at Springfield in June 1780: 'It may be considered a singular circumstance that the soldier above mentioned was wounded by the wind of a cannon-ball. His arm was fractured above the elbow without the smallest perceptible injury to his clothes, or contusion or discolouration of the skin'.[61]

War magnified the difficulties of surgery. Casualties of the Revolutionary War all too often had an inappropriate operation performed at the wrong time by a poorly educated surgeon in dirty conditions with nothing more than the most rudimentary pain relief. Many procedures were carried out in cold and poorly lit buildings with an operating table improvised from a door or planks. There was no control of workload and little or no opportunity for sub-specialisation. Much of the surgery was heroic and speed was always vital. British army doctor Robert Hamilton rejected the view that soldiers were somehow immune to the horrors of surgery. Even the bravest warrior who would have unquestioningly charged the enemy could 'tremble at the sight of a lancet'.[62] Wars did, however, bring unprecedented opportunities for army surgeons to gain experience and the more talented among them — men such as John Hunter, John Jones, and John Ranby — were able to achieve surprisingly good results.

In gunshot wounds, the immediate priorities were to remove the ball and stop haemorrhage. Ranby recommended enlarging the wound and he favoured using his fingers rather than a probe or forceps. He was cautious when the ball was beyond the reach of a finger; 'I could never bring myself to thrust a pair of long forceps the Lord knows where, with scarce any probability of success'. In these cases, it was often better to leave the ball in situ. Ranby notes that over years some worked themselves to the surface and were very easily extracted.[63] Jones advised simple dressings such as dry soft lint.[64]

The belief that it was important to lessen inflammation and promote suppuration ('laudable pus') led to the use of antiphlogistic therapies. Jones managed his wounded patients with bleeding, laxatives, warm baths, and poultices.[65] Hunter particularly recommended bleeding by the lancet or the application of leeches but he cautioned that these should be used sparingly in gunshot wounds accompanied by fever and systemic upset.[66]

Jones decried the traditional approach to simple fractures which, he says, was performed with 'more or less violence'. The objects of management were 'to reduce the broken extremities, as nearly as possible to their natural situation, and to retain them when there, by the most easy, simple and effective means'. He makes specific recommendations for the reduction of the fracture and the subsequent bandaging and splinting. Compound fractures, where the broken bones extended through the skin, often required removal of the limb.[67]

Amputation was the archetypal surgical operation of war. In the mid-eighteenth century there was controversy as to the indications, timing, and technique. Frederick the Great forbade amputation in his army except in fully developed gangrene.[68] The following passage, written by American army surgeon James Tilton, suggests a relatively conservative approach during the Revolutionary War.

> 'the longer we continued in service, amputation and cutting generally became less fashionable. From obstinacy in the patients and other contingencies, we had frequent opportunity of observing, that limbs might be saved, which the best authorities directed to be cut off.'[69]

Nevertheless, it was obvious that where there was very extensive damage to bones, joints, nerves, and soft tissues that limbs would have to be sacrificed to save life. Jean Faure, a French military surgeon, conducted a small trial in the British wounded at the Battle of Fontenoy in 1745. He concluded that delayed amputation was preferable.[70] Opinions remained divided at the time of the American Revolution. Ranby favoured early amputation before inflammation set in.[71] Hunter advocated some delay, only resorting to amputation on the battlefield where it was difficult to move a soldier with a shattered limb.[72]

Jones gives a detailed account of the operation and the necessary preparations. The equipment included a tourniquet, tape, an amputating knife, a catlin (long double-bladed surgical knife), a saw, a tenaculum (type of forceps), needles, ligatures of waxed thread, and scissors. If the leg was to be removed, the patient was ideally laid on a firm table and covered with blankets with a pillow to support his head. After the initial skin incision, the muscles were divided and the bone sawed through. The main arteries were then secured, the tourniquet removed, and the stump dressed with lint and linen and bandaged. The patient then rested in bed, his thigh a little elevated and the knee bent.[73]

American doctor Charles Gillman described administering opium and rum to amputation patients. Their ears were covered, and with a sharp knife and saw, 'the result was little discomfort to the man'.[74] Only a minority of soldiers of any nationality would have received this quality of surgical care. Uzal Johnson, a loyalist surgeon, made the following entry in his diary for Saturday, 2 September 1780.

> 'I went to see a Militiaman that was in the Skirmish at Cedar Springs the 8th of August. He got wounded in the Arm. It was taken off by one Frost, a Black Smith, with a Shoemaker's knife and Carpenter's saw. He stopped the Blood with Fungus of W[hite] Oak.'[75]

Penetrating wounds to the chest by sword or bayonet were routinely managed by enlargement of the wound to allow the discharge of blood. Jones advised 'large and repeated venesections' where there was prolific haemorrhage. Musket ball wounds required only superficial dressings.[76] Hunter divided abdominal wounds into those simply penetrating the cavity and those affecting viscera. In the former, recovery was common but in the latter, there was likely to be peritonitis and he admitted that there was no surgical solution, only 'a good deal of art'.[77] The main invasive procedure in wounds of the head was trephination, the making of one or more holes in the skull with the intent of relieving pressure on the brain and reducing inflammation of the membranes. Jones does not refer to scalping but there are a few anecdotal accounts of successful treatment by boring of the skull and a gradual healing over of the wound. Cranial wounds were also managed with vigorous antiphlogistic measures.[78]

Post-operative infection was routine but the more specific and mostly fatal complication of tetanus was feared by army and navy surgeons. Of nineteen men who underwent amputation in the British hospital at Bermuda in 1789, nine died of tetanus.[79] Ranby describes it in a patient; 'three or four days after the amputation (his jaw being fixed by a convulsive attack, and his countenance greatly distorted) he expired'.[80]

Beyond systemic infections, patients were vulnerable to dehydration, hypovolaemic shock, and gangrene. The antiphlogistic interventions were likely to exacerbate all these complications. It is difficult to generalise regarding surgical mortality rates. Jones observes that those undergoing operations in the country private practice of small towns did better than those admitted to the overcrowded hospitals of the cities.[81] Precise figures are, however, more elusive, and not necessarily representative.[82] Individual surgeons published surprisingly good results. In 1737, Alexander Monro of Edinburgh claimed that his special amputation technique had resulted in only nine deaths in 99 patients.[83] It is inconceivable that similar results were obtained in war. The mortality rate for amputation at mid-thigh was likely to be in the order of 50 per cent.[84] Reporting on amputations performed at Haslar Hospital between 1772 and 1778, the British naval physician Gilbert Blane documented ten deaths in twenty-seven leg procedures. Amputation of the arm was generally a safer undertaking, with Blane describing two deaths in nine patients.[85]

In his ground-breaking work on military medicine published in 1764, British physician Richard Brocklesby asserted that army life was 'every instant obnoxious'. Disease, he claimed, laid greater waste in all who followed an army than it did in any other class of men.[86] John Pringle agreed, broadly attributing this to soldiers 'being more exposed to the injuries of the weather and always crowded together in camps, barracks and hospitals'.[87] The Revolutionary War also brought an increased risk of pestilence to the civilians of the colonies and to the American Indian population.

In considering the diseases of the War, it is reasonable to start with typhus, the history of which can be regarded as the 'history of human misery'. Epidemics have long been associated with conflict and there were to be significant outbreaks during the Revolution, especially on the American side. The disorder is cause by *rickettsia*, a type of highly pleomorphic bacteria. In epidemics, the disease is transmitted to humans by the human body louse. Characteristic symptoms and signs include malaise, headache, the appearance of small haemorrhages in the skin (petechiae) and gangrene of the extremities. Fatal cases develop increasing drowsiness and coma.[88] Common contemporary terms for the disorder, reflecting its connection with overcrowding, were 'jail distemper', 'jail fever', 'ship fever', 'camp fever', 'hospital fever', and 'putrid fever'.[89] The unhygienic eighteenth-century soldier was an ideal carrier, the threat of infection increasing when the men huddled together in winter quarters. The disease was less common in an army on the move. It was managed with dietary modifications, bleeding, laxatives, emetics, blisters, wine, bark, and other components of the antiphlogistic arnementarium.[90] Mortality rates varied from 5 to 25 per cent although in extreme circumstances this might reach 60 per cent.[91] In interpreting contemporary writings, it is often difficult to distinguish typhus from typhoid, a disease caused by organisms in contaminated water. Typhoid was generally less seasonal and less deadly.[92]

Although not as notorious as typhus, army returns confirm that dysentery was the commonest disease of the War, regularly affecting all armies. This depressing affliction is caused by a variety of bacteria and is associated with the passage of bloody diarrhoea. In more severe cases there is profound weakness and dehydration.[93] It was commonly referred to as the 'flux' or 'bloody flux' but, confusingly, in America it was also called 'camp fever' or 'camp distemper', terms that in Europe were applied to typhus.[94] Gerard Van Swieten, an Austrian physician whose textbook was translated and published in Philadelphia in 1776, thought the disorder to arise either spontaneously or to progress from chronic diarrhoea.[95] It was not commonly fatal in itself but it complicated other infectious complaints. In James Tilton's words:

> 'The putrid diarrhoea was generally the result or dregs of other camp and hospital diseases; and was the most intractable disorder of any we had to deal with.'[96]

Treatments were typically futile although the warm baths and opium prescribed in some regimens may have given the patient succour.[97] In soldiers disabled by the depravities of army life and weakened by co-morbid conditions, the mortality rates were significant. Tilton describes 'multitudes wasting away'.[98]

Smallpox has been alluded to in the context of quarantine and inoculation. When this dangerous and disfiguring disease was contracted naturally it usually started with flu-like symptoms and increasing debility. The first smallpox sores appeared on the neck, throat and nose on about the fourth day. The rash then spread rapidly, sometimes associated with a fulminant course and an early death from internal haemorrhage but more commonly manifesting itself as pustules particularly affecting the soles of the feet, the palms of the hands, the face, neck, back and lower arms. The pustules emitted an offensive smell, and the sufferer was likely to become dehydrated. Death, when it occurred, was often after ten to sixteen days of distress.[99] Contemporary treatments were unhelpful, with the bleeding resorted to in severe cases only likely to shorten life.[100]

Mortality rates varied widely. A key factor was acquired immunity due to previous exposure. In eighteenth-century America, smallpox was less prevalent than in Britain and thus immunity was lower. It was also lower in country dwellers compared with their city brethren.[101] In seventeenth-century London, fatality rates were around 7 per cent, lower than in the 1721 Boston epidemic in which 15 per cent of patients died. However, rates of 30 per cent were reported in epidemics in both Britain and America in the eighteenth century.[102] Brocklesby collected information from British regimental surgeons and concluded that in the earlier wars of the century a little more than 1 in 4 soldiers did not survive the disorder.[103] American Indians were especially vulnerable, many dying before the tell-tale skin eruption appeared. Britain's American Indian allies carried the disease to their homelands in the west.[104] Government records suggest mortality rates of 55 to 90 per cent.[105]

Malaria was present in most of the colonies, but it was particularly prevalent in the hot summers of the American south where it caused great suffering in Cornwallis's British army. The aetiology of the disease was not understood. When Lieutenant Colonel Nisbet Balfour wrote from his camp at Charleston that he was 'in perfect health, excepting the amusement of a few muskettoes and rattlesnakes', he had no conception that it was the insects that were man's worst enemy.[106] The marshes and rice fields of the south provided ideal conditions for the breeding of the mosquitoes which carried the organisms (plasmodia) which caused malaria.[107] The classic symptomatology was of an intermittent high fever with associated rigors and exhaustion. Army doctors referred to the disease as 'intermitting' or 'remitting fever' while the soldiers complained of 'swamp fever' and 'ague'. Unlike other systemic infectious diseases, there was a potentially effective treatment in the form of Peruvian bark, the cinchona from which quinine was later to be extracted.[108] Robert Jackson, whose regiment was badly affected, extolled the use of bark but also pointed out that it had to be of good quality and given in sufficient amount; 'Three or four ounces seldom failed of checking progress of the most formidable fevers of America; one or two frequently did not produce any sensitive effect'. Jackson noted that some British surgeons and most German surgeons were not convinced of the efficacy of bark and that the mortality from fever in their regiments was a quarter to a third compared with less than one in twenty when bark was freely administered.[109]

Scurvy, caused by a deficiency of Vitamin C, is generally regarded as a disease of the navy; between 1600 and 1800 it killed more than a million sailors.[110] It could, however, also affect armies, especially where supplies of fresh produce broke down and soldiers were limited to 'salt rations'. Van Swieten graphically describes the onset of the disorder.

'the skin is stained with spots of different colours, the mouth begins to smell, the teeth loosen in the sockets, the gums swell, itch, grow painful and bleed at the least touch.'

He was convinced of the restorative effects of fruit and vegetables but, immersed in the contemporary theories of disease, he was reluctant to accept that simple deficiency could be the cause, also invoking the role of 'noisome vapours arising from marshy grounds'.[111]

'The Itch' or scabies, an irritating skin disorder, was extremely common in the armies of the eighteenth century. Pringle thought it to be a contagious disease and not due to 'effluvia'. He recommended sulphur as a safe and effective cure.[112] Venereal disease was also ever-present. Robert Hamilton commented that among the soldiers, 'it is so prevalent that no reproach follows it, either from their comrades or from any of the officers'.[113] The 'pox' was a mixture of syphilis and gonorrhoea although the two disorders were not well differentiated in the eighteenth century. Mercury was widely prescribed. Probably because of its toxicity and lack of efficacy there were many panaceas on offer. 'Keyser's Famous Pills' were a favourite colonial nostrum of the 1770s. In severe cases where passing urine became difficult surgical options included probing, irrigations, and reopening the urethra by pounding the penis with a mallet.[114]

French Physician Jean Colombier, in his '*Précepts sur la Santé des Gens de Guerre ou Hygiene Militaire* of 1775, divides the harmful effects of alcohol into drunkenness, the accidents that occurred as a result, and the toxicity to the body. The latter would include chronic alcoholic liver disease.[115] Drunkenness was endemic in the British Army, most soldiers supplementing their rum ration by purchasing liquor from suttlers.[116] That the Continental Army was no different is obvious from the words of Major Joseph Bloomfield of the 3rd New Jersey Regiment.

'It is strange that when men have Money that are fond of Drink, what Pains they will take to stupify themselves & then when in Liquor murder their best Friends if denyed the pernicious Liquor.'[117]

Other physical disorders stalking the soldiers of the Revolution included respiratory infections, tuberculosis (consumption), musculoskeletal ailments ('rheumatism'), heatstroke, frostbite, hookworm, and various eye complaints.

Yellow fever is a notable exclusion from this list as it appears to have been absent from North America between 1763 and 1793 with the possible exception of a local outbreak in Virginia in 1773.[118]

There was also malingering. A few soldiers resorted to self-mutilation to avoid serving in the War. The author of the outrageous *Advice to the Officers of the British Army* advises the private soldier, 'If the duty runs hard, you may easily sham sick by swallowing a quid of tobacco'. Another favoured gambit was the feigning of rheumatism which was 'an admirable pretence, not easily discovered'.[119] There was also genuine mental illness in the ranks although there are limited allusions to this in contemporary medical texts and soldiers' memoirs. Van Swieten observes that a soldier once removed from his family might become 'melancholy'.[120] This syndrome, often termed 'nostalgia', presumably ranged in severity from mild homesickness to severe depression.[121] In 1778, nostalgia was reported to be frequent among the American militia and recruits from New England.[122] The eighteenth-century entity of 'cannon fever' which affected men much exposed to battle is likely to have overlapped with the more recent diagnoses of 'shell-shock' and post-traumatic stress disorder.

Preventative medicine in the army, commonly referred to as 'military hygiene', was proposed by John Pringle, Richard Brocklesby, Donald Monro, and Jean Colombier. Their works were pioneering but not entirely innovatory. They drew heavily from the lessons of antiquity, Pringle freely quoting the measures adopted by the Romans.[123] Colombier noted that the ancients understood the power of prevention whereas, '*nous au contraire, nous cherchons principalement à guérir.*'[124] As these medical men had first-hand experience of the common diseases of campaigning, their views were credible. Benjamin Rush, a fervent advocate of prevention, understood the centrality of army officers in applying the dictums of military hygiene.

> 'Soldiers are but little more than adult children. That officer, therefore, will best perform his duty to his men, who obliges them to take the most care of their HEALTH.'[125]

Practical steps taken by both armies (often advertised in general orders) included the encouragement of scrupulous personal cleanliness, the healthy location of campsites, more spacious accommodation, the fumigation and ventilation of barracks, the proper management of latrines, better clothing, strict discipline and the provision of good food and clean water. A British hospital report from Halifax in 1782 concluded that epidemics were best prevented by 'Space, good Air, and Cleanliness'.[126] As will be seen in subsequent chapters, it often proved difficult to apply these standards.

Another potential step forward in army medicine was the more frequent collection of data pertaining to disease and wounds. This arithmetic methodology reflected the emergence in the eighteenth century of a climate of 'rational empiricism', an emphasis on observation rather than theory. Ulrich Tröhler argues that this more critical and quantitative approach to medicine was fostered in Britain in the second half of the century.[127] War was a good testing ground for novel initiatives. In his *View of the Diseases of the Army*, Thomas Dickson Reide stresses the usefulness of 'military medical returns'; the doctor 'cannot, without their assistance, judge accurately of the effects of the medicines he prescribes, nor of the method of cure he adopts'.[128] Reide routinely collected his regimental medical data but the practice was not formalised in the British army until the Peninsular War.[129] British army returns including sick rates are available for the American Revolutionary period although these are not comprehensive, representing about 50 per cent of the army's service between 1775 and 1781.[130]

Legislation enacted at the end of 1776 demanded that American hospital surgeons provide weekly reports of the number and condition of men under treatment.[131] Washington understood the importance of this record keeping. In April 1781, he wrote to Director General John Cochran asking for more accurate hospital returns. In the same month, several army doctors commented that they had no paper and so could not submit them.[132] Despite the inevitable gaps and inaccuracies in the data, the collection of medical returns measured the human cost of the War and would eventually result in a better understanding of the diseases which afflicted armies.

Chapter 2

The Medical Services of Britain and its Allies

They [the British] hate us in every Shape we appear to them. Their care of our wounded was entirely the effect of the perfection of their medical establishment.

Benjamin Rush, October 1777

The origins of the British Army's medical services are obscure. From very early times, a physician or surgeon was appointed to the commander-in-chief when he went on campaign. Surgeons were attached to the regiments of Cavaliers and Roundheads in the English Civil War and, from 1660, a physician general and surgeon general exerted control in peace and in war.[1] Medical services in the field were dominated by the general hospitals. By the 1740s, the term 'general hospital' was widely used to describe the staff of the medical department rather than a particular facility. During the War of the Austrian Succession and the Seven Years War on the Continent, the general hospitals were commonly closed at the end of each campaign. However, in North America during the Seven Years War (the French and Indian War 1754–1763) the major hospitals accepted patients all year round. This practice continued in the American Revolution.[2]

The army's commander-in-chief had ultimate authority over the medical department. Hospital supplies, medical personnel, and the responsibility for the daily functioning of the service were all under his jurisdiction. In practice, commanders seldom interfered, no doubt preoccupied by purely military matters. The War Office actively encouraged a policy of non-intervention. In March 1778, the secretary at war informed General William Howe of the planned appointment of James Napier as superintendent of hospitals in North America.

'Upon the whole, Sir, as Mr Napier [who, in the event, did not accept the post] is acknowledged to be fully informed in every Branch of the Hospital Department, and as his Opinion when ratified by your approbation will be decisive on any Difficulties which may arise among the several members of it, I should hope that this Service will be conducted in a manner to give you the least Trouble.'[3]

There was little change in the governance of the medical department between 1660 and 1750.[4] At the onset of the Revolution in 1775, the physician general was Sir Edward Wilmot and the surgeon general, David Middleton. Longevity was no bar to high office. Wilmot held the post for forty years up to his death at ninety-three.[5]

There was a short-lived attempt to form a medical board in 1756 but the more crucial change in the same year was the creation of the post of inspector of regimental infirmaries. The appointee, Robert Adair, had originally joined the army as a staff surgeon in 1742. The duties of his new post, which he was to occupy for thirty years, were wide. During the American Revolution, he effectively acted as a surgeon general, corresponding with the army's commanders, ordering supplies of hospital equipment and medicines, and nominating surgeons and mates. He was responsible for professional standards and the state of the department's finances. His own inflated pay, 30 shillings a day, compared with twenty shillings for the physician and surgeon generals, reflected both the importance and the full-time nature of the role.[6] Adair was capable, energetic, and charismatic. He was also pre-occupied by the perceived need to economise and many of his initiatives culminated in cost-cutting.[7]

While Adair supervised affairs from London, there was a proliferation of inspectorial posts designed to lead the department through the Revolutionary War. For instance, in 1777 Michael Morris was appointed 'inspector of hospitals' and Hugh Alexander Kennedy became 'inspector of regimental infirmaries in North America'.[8]

The most important new post was that of 'superintendent general of hospitals for British forces in North America', created in April 1779 with the objective of centralising authority.[9] Once James Napier had withdrawn from consideration, the two candidates were John Mervin Nooth and Jonathan Mallet, both experienced medical officers already serving in America. The British army medical department was not afflicted by the intense infighting which characterised the American service but there were rivalries and ill-feeling. Nooth and Mallet both had their supporters, and both lobbied the War Office, the keen competition evolving into a feud. Two years after Nooth's appointment, Mallet was still having to be placated by the secretary at war, who assured him that 'no injustice' had occurred.[10]

Nooth's responsibilities were mostly clerical and supervisory in nature. His correspondence suggests that he was an ineffective leader. He complained to Adair from Philadelphia of the heavy drinking of wine by patients and, perversely, of the excessive consumption of vegetables. A hospital garden would not be big enough if the 'rage' for vegetables persisted. There were also issues with the funding of hospitals. Adair agreed with Nooth that wine consumption was too high, and he weighed in that there were too many hospital mates and servants in employment. When instructed by Adair to supervise the Hessian hospital in the city, Nooth did so with ill grace.[11]

At the start of the eighteenth century, the total medical staff in the British Army did not exceed around 170 officers.[12] The first proper hospital in North America was formed in 1754, the number of officers increasing during the French and Indian War. Reduced in 1764, the department was revived in 1775.[13] It is difficult to quote a definite strength for the medical department in America in the years of the Revolution. Entries in Drew's impressive but not entirely comprehensive *Commissioned Officers in the Medical Services of the British Army* allow the following computation: eleven inspectors; eight physicians; twenty-three staff surgeons; fourteen apothecaries; three purveyors; eighty-three regimental surgeons. These 140 posts exclude hospital mates and regimental surgeon's mates as they were only warrant officers. One analysis of regimental returns for the War suggests that there were approximately 230 soldiers per regimental surgeon or mate.[14] Towards the end of the conflict in 1782, the hospital staff in America was made up of the superintendent general, six physicians, thirteen staff surgeons, eight apothecaries, and seventy hospital mates.[15]

To define these medical roles, it is important to understand that, beyond the most senior inspectorial posts, there were two very broad groups of medical officers, the hospital staff, and the regimental contingent. The former included the physicians, staff surgeons, apothecaries, purveyors, and hospital mates whereas the latter were the regimental surgeons and surgeon's mates.

The physicians were commissioned on the recommendation of the physician general and were regarded as the elite of the army medical profession. They were few, only ten being employed at any one time in North America and the West Indies.[16] Most were appointed directly from civilian life, but some were promoted from the ranks of apothecaries and staff surgeons. Always highly qualified, many were in possession of university degrees or were licentiates, members, or fellows of the College of Physicians of London. Physicians exerted considerable influence despite their rarity and frequent lack of previous practical experience.[17] In September 1775, the secretary at war wrote to General Thomas Gage regarding their role.

> 'The Physicians to the Hospital, and the chief Surgeon are to be considered as the Principal Officers of the Hospital. The Senior Physician by appointment is to attend the General Hospital, to visit the sick, and prescribe for them such diet and Medicines as he shall judge most proper, to give Directions to have them conveniently lodged in Wards with a free Air, kept clean and not crowded, to assign the several parts of duty to the other Physicians who may be employed, to the Master Apothecary, and the Mates.'[18]

They were very unlikely to get involved in manual tasks such as cutting, dressing, and bleeding.

The formal relationship between physicians and surgeons was blurred. A regulation stipulated that operations could be performed only with the consent of both a physician and surgeon although it is very unlikely that this was applied after a major battle.[19] At least some physicians despised their medical 'inferiors', viewing surgeons as mere artisans and apothecaries as shopkeepers.[20] This was not conducive to the smooth functioning of the department. In 1782, Adair complained of disputes between physicians and surgeons, the whole corps therefore 'rendered contemptible'.[21]

Staff surgeons were all those surgeons not belonging to regiments. They were selected and recommended by the surgeon general and employed in the field, in a general hospital or in a garrison. Their numbers increased in war. During the American Revolution, there were at one time twenty-one surgeons attached to the hospitals in North America and the West Indies. Some received direct commissions from civilian life while others were promoted from hospital mates, apothecaries, and regimental surgeons.[22] Whereas the physicians were admired for their qualifications and theoretical knowledge, the staff surgeons were valued for their practical experience and surgical skills.[23] They were expected to be flexible. Staff Surgeon Thompson Forster served on a hospital ship at the Battle of White Plains in 1776 and described his duties in his diary.

> 'Upon all Expeditions of this sort we act in the threefold capacities of Physician, Surgeon and Apothecary; Physicians or Apothecaries are never detached, but remain in Garrison, I have frequently had more Physical cases than Surgical, which was the case here.'[24]

These men of action often won the respect of military officers.

Hospital mates were on the lowest rung of the general hospital's medical hierarchy, their job being to carry out the instructions of the physicians and surgeons. They were warrant officers, those intended for medical duties being appointed by the physician general and those with a surgical role by the surgeon general.[25] Many were of poor quality, and they were widely criticised. When their remuneration was increased in 1781, the authorities in London were reminded that 'many serving in North America are not deserving of such an increase of Pay'. Commander-in-Chief Henry Clinton was instructed by the secretary at war that all the mates should be examined by the physicians and surgeons of the hospitals and dismissed if found to be incompetent. In future, the mates would have to pass a proper examination.[26]

There are anecdotes of low calibre hospital mates. A Mr Prendergast, a mate in Canada, was said by his overworked colleagues to have 'remained at his ease in Three Rivers for upwards of two Years'. He was refractory to correction, a military officer later commenting that 'the Service was very little indebted to him for his attendance'.[27] Hospital Mate James Connor was placed under arrest at Niagara in 1783 after having 'insulted, beat and abused' a ship's captain to obtain grog.[28]

There were also good hospital mates.[29] Some were promoted to surgeons. However, such promotions were uncommon and the hospital mates' reputation for mediocrity may have been in part attributable to their low morale. Even ambitious well-educated men had no guarantee of progress, often remaining in the rank for many years.[30] Furthermore, as they only held warrants and not commissions, they could be discharged at any time without compensation or the prospect of half-pay.[31]

Purveyors were effectively commissariat officers to the hospital, responsible for the distribution of food and medical comforts and all the connected accounts.[32] Apothecaries took care of medicines and medical stores. They were largely appointed from hospital and surgeon's mates and in the hospital hierarchy were placed somewhere between the mates and the staff surgeons. They were variably qualified. At least a few were well educated and could aspire to eventual promotion to physician. The senior apothecary to a general hospital or a force in the field was designated 'master-apothecary' although this role fell into disuse during the Revolutionary War, the last incumbent being Surgeon Arthur Edwards who was appointed in North America in 1778.[33]

We now come to the largest group of medical officers, the regimental surgeons and mates. This was a diverse group of men, but it is possible to reach some conclusions regarding their background, method of recruitment, qualifications, training, competence, and status.

Each cavalry regiment had a surgeon. The infantry regiments in America had a surgeon and one or two mates.[34] Regimental surgeons received their commissions from the secretary at war or from the commander-in-chief in the field. They were expected to have previously passed an examination at Surgeon's Hall although this was not universal. A few were in possession of medical degrees, especially from Edinburgh and Glasgow.[35] The sale of medical commissions was forbidden but this did not prevent some clandestine trading. When the War Office discovered a surgeon's commission in New York to have been obtained by deception it was rescinded. In 1774, James Latham of the 8th Foot offered his surgeon's post for £340, '£60 less than the usual price'.[36]

Regimental mates gained their position via a warrant signed by the colonel of the regiment. As for the hospital mates, there were growing demands for them to be examined but many will still have entered the army with scant knowledge of medicine. Some had spent a year or two assisting a country surgeon or apothecary while others were raised from private soldiers who had some aptitude in simple tasks such as bandaging. Conversely, there were a number of medical school students and even university graduates, who were determined to use the army as a training opportunity for a future career in medicine.[37] Most mates were young, often between sixteen and twenty-five years of age at the time of recruitment. Their promotion was generally dependent on merit. About half of British army surgeons in the Revolutionary War had originally served in the lower rank.[38]

Surgeons and their mates were exempted from routine duties such as mounting guard and attending courts-martial, their charge being the care of the sick and wounded. The surgeons were expected to man the regimental hospitals, examine recruits, and supervise punishments such as flogging.[39] The mates commonly carried out many of the surgeon's duties and might have to quickly fill their shoes in times of war. When a regiment was split into detachments the mate routinely accompanied the smaller unit.[40]

In times of peace, medical responsibility for a regiment of perhaps 300–500 men was not unduly onerous but in war it was different. The surgeon might have upwards of 700 lives in his hands. A major battle or epidemic could rapidly lead to an overwhelming workload.[41] John Peebles, an officer in the Black Watch, witnessed a violent outbreak of disease in New York in the autumn of 1779. On 1 September:

> 'more men fell down, 15 sick today, the sick of the Battn (about 120) are lodged in two Barns, only one surgeon to attend them.'

The situation had not improved a month later with apparently no regimental doctors available.

> 'their great numbers [sick] does not admit of that care, treatment & attention that is necessary, only one Hospital mate to attend 130 or 40 Sick & few comforts.'[42]

To perform such duties, mates were paid 3s 6d a day and surgeons 4s.[43] This was around three shillings after stoppages.[44] This low rate of remuneration tempted surgeons to manipulate the 'medical money', £80 per annum provided to purchase medicines and other supplies. As any surplus ended up in the surgeon's pocket, allegations of corruption were predictable. At least some surgeons did deliberately minimise the outlay. A surgeon's mate who was generous with medicines was unlikely to be appreciated by his senior colleague.[45]

How competent were the British regimental surgeons and mates of the Revolutionary period? In the eighteenth century, senior politicians and medical officers were mostly critical of the regimental medical men. Adair advised the secretary at war, Charles Jenkinson, that medicines should not be allocated directly to regiments as the physicians 'are supposed to understand the internal Diseases of the Soldier better than a Regimental Surgeon'.[46] This was not surprising, but even their surgical skills were doubted. In September 1775, William Howe, the commander-in-chief, ordered that 'No Amputation or other Intricate Operation [was] to be Undertaken by any of the Surjeons without Consultation first hand, with the Surjeons and Physicians of the General Hospital'.[47] When staff surgeon vacancies became available in New York, the War Office refused to fill them with regimental surgeons as the latter had 'very rarely had opportunity of acquiring great skill to perform the great operations of surgery or sufficient judgement to decide upon the necessity of performing them'. Writing to General Clinton in 1781, the secretary at war suggested that they were also ignorant of the nature of disease; 'it is well known that the Company's surgeons have very little physical knowledge and are totally ignorant of medicine and the proper method of treating dysenteries and intermittent fevers'.[48]

Robert Hamilton, whose *Duties of a Regimental Surgeon Considered* was first published in 1787, wished that the post might 'become more respectable'.[49] According to Hamilton, too many surgeons were careless in their duties.

'Is it to be supposed the surgeon who passes his morning in walks of recreation, or the day in sports, and the evening, when the bottle does not intervene, at cards, billiards, or back-gammon, can have the complaints of his sick soldiers much at heart?'[50]

As for the lower grade, Hamilton reached the sad conclusion that 'almost any person may be a surgeon's mate'.[51]

Attempts to screen out incompetents by examination were confounded by the facile nature of the testing and the examiners' leniency. In March 1776, at the height of the Revolutionary War, seventy-four candidates for various army medical appointments and diplomas were all passed.[52]

There were some examples of undoubted individual excellence. Hamilton acknowledged that several eminent men had been and still were in the post of regimental surgeon.[53] He might have included himself, as his humble service as a surgeon's mate in the 10th Regiment of Foot between 1780 and 1785 did not prevent him eventually rising to the rank of physician. In her cogent defence of the British regimental surgeons of the Revolution, Tabitha Marshall also quotes the cases of James McCausland, Robert Jackson and Thomas Dickson Reide, all veterans of the American War. McCausland, surgeon to the 8th Regiment, served at Fort Niagara in 1779. Unable to obtain medical supplies from Quebec, he ordered them from Europe at his own expense. Jackson, who served as a surgeon's mate in the South, became a highly respected and influential medical author. Reide, surgeon to the 29th Regiment in Canada, was a pioneer in the collection of medical statistics.[54]

The low status of army surgeons and mates in society was made obvious when George III reviewed the troops in 1779; 'no surgeon was allowed to kiss his hand'.[55] The credibility of regimental surgeons and other doctors in the army was closely connected to military officers' perceptions of their abilities. This was not simply an egotistical consideration. Doctors' advice on the prevention of disease and other medical subjects was unlikely to be followed unless they commanded respect. Some military officers were dismissive of medical recommendations. Hugh Alexander Kennedy, physician to the hospital at Quebec, complained to his new commander-in-chief Guy Carleton in 1782 that he had suffered four years of 'oppressive servitude' under General Frederick Haldimand.[56] If a physician was treated so poorly, it must have been a commonplace experience for regimental surgeons. Some officers were very ready to compare regimental doctors adversely to hospital staff. Conversely, there are many general orders issued during the War which suggest that senior military officers had a genuine concern for the wellbeing of the sick and wounded.[57]

The status of army medical officers was not helped by the blurring of distinctions of rank and qualification at the bottom of the medical hierarchy. The elevation of ordinary soldiers to the rank of surgeon's mate has been referred to. The author of *Advice to the Officers of the British Army* takes aim at this transaction.

> 'As the soldiers are apt to be extremely troublesome to the surgeon of a regiment and your mate may be ignorant, or too much of a gentleman, take a private man out of the ranks, and instruct him to act as your deputy. The principal part of his business will be to bleed and dress sore backs.'[58]

These men had no formal training. The best-known example is that of Roger Lamb who acted as a doctor to the 9th and 23rd Regiments. His *Journal* and *Memoir* of the American War are vital eyewitness accounts. Lamb was doubling up, retaining his military role. In a later petition, he described his duties. At the Battle of Camden, he carried the regimental colours:

> 'and immediately after was appointed temporary Surgeon to the Regiment, having had some little knowledge of physic, and received

the approbation of all his Officers for his care of the sick and wounded.'[59]

Elsewhere, Lamb describes his role as being that of 'assistant surgeon', a term that was eventually to replace that of surgeon's mate.[60] His story illustrates the difficulty of making generalisations regarding the educational status, competence, and credibility of regimental surgeons.

There were three basic types of hospitals in the eighteenth-century British army at war. The general hospital was the largest facility, typically having around 400 beds for an army of 20,000 to 30,000 men. On campaign, one would be necessarily opened in convenient buildings, perhaps a church or factory, in a town or city not too distant from the action. During the Revolutionary War, there were general hospitals at Boston, New York, Philadelphia, Quebec, and other key strategic sites. The staff would routinely include a director, a purveyor, a physician and two mates, a staff surgeon and mate, and an apothecary.[61]

The 'flying hospital' was designed to follow in the rear of the army, always ready to receive the sick and wounded and to transfer them on to the general hospitals as needed. The regimental hospital was set up by the regiment's surgeon. Wherever his unit encamped, he commandeered local houses or erected tents to accommodate patients with more minor illnesses or wounds.[62]

There was great controversy as to the relative roles of the hospitals, particularly the general and regimental types. The secretary at state issued regulations for the management of the general hospitals in North America in 1775.[63] These were well-intentioned and reflected best practice. However, the army's general hospitals had long been castigated in the medical literature. John Pringle attributed the spread of diseases to the 'foul air' of the crowded hospital wards. 'The sick', he warned, 'should not be sent to one common hospital'.[64] Surgeon John Ranby concurred that this 'miserable confinement' led to the loss of 'an abundance of valuable lives'.[65]

Robert Jackson was a particular critic; 'it is unfortunate that the mode, too frequently pursued, of collecting sick soldiers into general hospitals, so multiplies the causes of disease.'[66] Jackson and others claimed that soldiers recovered from illness more quickly if left in the care of their regimental surgeons, often in two weeks rather than the six weeks or more for those admitted to the general facilities. Sick men might not even reach the general hospital, dying in transit.[67] These arguments held sway in high places. Adair agreed that regimental hospitals were 'better adapted' to receive the sick.[68] His view was undoubtedly influenced by the greater expense of general hospitals. There was a determined effort to reduce the number of general hospitals in North America towards the end of the War, especially in Canada. General orders repeatedly reminded officers that soldiers with more minor disorders should be kept with their regiment.[69]

This wave of support for the regimental hospitals overlooked the reality that they were often poorly sited and staffed by clumsy surgeon's mates. Brocklesby warned that seventy to eighty sick soldiers crammed into a small house were in no better a situation than in a larger crowded hospital.[70] In November 1779, Mervin Nooth reported to General Clinton that he had visited regimental hospitals where ill men had been abandoned on lice-infested straw until they, 'are frequently so shamefully nasty and lousy and so much in want of necessaries that it is out of the power of the persons attending them to clean them'.[71] Even more than in the general hospitals, soldiers in the regimental hospitals were vulnerable to negligent medical care. The debate continued into the Napoleonic period with the inevitable conclusion that both types of hospital were necessary. A major battle or epidemic required the greater capacity of the general hospitals.[72]

Distressing accounts of sick soldiers lying in their own filth brings us to the subject of army nursing care in the Revolutionary period. Female nurses are often overlooked, as if they only appeared at the time of Florence Nightingale. As is well described by Paul Kopperman, it was the case as early as 1750 that the term 'female nurse' was redundant as almost all nurses were female. These women filled diverse roles in British eighteenth-century general hospitals, acting both as nurses and also as laundresses, cooks and matrons. The latter post was at the top of the nursing hierarchy, the matron being the most respected woman in the army.[73]

Compared with the forces in Europe, the British Army in America was poorly provided with nursing staff. Rather than sending out experienced nurses, there was a reliance on untrained soldiers' wives who were recruited opportunistically.[74] Periods of intensive campaigning culminated in hasty advertisements for nurses being placed in general orders and in local newspapers.[75] Pringle and Monro both emphasised the importance of nurses in the maintenance of standards in general hospitals.[76] The shortage of experienced nurses in the Revolutionary War was a significant contributor to the shortcomings of the general hospitals, described as 'death traps' by Neil Cantlie, the historian of the British Army medical department.[77]

Published in 1780, the second edition of Monro's work on the health of soldiers makes pragmatic suggestions for the management of wounded in battle. The regimental surgeons and mates were to be placed in the rear of their own regiment where they could safely provide first aid and perform urgent surgery. After the battle, the wounded were to be removed to the flying hospital or the nearest general hospital. Several staff surgeons were also to accompany the army into action. They were attached to the suite of the commanders of brigades and were given wagons to carry the surgical supplies and to evacuate the wounded.[78]

The reality was often different. Monro's writings suggest a central role for the flying hospital. Cantlie makes several allusions to their use in the War, but Kopperman insists that the term was little used after 1770.[79] The temporary hospitals which were quickly opened around the edges of battlefields would now more commonly be referred to as 'field hospitals'. Examples include the use of the farm stables at Germantown and the local meeting house at Guilford Courthouse. Wounded soldiers were usually carried to these makeshift hospitals by their comrades or the musicians of the regiment. The latter were routinely instructed to remain with their companies to give this assistance.[80]

These arrangements left much to chance. In July 1777, Burgoyne's army clashed with the rebels at Skenesborough. Roger Lamb, acting as a surgeon's mate, was soon surrounded by wounded men. He had nothing to dress them as the medicine box was with the regimental surgeon behind the lines. He ripped up his own shirt and, with the help of a soldier's wife, fashioned bandages to stem bleeding. The wounded were carried in blankets to a small hut, two miles in the rear.[81]

Staff Surgeon John Macnamara Hayes arrived at Skenesborough later in the day:

'Most of [the wounded] are in sheds made of Boughs which are no defence from rain, now w[hi]ch unfortunately set in these three or four days almost constantly... I never experienced more uneasiness at seeing the Wounded Suffer, nor do I wish to be in so disagreeable a Situation again. Had I the Common Necessaries for their relief, I sh[oul]d not Complain, but without them, how great must Man's feelings be; My hand embrued in Blood, My face as dirty & my beard as long as a Capuetien fryar with every thing filthy on me is my pres[en]t Situation, nor can I help it, as my things are 25 Miles off.'[82]

The inadequacies of battlefield medicine were more due to a shortage of medical officers and supplies than to a lack of humanity. Wounded soldiers around the field commonly fell into the hands of the enemy. In the Revolutionary War they were usually well treated. Enlightened military officers such as Burgoyne and Gates ensured this. After the Battle of Freeman's Farm, Burgoyne asked his adversary for protection of the 300 wounded he was leaving behind; this was something he would 'show to any enemy in the same case'. Surgeon Hayes acted as the go-between, receiving the reply that the American general would respect the conventions of war.[83]

Lamb's account of injured soldiers being carried in blankets reflects the absence of a proper service to evacuate the wounded. This applied equally to their immediate removal from the field and their subsequent carriage. There was always the need to transport invalids between regimental hospitals when the army was on the move and to move them between general hospitals as these were opened and closed.

Where available, water transport was used, for instance after the Battle of Germantown. Wagons were more commonly relied upon. These were not specially designed vehicles. They were drawn from the multiplicity of wagons which accompanied the army.[84] A few 'hospital wagons' would be allocated for the use of the medical corps. A general order of January 1781 stipulates that the sick were only to be carried in the wagons if they had a certificate from a surgeon testifying that they could not walk or ride on horseback.[85] This reflected the chronic shortage of vehicles. The problem was most acute when the army was on the march and sick rates were high, such as occurred during Cornwallis's campaigning in the South. Military priorities trumped medical ones. In January 1781, the commander took the fateful step of burning the wagons as they were slowing his progress. The 23rd Regiment had originally been given three large wagons, but this was later reduced to a single four-wheeled carriage 'intended for the conveyance of their medicine chest, sick men, forage or any other necessary purpose'.[86]

Men who were severely wounded or chronically sick and judged to be unfit for service were sent back to England. This final evacuation was not without danger. Transports carrying the invalids were preyed upon by privateers and at risk of shipwreck. The *Henry and Ann* was captured by a French privateer in 1779 and the sick on board imprisoned for two years. The leaky *America* transport took invalids from Philadelphia the same year and had to be rescued after foundering off the coast for two months. An investigation was ordered into the 'shameful inattention to the safety of men who have suffered in His Majesty's Service'.[87] Such an inquiry might have been reasonably extended to all the army's arrangements for the transport of its most vulnerable soldiers, a sad situation which was to persist during the Napoleonic wars.

The British had to import the bulk of medicines and other medical supplies from England. These shipments were substantial. In March 1778, the following arrived at New York: 217 bales of bedding; hospital utensils; provisions; twenty hospital and thirty surgeons' tents; thirty-six chests of medical stores. Additional supplies arrived later in the year and in the following March.[88]

Jackson comments that there was commonly a 'superfluity' of medical supplies at the army's American headquarters.[89] There are, however, reports of shortages at particular periods and of specific items. An epidemic of disease in New York in 1779 led to a dearth of medicines and the need to appropriate supplies intended for the West Indies.[90] In the South there were drug shortages in 1780 but the problem was less obvious in 1781.[91] Shortages of specific drugs led to price inflation and the need to adapt. Both British and Americans were forced to use substitutes for Peruvian bark, including wine and local botanicals such as Virginia snakeroot.[92] Each non-commissioned officer and private soldier made a weekly payment to the regimental surgeon to purchase medicines and supplies but, as has been referred to, unscrupulous surgeons were tempted to embezzle the funds or to buy inferior medicines.[93]

What conclusions can we reach regarding the quality of the British Army medical department in the Revolutionary War? There are negatives. Officials in the higher echelons of the department were prone to bickering. At the lower end, the mates were often poorly qualified and little trained. Organisational shortcomings, notably the lack of suitable transport for sick and wounded and the overcrowding in general hospitals, were not resolved. Attempts at improvement on the ground were often undermined by the parsimony of Adair in London.

On the other hand, there was a rational organisational structure and many of the hospital staff, especially the physicians and staff surgeons, were highly competent. Even the humbler regimental surgeons and mates sometimes demonstrated surprising abilities, rising through the medical ranks. There was at least a semblance of what now would be referred to as 'clinical governance': formal arrangements for the supervision of inexperienced doctors. To 'do no harm', the staff of the general hospital oversaw the activities of the regimental personnel.

Robert Jackson concluded that the medical department of the American War was 'well conducted'.[94] It must be judged by the standards of the time and the doctors of other nations were mostly admiring. When Benjamin Rush made plans for the Continental Army's embryonic medical corps, he emulated the British.[95]

The Hessian (German) soldiers who fought for the British in America had their own medical service. This autonomy is confirmed by Article XII of the treaty between George III and the Landgrave of Hesse-Kassel:

> 'Sick members of the Hessian Corps shall remain under the care of their physicians, surgeons, and other persons appointed for that purpose, under the orders of the general commanding the corps of that nation, and everything shall be allowed them that His Britannic Majesty allows his own troops.'[96]

On the list of 'Hessian Troops placed at the disposal of the English Crown' in 1776 are 100 'field surgeons'. This is a very approximate figure which excludes some of the hospital staff. Referrals to ranks of physicians, surgeons and apothecaries suggest a similar organisational structure to the British service.[97]

The Hessian hospitals were of low quality. Captain Johann Ewald describes the state of the hospital after the surrender of Yorktown:

> 'Our poor sick and wounded lay without medication or food, in conditions pitiful enough to soften the hardest heart. Their nourishment consisted of stinking salted meat, a little flour, or worm-infested zwieback biscuits. These wretched people were dying like flies.'

The Hessian hospital ships were ordinary transports and especially unsuitable for medical care. The adjutant general, Major Baurmeister, complained that the ships had killed many of his men.[98]

At the first Battle of Trenton, the Hessians suffered heavy casualties and had their own field hospital. Again, there was an air of helplessness and lack of provision, the Americans having to supply the Hessian surgeons with surgical instruments.[100]

Brocklesby had a very low opinion of the German service. Their military hospitals were 'neglected', and their doctors were 'rude and barbarous'.[101]

They were still barbers, expected to shave the officers.[102] Training was often inadequate or non-existent. In October 1780, we find the following in an army list.

'On the first of the month, Frantz Vierbach from Munich in Bavaria, serving as a private soldier in Major von Stanford's company, left here, since he had been ordered to serve as an apothecary with the German troops.'[103]

James Thacher was impressed by the dexterity of the British surgeons after Saratoga:

'but the Germans, with a few exceptions, do no credit to their profession; some of them are the most uncouth and clumsy operators I ever witnessed, and appear to be destitute of all sympathy and tenderness towards the suffering patient.'[104]

Some Hessian army doctors chose to stay in America after the War. When his enlistment expired in July 1783, medical officer Christoph Prechtel went to Philadelphia 'to try his fortune'.[105]

The American loyalist regiments which fought for the Crown had their own surgeons. One such man was Uzal Johnson, who defected from the rebel cause to be commissioned surgeon to the 5th New Jersey Volunteers in March 1777. He participated in the Battle of King's Mountain, attending to both loyalist and enemy wounded.[106] In the South, the British relied on local doctors to fill their medical ranks. Perhaps as many as half the hospital mates in Cornwallis's army were loyalists. On campaign, some of these men were detached to the regiments, most as surgeon's mates.[107]

Physicians and surgeons had been attached to British naval expeditions since the age of Cromwell. Early in the eighteenth century, the navy's medical affairs were in the hands of the 'Sick and Hurt Board' which was composed of medical and lay members. The quality of medical care was poor with little attention to education or the status of the service. Two pioneering naval physicians, James Lind and Gilbert Blane, emphasised the importance of pragmatic measures to preserve the health of seamen.[108] Unfortunately, they were unable to reverse the malaise at the top of the organisation. The historians of the navy's medical department assert that 'the state of the navy from a medical point of view was so bad between the years 1778 (when the [American] war became general) and 1783 that it must be accounted partly responsible for the defeat which Britain suffered'.[109]

In 1780, at the height of the conflict, the number of British naval surgeons rose to 370, further increasing to 450 by 1783.[110] These men were warrant officers along with the master or purser. As they had no commission, they had no uniform until 1805.[111] Despite the deficiencies of the wider service, they were probably of higher quality than the army's regimental surgeons. Historian Richard Blanco speculates that this perceived superiority was due to a combination of factors but particularly that the naval surgeon was energised by his isolation, forced to take a pragmatic approach to the health of the irreplaceable crew. If staff surgeons on land had multiple roles, this was even more so for the surgeon of a ship of war who effectively acted as physician, surgeon, and apothecary.[112]

Official regulations gave guidance as to the optimal care of the sick and injured on board. Under 'other duties specified' is the following:

> 'to prepare dressings before an action; to instruct the crew in the use of tourniquets; to keep the sick berth stove alight; to use carpenters' saws if his own instruments are insufficient.'[113]

A contemporary work by naval surgeon William Northcote gives more detail:

> 'When the enemy is in sight and you are like to come to an action, as soon as all hands are called to quarters (if your cockpit is not sufficiently large) you must desire the first lieutenant, with the captain's permission, to order the carpenters to lay a platform for your wounded men; if the cables will not be wanted, in one of the cable tires, or otherwise in the after-hold, by clearing of all manner of lumber out of the way. On top of a smooth and even tire cask, let there be deals and planks laid close together, over them an old sail, and upon that some seamen's bedding from the purser's store-room (for which you are to have the captain's order if he will not otherwise deliver them) ready made up, and laid one by another to place your wounded men on after they are dressed, thus they may lie quiet without being disturbed.'

Ideally, the space for the reception of wounded, operations and dressings was to be eight to twelve feet square. Northcote gives advice on the selection of the surgical instruments and other vital supplies including wine, punch, grog, and vinegar. Candles provided illumination. The surgeon was to ensure that he had enough helpers available 'that he may want no assistance in the day of battle, however bloody the engagement may be'.[114]

A number of vessels were adapted to be 'hospital ships'. Examples in the Revolution included the *Tiger*, *Cambridge* and *Union*. They were not always fit for purpose, the Board complaining that in a two-decker only one deck could be devoted to the sick resulting in them being indiscriminately mixed together. Other vessels were converted to 'convalescent ships'. These might be moored close to the hospital ships, allowing the invalids to be kept off land where they might misbehave.[115]

More seriously wounded or sick sailors were returned to England where the major hospital was at Haslar on the south coast. In 1776, this was described as 'excellently adapted to purpose' but by 1780 it was overcrowded, and Forton Prison was used as an overflow. A new phase of building created two operating theatres and increased the hospital capacity in the Portsmouth area to 3,000 patients.[116]

Chapter 3

The Medical Services of America and France

No less attention should be paid to the choice of surgeons than other officers of the army.

George Washington, 24 September 1776

When the American Revolution erupted in 1775, the colonial militias were not equipped with a proper medical corps. Some civilian doctors had entered the citizen armies as officers, but the medical needs of the soldiers were in the hands of a few physicians who had no formal appointment. Most provinces established temporary medical services, staffed by local doctors working part-time.[1] The first stirrings of a more organised medical department for what was to become the Continental Army were in the Colony of Massachusetts Bay. With commendable common sense, the authorities made the following order on 8 May 1775:

'That the President *pro tempore*, Doctor Church, Doctor Taylor, Doctor Helten and Doctor Dunsmore be a committee, to examine such persons as are, or may be recommended for surgeons for the army, now forming in this colony.

Resolved, That the persons recommended by the commanding officers of the several regiments, be appointed as surgeons to their respective regiments, provided they appear to be duly qualified, on examination.'[2]

There was no formal medical provision at Lexington or Concord in April but after the carnage of Bunker Hill in June, the need for a permanent administrative structure for medical care became obvious. On 21 July, the Continental Congress approved the Hospital Bill, creating a medical department for the Continental Army. The task faced by the new organisation was daunting. In the words of the department's historian, Mary C. Gillett:

> 'A staff for the most part totally unfamiliar with military medicine, handicapped by a serious and chronic shortage of drugs and by confused and inadequate legislation, was expected to provide uniformly competent care for an untrained army whose health was jeopardised by poor hygiene and frequently inadequate food and clothing.'[3]

The new bill was well meaning. The 'Hospital' (in modern terms, the medical department) for an army of 20,000 men was to be staffed by physicians with no military rank. Unfortunately, the legislation was necessarily drawn up in haste and it lacked the required specificity. There was confusion relating to the relationship of the new department and its director to the pre-existing regimental system used by the individual colonies. Also, there was no clear line of communication with the Continental Congress.[4] It was an inauspicious beginning.

We will briefly summarise the subsequent organisational steps which shaped the department during the War. In September 1775, the Medical Committee was created. This allowed Congress some jurisdiction over medical affairs. The stimulus for the creation of the committee was the acute shortage of drugs but its authority was gradually extended such that it appointed personnel, undertook inspections, and resolved internal disputes. It remained in existence until May 1781 when its functions were transferred to the Board of War.[5]

To improve the coordination and increase centralisation of the medical services, Congress approved a sizeable reorganisation in April 1777. The new 'Hospital' was separated into four districts which corresponded to the military divisions of Washington's army. The districts were managed by deputy directors who were answerable to the director general who acquired wide-ranging powers. The army's senior doctor had authority up to the Virginia–North Carolina boundary and was in control of medical recruitment, the establishment of hospitals, and the enforcement of regulations. A suggestion to create the post of purveyor was not enacted so the management of supplies was also in the director general's hands.[6]

Congress was nervous of the director general's hegemony and in February 1778 it amended the earlier act to decentralise authority. A purveyor general was appointed, and the district directors were given almost complete autonomy.[7] This created a leadership vacuum much as had occurred at the outset of the War and the legislation of September 1780 restored the director general's administrative powers.[8] In the following March, the southern states were finally included in the jurisdiction of the medical department.[9] Congress remained uneasy and in 1782 it established the Medical Board to assist the director general. This supervisory board was made up of senior doctors and military officers. It reported directly to Congress.[10]

This short account of the organisational arrangements demonstrates Congress's dilemma. It vacillated between strong leader and weak leader models for the medical department. Both plans attracted constant objections and the inconsistency resulted in confusion and a lack of momentum. Congress's inability to decide how to supervise the department was linked to its innate distrust of army doctors. Any medical expenditure was intensely scrutinised and medical officers felt belittled; 'The dirtiest and basest actions are everyday depreciating the profession...till the very appellation [of doctor] has become a butt of satire, ridicule and contempt.'[11]

The best antidote to the impasse between Congress and the Hospital Department would have been high quality and constant leadership provided by the four men who filled the post of director general between 1775 and 1781, the years of fighting. The first director general, Benjamin Church, was appointed at the creation of the department in 1775. He was a talented and well-educated physician and surgeon and apparently a committed patriot. Church was soon embroiled in a dispute with the recalcitrant regimental surgeons (see later). Before he was able to impose his will, he was accused of 'criminal correspondence with the enemy' and summarily dismissed for treason. His guilt remains doubtful. The unfortunate doctor was lost at sea en route to the West Indies after his release from jail.[12]

John Morgan replaced Church in October 1775. He had served as a surgeon in the French and Indian War and studied in Europe with the celebrated surgeon John Hunter. Morgan's experience and intellect were undoubted, but his character divided opinion. John Adams applauded his conscientiousness and morality, and others acknowledged his sound judgement. Conversely, James Boswell, who encountered him in earlier life, believed him to be a conceited fool. Some regarded him as a revengeful man.[13] William Shippen, the third director general, replaced Morgan in April 1777, much of the reorganisation of this time having been his recommendation. Like Morgan, Shippen was trained in Edinburgh and London. He was a skilful teacher and physician and was blessed with elegant manners. However, his qualifications for the role were limited; he had no previous military experience and knew little or nothing of camp life or hospital sanitation. Historian Louis Duncan describes him as more of a 'scholar' than a 'doer'.[14]

The final director general of the years of conflict was John Cochran, who was appointed in January 1781. Cochran was a well-respected practitioner and, crucially, was an able administrator. He had not graduated from a medical school, having been entirely apprentice trained. He had military experience as a surgeon's mate in the French and Indian War. He lacked the ambition and quarrelsome tendencies of his predecessors.[15] Although Benjamin Rush did not rise above the rank of surgeon general to the Middle Department, he can be conveniently introduced at this point. Educated in Europe, Rush gained a stellar reputation as a patriot, author, teacher, and physician. He frequently influenced events in the upper echelons of the American hospital department.[16]

The role of the director general was challenging enough but during the early and middle years of the Revolution it was rendered almost unviable by the intense feuding between John Morgan and William Shippen. Long-standing medical rivals, the men became implacable enemies, each bent on the other's destruction. The grudge first arose when the two protagonists competed for academic status at the first American medical school in the 1760s.[17] When Shippen was appointed chief physician of General Hugh Mercer's flying camp in the summer of 1776, Director General Morgan was immediately suspicious of his old rival. Congressional failure to define the relative authority of the two men fanned the flames.

Despite his considerable efforts, Morgan's department was increasingly criticised and his dismissal by Congress became inevitable.[18] The director general had not been formally charged or given any opportunity to defend himself and, in 1777, he published a long and passionate *Vindication* of his actions. He was in no doubt as to the cause of his fall:

'Is it not manifest, that the Director [Shippen] and his attachments, have from his first coming into the service, pursued such measures, as they conceived were best calculated to raise him over the shoulders of every man, and to constitute him Head of the department. How truly Machiavellian has been his conduct and those who have assisted him.'[19]

Two and a half years after his cursory sacking, Congress resolved that Morgan should be exonerated. This allowed him to devote all his energy to the pursuit of Shippen. The adversaries spent the winter of 1779–80 gathering testimonies to support their respective positions. The toxic dispute undermined the whole department. Complaints multiplied and, in January 1780, Washington commanded that Shippen be placed under arms and brought to trial, charged on five counts of fraud, speculation in hospital supplies, corrupt financial practices, neglect of duty, and 'indecent and infamous conduct unbecoming an officer and Gentleman'.

Rush was Morgan's principal ally, and, during the two months of the trial, he marshalled the prosecution witnesses. These disclosed appalling conditions in army hospitals and alleged that Shippen was indifferent to the plight of the sick and wounded and that he had traded in wine and sugar from the public stores. In August 1780, the court acquitted Shippen of all charges but still censured his conduct. He briefly returned to his post, but this was now untenable, and he finally resigned at the start of 1781.[20] The quarrels continued, with letters from each side published in the *Pennsylvania Packet*. Rush was opposed to any attempt to rehabilitate Shippen, writing directly to his enemy

> 'Your reappointment... after the crimes you have committed is a new phenomenon in the history of mankind. It will serve like a high-water mark to show posterity the degrees of corruption that marked the present stage of the American Revolution.'[21]

The appointment of Cochran as the fourth director general brought an end to the acrimony at the top of the department. He was popular and had the support of his fellow physicians and Washington. His main challenges were to restore the morale of a dispirited and fragmented medical corps and to attract adequate resources in the face of an increasingly penurious Congress.[22]

Cochran was the only successful director general of the War, always acting for the good of the service and in the best interests of the doctors under his command. Many of these men very likely joined the rebel cause for a mixture of patriotic and personal reasons. Surgeon James Thacher heard the call to arms in April 1775; 'Never was a cause more just, more sacred than ours... We are not born to be slaves.' Later in his journal, he admits that he joined the conflict from 'motives of patriotism and private interest'. He ignored his friends' warnings that this was a civil war and that he would end up on a British gallows.[23]

The educational achievements of American doctors on the eve of the Revolution have been referred to in Chapter 1. The majority were apprenticeship trained at most, but some were university graduates and highly accomplished. Dr John Warren had mastered Dutch and was able to converse with European physicians in Latin.[24] A handful of doctors had previously gained limited experience in military medicine in the French and Indian War.[25]

Examinations were used throughout the War to screen out ignorant practitioners and quacks. Morgan followed the example of the Massachusetts army during the siege of Boston in initiating a system of examination for both the hospital mates and the regimental surgeons and mates. Those not willing to submit to this testing of their qualifications were dismissed.[26] Candidates were expected to have knowledge of anatomy, surgery, physiology, and medicine, and to exhibit good eyesight and dexterity. Most of the army surgeons of the War were examined by the director general and his deputies.[27] Thacher describes his examination in 1775 as 'close and severe'; six of the sixteen candidates failed. One of his fellows, when asked how he would induce a sweat in a patient with rheumatism, replied 'I would have him examined by the medical committee'.[28] In times of staff shortages, these rigorous standards were relaxed.

There was no formal military medicine training in America before the Revolution and the training that medical officers received during the campaigns was more opportunistic than concerted and more dependent on individuals than legislation. Physician General William Brown organised a course of lectures on 'the practice of physic', anatomy and surgery during the Middlebrook winter and spring encampment of 1778–79.[29] During the fighting, the more astute surgeons also learnt from the actions and writing of their more experienced British colleagues. John Ranby's surgical work was often quoted.[30]

As was the case for the medical departments of other armies at this period, the quality of Washington's doctors varied enormously. Some regimental surgeons and mates escaped examination, appointed directly by their colonel.[31] Such men were little respected by rebel soldiers such as Joseph Plumb Martin:

> 'I saw our surgeon's mate close by, endeavouring to cook his supper, blowing the fire and scratching his eyes. We both stepped up to him and he felt my pulse, at the same time very demurely shutting his eyes while I was laughing in his face. After a minute's consultation with his medical talisman, he very gravely told the sergeant that I was unfit for duty, having a high fever upon me. I was as well as he was: all the medicine I needed was a bellyful of victuals.'[32]

When Martin was later wounded in the ankle, the regimental surgeon had to be dragged away from the backgammon table.[33]

In contrast, there were experienced and dedicated army doctors such as John Cochran and Jonathan Potts. Cochran returned to his medical duties in 1777 less than one week after the death of his son from a fall.[34] General Anthony Wayne, Potts' friend, commented in 1780 that, 'I do not recall a single instance but what these doctors contended in the field of battle to dress the wounded – frequently in the eye of danger to save the life of a brave officer or wounded soldier.'[35]

The Hospital Bill of 1776 specified that there should be one surgeon and five mates for every 5,000 men.[36] Each regiment had already been allocated a surgeon and a mate.[37] How many doctors actually served with the rebel army? Duncan compiled a list of 1,400 medical officers who participated in the Revolution.[38] Despite this impressive number, there were many instances of inadequate manpower, battalions having neither surgeons nor mates.[39] In 1778, Cochran attempted to make a direct comparison between the staff of the British and American hospital departments. This was confounded by a lack of equivalence in some roles (see below), but he concluded that his own service was relatively underprovided with hospital mates.[40]

The duties of American medical personnel were elaborated in the Hospital Bill. The surgeons and apothecaries were to visit the sick and to answer to the director general. The surgeon's mates were to administer care to the sick and to obey the instructions of the surgeons and apothecaries.[41] Morgan was keen to maintain flexibility in these roles; 'I call all mine 'Hospital Mates' & not merely 'Surgeon Mates' because I will not suffer names to mislead, or allow any of them to refuse that Duty, under a notion that they are 'Surgeon Mates' and that it is no part of their Duty to assist the Apothecary.'[42]

There was a subtle difference in the status of British and American army medical men. As has been alluded to in the previous chapter, British hospital and regimental mates were not commissioned but were only warrant officers. In the American service, Congress instructed that both surgeons and mates be commissioned, implying the status of officers.[43] A listing of the establishment of the American medical department made in April 1777 shows posts ranging from the director general at the top to regimental surgeon's mates at the bottom.[44] Most had functions similar to the British service. One exception was the role of apothecary which in the American service was less distinct and more subsumed into the duties of hospital physicians and surgeons.[45]

Discord was not confined to the higher ranks of the Continental Army's medical department. Regimental surgeons were soon discontented with their pay and what they perceived to be poor treatment compared with their colleagues in the general hospitals. The infighting was exacerbated by shortages of medicines and hospital supplies and the necessarily limited release of resources from the general hospitals to the regimental surgeons. In what was to develop into an overt competition between regimental and hospital doctors, the former received support from their colonels.[46]

Church and Morgan strove to support their hospital services and to gain the upper hand over the regimental surgeons who were treating the general hospitals as storehouses from which they could order anything they wanted. Some refused to transfer their sick men to the general hospital. The exasperated Morgan attacked the surgeons, describing them as 'unintelligent, ignorant, crude to a degree scarcely to be imagined.' Some, he alleged, had never seen a surgical operation.[47] Washington eventually stepped in to support his director general, writing the following to Congress on 25 September 1776:

> 'The Regimental Surgeons I am speaking of – Many of whom are very great Rascals, countenancing the Men in Sham Complaints to exempt them from duty, and often receiving Bribes to Certify Indispositions with a view to secure discharges or Furloughs.'

The commander advised Congress that there would be 'constant bickering' from the regimental surgeons 'till [they are] made to look up to the Director

General of the Army as a Superior'. He accused them of trying to break up the general hospitals by their exorbitant demands for supplies.[48] Legislation enacted at this time subordinated the regimental surgeons to the heads of the divisions of the Hospital Department.[49] This did not resolve the ill-feeling and the unhappy relationship between regimental surgeons and hospital medical officers persisted during the directorships of Shippen and Cochran.

As was the case in European forces, the Continental Army's general hospitals were opportunistically opened in houses and public buildings. The latter were usually barns, churches and college halls and they all had disadvantages, often being cramped, dirty and poorly ventilated.[50] Attempts were made to regulate these institutions; the instructions issued by Morgan regarding the general hospital at Long Island in June 1776 are typical, emphasising the importance of adequate returns, supplies, diet and staffing.[51] At the outset of the War, the hospitals' nurses were mainly soldiers but, in June 1777, Washington tried to replace them with females, releasing a general order that women should attend the hospital in numbers proportionate to the sick in each regiment. There was theoretically one nurse for every ten patients. Nursing staff were answerable to the matron.[52]

Regulations and orders were backed up by a system of inspection. However, it was near impossible to visit the hundreds of medical institutions located in the thirteen states.[53] Many American general hospitals were of low quality. There were increasing complaints of poor care and the dissemination of infectious diseases. At Lancaster in late 1777, 500 men spent six weeks on cold floors without straw or coverings. At Ephrata in early 1778, there were only ten blankets for the 180 patients.[54]

Both senior doctors and ordinary soldiers were disillusioned. Rush wrote to Washington in December 1777 stating that there were 5,000 sick in the general hospitals:

'There cannot be a greater calamity for a sick man than to come into our hospital at *this season* of the year. Old disorders are prolonged, and new Ones contracted among us. This last is so much the case that I am safe when I assert that a *great majority* of those who die in our hands perish with fevers caught in our hospitals.'

He added that he had seen twenty sick men in a room only large enough for six to eight and that the hospitals' surgeons were also dying of infection.[55] When James Fergus of the Pennsylvania Militia fell ill at Charleston in the summer of 1779, he informed his surgeon that 'I had seen the hospitals in Philadelphia, Princeton, and Newark and would prefer dying in the open air of the woods rather [than] be stifled to death in a crowded hospital'.[56]

There were two laudable initiatives. The general hospital at the spa of Yellow Springs was unique. It was permanent and specially constructed rather than being temporary and requisitioned. The three-storey building had broad porches with kitchen and bathing facilities. It was the largest military hospital in Pennsylvania, and it had a good health record compared with the hospitals in Bethlehem and Lititz. It remained the only army hospital built by an order of Congress.[57]

Surgeon James Tilton believed that 'the cardinal point or principle to be observed in the direction of all hospitals is to avoid infection'.[58] His 'Tilton Huts' were relatively spacious and amply ventilated with the separate wards fumigated by smoke. They were used at Morristown in the winter of 1779–80 but, as for the Yellow Springs project, this potential improvement was not more widely implemented.[59]

The American authorities could not assume the unconditional help of local communities. At least some citizens were averse to the proximity of sick soldiers, and they resisted the conversion of their public buildings to general hospitals. Examples included Newark, Fishkill, and even the College of Philadelphia.[60]

Regimental hospitals were often set up in houses when the Continental Army was in urban areas. In the field, they were established in camp, generally in tents in the summer and in wooden huts in the winter.[61] Controversy regarding the role of the regimental hospitals contributed to the rancour between the hospital and regimental surgeons. As detailed in the previous chapter, these disagreements were not limited to the American service. Legislation in the earlier years of the War implied a subsidiary role for the regimental facilities. They were forbidden in the neighbourhood of a general hospital and all American soldiers requiring more prolonged attention for their wounds or disease were to be treated in the general hospital wards.[62] It took time to open general hospitals and regimental hospitals remained indispensable on the ground.[63] Washington acknowledged as much in May 1782 when he supported the issue of hospital tents to regiments, albeit 'Under proper Regulations and Restrictions'.[64]

As in the British Army, the term 'flying hospital' was loosely used. It was most often comprised of tents although wooden huts might be substituted when the army was camped for several months.[65] Cochran organised two for each brigade.[66] The flying hospital was most useful when a battle was fought a great distance from any general hospital and there was limited transport. It accommodated soldiers who would soon return to duty or who would be later transferred to a general hospital. The mobility of the flying hospital provided the rationale for its use, but it was also a weakness. The constant movement was detrimental to the patients' health, its presence slowed the army, and it was vulnerable to enemy fire and capture.[67] Tilton thought that it should be temporary and regarded as a branch of the general hospital.[68] In reality, it often functioned as a larger and more formal version of the regimental hospital.[69] Disagreements regarding their function did not negate the impact of the regimental and flying hospitals; at Valley Forge in the spring of 1778 there were 3,800 men in the two facilities compared with around 2,000 in the general hospitals.[70]

In addition to these three major types of hospitals there were specialist hospitals whose roles are self-evident. Smallpox hospitals were opened soon after the outbreak of hostilities to isolate solders with the disease.[71] Convalescent hospitals were created to reduce the high rate of general hospital readmissions. Staffing levels were lower than in the general hospitals. The convalescent unit at Cambridge in 1775 had seventy to eighty patients, their care overseen by a physician and one or two mates. Officers' status as gentlemen meant that they were routinely treated for wounds and sickness in private houses rather than in the army's hospitals. On occasion, they took the regimental surgeon with them.[72]

The battlefield medical arrangements of the Continental Army were similar to those of European powers of the period and there were the same problems of poor organisation and inadequate manpower. Attempts were made to formalise the management of casualties. Director General Morgan issued the following instructions in July 1776:

> 'It being the duty of the Regimental Surgeons and Mates, in case of action, in the field, to attend the Corps to which they belong, in order to dress the wounded in battle; they are to take post in the rear of the troops engaged in action, at the distance of three, four, or five hundred yards, behind some convenient hill, if at hand, there to dress the wounded, who require to be dressed, on or near the field of battle.'

Morgan recommended that this immediate surgical treatment should include the prevention of haemorrhage, the removal of foreign bodies from wounds, the reduction of fractures, and the application of bandages.[73]

The director general also advised that the regimental surgeons should liaise with the officers of their corps to identify men to carry wounded from the field using 'wheelbarrows or other more convenient biers'.[74] The camp colourmen and musicians were sometimes assigned this duty.[75] Unless there was a general hospital very close by, the wounded were taken to field hospitals hastily adapted from buildings close to the action. William Hutchinson of the Second Delaware Regiment fought at Germantown:

> 'After the battle... [I] had occasion to enter the apartment called the hospital, in which the wounded were dressing and where the necessary surgical operations were performing and there beheld a most horrid sight. The floor was covered with human blood; amputated arms and legs lay in different places in appalling array.'[76]

The legislation of April 1777 stipulated that a 'suitable number' of wagons and litters be reserved for the transport of the sick and wounded.[77] Demand often exceeded supply and the difficulty of moving ill and injured soldiers over large distances to the general hospitals was one reason for the introduction of flying hospitals. Leaving these men in the hands of local doctors was often unsatisfactory as it was expensive, and the civilian physicians were of erratic quality and not easy to supervise. Despite the challenge of obtaining adequate transport, it was usual for the sick and wounded in a campaign to be taken to a general hospital when their number exceeded ten per cent of the total force. The convoy was routinely escorted by a platoon to give protection from the enemy and to discourage desertion.[78]

The purveyor and his staff were responsible for the procurement of hospital supplies and medicines. The apothecary received drugs from the purveyor and prepared and delivered them to the hospitals and regiments. Congress underestimated the scale of medical supplies needed for the conflict and there were chronic shortages. The problem was most acute in 1776 when many hospitals lacked medicines and provisions. These shortages were exacerbated by poor coordination and a lack of transport.[79]

Most drugs had previously been imported from England. During the Revolutionary War, some were obtained from local manufacture and from the capture of British ships by the American navy and privateers. The chaotic state of drug supply was not eased until the alliance with France early in 1778. Around a dozen commonly used agents were in critical short supply. The most valued of these was Peruvian bark of which tons were used. Its price more than quadrupled between June 1776 and September 1777. Lint was also hard to find and other equipment often in short supply included surgical instruments, glass vials, and mortars and pestles.[80]

Was the American medical service of the War fit for purpose? In the early years there were serious inadequacies. The most virulent criticisms were often made by army doctors. Shippen wrote to Congress in late 1776:

> 'I saw on my first entering the army that many more brave Americans fall a sacrifice to neglect and iniquity in the medical department than fell by the sword of the enemy. I saw directors but no direction; physicians and surgeons, but too much about their business, and the care of the sick committed to young boys, in the character of mates, quite ignorant, and, as I am informed, hired at half price, etc.'[81]

This attack may have been in part politically motivated, but it contained much truth. Some defects were never fully corrected. Medical appointments were made for reasons other than professional ability, there was excessive reliance on flying and regimental hospitals, and no proper system for evacuating the wounded. Procurement and distribution of hospital supplies and drugs lacked method for most of the War. Above all, there was confusion regarding authority and responsibility at the top of the department which led to damaging disputes.[82]

Progress was made. Towards the end of the conflict, the department was better led. There were gradual improvements in conditions in the general hospitals and the management of convalescents. Medical chests were more often filled, soldiers were inoculated, and the rudiments of hygiene were better enforced. Blanco, the best authority on the American medical services of the War, concludes that although the comparison was not straightforward, 'the level of medicine in the Continental army was roughly equivalent to that of Great Britain'.[83]

If this is true, then it was a considerable achievement for a service in its infancy. Arguably, the most powerful force in its growth was George Washington's patronage. The general had experienced illness – he contracted smallpox in Barbados in 1751 – and he was acutely aware of the need to protect his fragile army of Continentals and militiamen from the ravages of disease.[84]

Soon after he assumed command at Cambridge in July 1775, he wrote to the president of Congress:

> 'I have made enquiry into the Establishment of the Hospital, and find it in a very unsettled Condition. There is no Principal Director, or any Subordination among the Surgeons, of Consequence, Disputes and Contentions have arisen, and must continue until it is reduced to some system. I could wish it was immediately taken into Consideration, as the Lives and Health of both officers and men, so much depend upon a due Regulation of this department.'[85]

Washington's close involvement in the organisation and quality control of the medical department persisted throughout the War. In the summer of 1779, he replied to a line officer who had complained of an incompetent regimental surgeon, promising that he would raise the matter with the director general.[86] After the victory at Yorktown, he continued to inspect the remaining hospitals, urging that they be 'amply Supplyed with Medicines, refreshments and accommodations'.[87]

Washington's greatest contribution to the preventative medicine of the War was his support for mass smallpox inoculation. However, his steadfast promotion of good military hygiene – instructions to clean camps and maintain proper latrines are oft repeated in his general orders – must also have saved many lives. No doubt, his preoccupation with such measures was in large part a hard-headed strategy to maintain the strength of his forces; 'one good-seasoned and well-trained soldier, recovered to health, is worth a dozen new recruits.'[88]

Gordon Jones argues that Washington's good understanding of medical matters was a result of his other life as a Virginian slave-owner:

> 'When we consider their extensive libraries, we have little cause to wonder that the masters of plantations felt quite able to treat and nurse their families and slaves. This plantation-master medical competence showed plainly in George Washington's insight, as commander-in-chief, into the medical problems of his army... A New England farmer or a Philadelphia merchant would not have had Washington's insight since neither would have been experienced in the long-term care of 200 slaves and dependants.'[89]

The Continental navy was new, and its medical arrangements were basic. Fortunately, sick rates in American sailors were generally lower than in their British counterparts. Most colonial ships operated out of seaports and could quickly return, thus limiting the impact of scurvy, malnutrition, and infectious diseases.[90]

The American navy's surgeons were untested, and they had limited opportunities to gain experience of the management of casualties during the War. The only substantive battle between the British navy and a colonial fleet in North America was at Valcour Island on Lake Champlain in 1776. Surgeons were guided by contemporary surgical texts and a few regulations. Article 16 of the naval regulations called for a convenient place for the care of the sick and wounded. Casualties were to be moved there with their hammocks and bedding, carried by crew members who were also responsible for their care and cleanliness. Buckets were provided for 'expectoration, vomitus, and other products'.[91]

John Paul Jones, the most celebrated American naval commander of the War, made raids across the Atlantic. In September 1779, he fought a sharp action against British naval forces off Flamborough Head on the East Yorkshire coast. The Americans were victorious but suffered 300 casualties.[92] Nathaniel Fanning was among Jones's men, and he well describes the inadequate medical provision:

> 'Of the wounded, nearly one hundred of that number were thrown overboard from the vessels in the squadron, where they had been conveyed after the action. With regard to so many of the wounded having died [around 150 out of 300], it was probably owing to the unskillfulness of the surgeons who amputated them. The fact was, we had but one surgeon in the squadron who really knew his duty, and that was doctor [Laurence] Brooks, a Virginian; this man was as bloody as a butcher from the commencement of the battle until towards night of the day after. The greater part of the wounded had their legs or arms shot away, or the bones so badly fractured that they were obliged to suffer under the operation of amputation. Some of these poor fellows having once gone through this severe trial by the unskilled surgeons were obliged to suffer another amputation in one, two, or three days thereafter by doctor Brooks.'

The wounded were scattered about the ships of the squadron, and it was impossible for Brooks to visit them all.[93]

France formally recognised the United States on 6 February 1778 and French forces made two significant military incursions during the War. In 1778, Admiral Charles Hector Comte d'Estaing joined American forces in an unsuccessful attempt to seize Newport, Rhode Island. Two years later, the troops of Lieutenant General Comte de Rochambeau arrived. The French general's cooperation with Washington ultimately resulted in the capture of Yorktown by the American-French army.

The provision of medical care to d'Estaing's squadron relied on improvised hospitals in Newport, Boston, Savannah, and Charleston.[94] Rochambeau's army of 8,000 men required a proper *service de santé*. A document in the *Archives Historique de la Guerre* dated March 1780 lists the French hospital establishment for an expeditionary force of the period:

> '1 *régisseur* [manager]; 1 *directeur de comptabilité* [accounting]; 4 *directeurs d'hôpitaux*; 4 *garde-magasins* [storekeepers]; 1 *premier médecin* [physician]; 2 *médecins-ordinaires*; 1 *premier chirurgien* [surgeon]; 1 *chirurgien-major*; 8 *chirurgiens aides-majors*; 8 *sous-aides-majors*; 36 *élèves* [pupil surgeons]; 1 *apothicaire-major*; 4 *apothicaires-aides-majors*; 8 *élèves* [pupil apothecaries].'

The hospital staffing was completed by numerous clerical and financial posts and by 100 *infirmiers* who administered the routine care on the wards.[95] Each regiment had a *chirurgien-major* and each company was additionally provided with an auxiliary surgeon. The latter were raised from the ranks and were variably referred to as *fraters* and *garçons-chirurgiens*. They were comparable to the surgeon's mates of the British and American armies and were scorned by better-qualified medical officers; 'Because they can use a lancet and can boil senna, they regard themselves as equal to physicians'.[96] The whole medical department was managed not by doctors but by the *commissaires des guerres*, the agents of the French army's administration.[97]

Hospitals were opened for Rochambeau's army first at Newport and then on the route to Yorktown.[98] The *service de santé* was apparently well led and organised but it was prone to the same shortcomings as the other army medical departments of the time.[99] *Commissaire des Guerres* Claude Blanchard vents his frustrations at Yorktown in October 1781:

> 'It is nothing to see unfortunates when one can give them help; but it is cruel to be not able to help them and that's what I felt. The

hospital supplies and employees had not yet arrived and they were not likely to in view of the forced marches we had made.'

Blanchard was denied transport by a military officer and was forced to improvise. The generals, he complained, lacked 'foresight'.[100]

The most prominent figure in the French service in North America was *Premier Médecin* Jean-François Coste. When Rochambeau asked Coste to give the troops instructions to maintain their health, the physician emphasised the avoidance of '*cöits faciles*' to prevent venereal disease, abstention from strong liquors, the addition of vinegar to drinking water, avoidance of extremes of temperature, and regular changes of clothes.[101] Coste also wrote a *Compendium Pharmaceuticum*, published in Newport in 1780. The short work in Latin detailed eighty-eight drug treatments commonly employed in military hospitals and gave practical advice for their optimal use. The author stressed the value of simplicity.[102]

Coste was much respected by his American allies and for good reason. Whilst in Newport, he arranged inoculation for more than 3,000 people. He subsequently received honorary diplomas from the Colleges of Williamsburg and Philadelphia and his contribution to the American service after Yorktown was recognised by Washington.[103]

'Head Quarters, 7th October 1782

Your humane attention to the American Hospitals which were established in Williamsburg after the Siege of York[town] has been properly represented to me – I beg you to be assured, Sir, that I entertain a due sense of your kindness on that occasion, and take this opportunity of testifying how much I think myself and the public obliged to you.'[104]

Campaigns

Chapter 4

Lexington and Concord; Siege of Boston; Bunker Hill

April 1775–July 1776

A musket ball, death-winged, has pierced my groin,
And widely op'd the swift curr'nt of my veins.
Bear me, then, soldiers to that hollow space,
A little hence, just in the hill's decline.
A surgeon there may stop the gushing wound,
And gain a short respite to life, that yet
I may return, and fight one half hour more.

A Gentleman of Maryland, 1776[1]

Lieutenant Hamilton feigned illness on 19 April 1775. His place in Lieutenant Colonel Francis Smith's expedition was taken by volunteer Jeremy Lister. The 22-year-old ensign of the British 10th Regiment was unscathed at the skirmish at Lexington but on the subsequent British retreat from Concord he received a gunshot wound while under intense American fire at Meriam's Corner, a bend in the road near the farm of Nathan and Abigail Meriam. Lister's detailed account of his wounding and medical treatment foreshadows innumerable similar experiences endured by British and American soldiers (and their allies) in the years between Lexington and Yorktown. The chaos of the battlefield, the all too often improvised nature of medical assistance, the real prospect of no help at all, the fear of pain and dying.

The musket ball shattered Lister's right elbow. He made his way back to Lexington where he was examined by Mr Simes, surgeon's mate to the 43rd Regiment. As a mere warrant officer, Simes is not included in Drew's roll of British Army commissioned medical officers, so we have no knowledge of his qualifications. He may have had very little surgical experience or even have been an ordinary soldier acting up from the ranks.[2] Whatever, he succeeded in extracting the impacted ball from the bone. By now Lister was feeing faint due to a combination of blood loss, exhaustion, and hunger. He managed to obtain a little food and some water from a pond. The British force remained under heavy fire and Lieutenant Colonel Smith, perhaps remembering that Lister was a volunteer, lent the wounded man his horse. As the balls 'whistled so smartly' around his ears, Lister chose to dismount, first using the horse as a shield and then generously giving it over to more seriously wounded comrades.

Eventually, the beleaguered party arrived back at Bunker Hill at Charleston. The relief was palpable, particularly for the wounded. There were accusations of brutality. The bodies of British soldiers had allegedly been 'scalp'd, their Eyes goug'd, their Noses and Ears cut of[f]'. Lister, still lightheaded, was transported by boat to the main town of Boston where he reached his lodgings at nine o'clock in the evening after a march of sixty miles in twenty-four hours, twenty-four miles while wounded. The mistress of the house provided tea and he was attended by a surgeon of the town who dressed the wound. In the morning, he was visited by Arthur Edwards, surgeon of his regiment, and Purveyor Jonathan Mallet. These men had thirty years of military medical experience between them, so the patient was in good hands.[3] Some bone fragments were extracted, and it was decided that immediate amputation of the arm was not necessary. He was in great pain. He was given a light diet, the wound was dressed twice a day, and he was regularly dosed with Jesuit's bark, a typical antiphlogistic treatment. He remained weak but after two weeks was well enough to leave his bed.

On 9 May, three weeks following his wounding, Lister was visited by 'a large number of the faculty'. Some were keen to amputate but Mallet, the senior doctor, resisted; an opinion that was to save the soldier's arm. Lister only asked that should the operation become necessary, he be given some notice to prepare himself. Without antisepsis or antibiotics, his stormy clinical course continued. The surgeons opened up the wound to the bone twice more, on the 10th and 21st of May, while the pain and debility persisted. In early June, he remained so weak that he needed the help of his servant to leave his bed. His friends were pessimistic but by 17 June, the day of the Battle of Bunker Hill, he was apparently improved, dining with fellow officers. He was able to use his hand. A month later, he reassured his father that he was getting stronger each day although it was unlikely that he would ever be able to bend his elbow. His surgeons were cautious and on 19 August he became unwell again with some deterioration in the wound. Thankfully, this relapse was self-limiting and by mid-September he was able to walk outside. He was eventually evacuated to England in December, arriving at Portsmouth in January 1776. He later served in the recruiting service, a common haven for soldiers convalescing from wounds or sickness.[4]

Casualty figures for the Battle of Lexington and Concord vary. The American force – made up of volunteers, minutemen, and militia – probably lost less than a hundred men from 3,500 to 4,000 combatants; half of these were killed. The British inevitably suffered more, losing fifteen per cent of their men with more than seventy dead. Considering their extreme exposure to enemy fire during the retreat, even this number might be regarded as low.[5] According to Smith, his force was under enemy fire 'without the intermission of five minutes altogether, for I believe upwards of 18 miles'. A British officer admitted that they had been forced to dance to the 'tune of Yankee Doodle'.[6] Some had lucky escapes; a marine had his hat shot off three times, two balls through his coat, and his bayonet blown from his side.[7] One theory invoked to explain the relatively low British losses was that the buckshot used by many of the patriots was smaller than conventional eighteenth-century musket balls.[8]

We have other eyewitness accounts of both British and American wounded. Lieutenant Thomas Hawkshaw was shot in the cheek, a matter of particular regret as he had been judged to be the most handsome man in the British Army. Lieutenant Frederick Mackenzie meticulously documents the wounds in seventeen fellow officers. Five, including Lister, were wounded in the arm or hand; four in the leg or foot; two in the head or neck; two in the chest; four more slightly and the site not specified. A further two officers had fatal wounds, one poorly documented and the other 'in the body and 2 other places'.[9]

There were some remarkable survivals among the American wounded. Samuel Whittemore, reputedly 80 years old, would live another eighteen years after receiving treatment for bayonet wounds and a gunshot injury to the face.[10] John Tolman was left for dead after receiving a shot in the back but was later able to write his memoirs in old age.[11] One of the more detailed accounts of a wounding has been left by Daniel Hemenway of Framingham who, like many others, had voluntarily turned out with his musket and who later petitioned the Massachusetts General Assembly.

> 'And on the 19th Day of April last Your Petitioner by alarm with the Company he belonged to engaged the British troops: At Lexington &c in which engagement was wounded at Cambridge, received a ball from the enemy that first passed through his right thumb & broak the bone to shivers that penetrated his body at the lower part on the rib & made its way through the midriff & was cut out at his back, which after hath put him into great pain, his being at such a distance from his Family when wounded; the pain & expense of getting home, his cost for providing necessary comfortable things for his support, the constant attention Day & Night in the time of his extremity, the entire loss of four months' time in a Season of the year when everything for the Support of a large Family is depending, the Surgeons Bills. Doctr. Hemenway for dressing his wounds seventy-seven times & necessary Topical and Internal remidies. Charges Ten Pounds eight shillings. Doctr. Stone for advice, Dressing &c Three Dollars and although the wounds are healed, at the present time is unable to perform any hard service, & is ever likely to have the misfortune in a good measure to lose the use of his right thumb &c.'

Hemenway was successful in his petition: his medical bills to the sum of £17 12s 6d were paid out of the public treasury. More than six pounds of this amount went to his brother, Dr Ebenezer Hemenway.[12] Nathaniel Cleaves of Beverly and Israel Everett of Dedham both paid the more modest sum of three shillings for their wound surgery.[13] The receipt of medical bills by patriot soldiers at the inception of their fight for liberty underlines the lack of any formal army medical service at Lexington and Concord. The care of the American wounded was opportunistic or even accidental.[14] Injured men were carried off by comrades in blankets, carts, and wheelbarrows. Dr William Aspinwall, an expert on smallpox inoculation and a volunteer with the soldiers from Brookline, later testified that he and medical colleagues cared for wounded soldiers from 19 April to 12 August, 'before the Regular Appt.mt of surgeons to ye Reg.mts'.[15]

Of the thirteen American doctors present at the fighting, six were combatants and seven served only in a medical capacity. The former included the influential patriot Joseph Warren, president of the Provincial Congress of Massachusetts and chairman of the Committee of Public Safety. All these men survived the battle although Warren had a lock of hair shot off in one of the skirmishes. Seven of the doctors subsequently became surgeons in the Massachusetts or Continental armies.[16]

On the eve of the battle, the Congress had directed the placement of medical chests and linen in Concord and the surrounding towns and villages.[17] Local buildings along the Boston to Concord road served as temporary hospitals. Cooper's Tavern, situated by a crossroad to Woburn, was staffed by at least three doctors.[18] On the evening of 19 April, a temporary American field hospital was opened in the Anglican church at Cambridge. A second hospital was established two days later. Other wounded were taken to private houses.[19]

In contrast, the British medical services of April 1775 were well established and organised along traditional lines (see Chapter 2). Allowing for one surgeon and one surgeon's mate attached to each regiment, there should theoretically have been around thirty regimental doctors in Boston; in reality it was probably much less. There would also have been a limited number of non-regimental army medical staff and the informal help of local physicians, at least some of whom would have had loyalist sympathies. There was a hospital ship in the harbour but at this stage no general hospital in the city.[20] In the event, British medical resources were only slowly employed. They were not anticipating so many casualties.[21] It seems that only Surgeon's Mate Simes accompanied the original detachment of 700 men under Smith. It is likely that more regimental surgeons and mates were with the British reinforcements under Brigadier Hugh Earl Percy. They, like their American cousins, were not well equipped. Two wagons of medical stores had lost contact with Percy's force and were later captured at Menotomy (now Arlington).[22]

There was no proper arrangement for the evacuation of the wounded, a particular problem for soldiers in rapid retreat. At Concord, some British casualties were tended to by local doctors and the more seriously injured were left behind. Two chaises, bedding and horses were confiscated to carry off the less seriously wounded. Once the advanced party was reinforced by Percy's fresher troops, the wounded were moved in wagons in the centre of the retreating force, or they were on horses or on foot. At Lexington, they were allowed a short respite, taken to William Monroe's tavern where they were given rum. Many had their wounds dressed in the parlour.[23]

At the end of the humiliating and exhausting retreat, Frederick Mackenzie simply noted in his diary, 'We brought off most of our wounded men'.[24] In Boston, the lack of any general hospital meant that the medical work was in regimental facilities and in private homes.

Lister was not the only soldier to hear rumours of atrocities. Reports of scalping were common.[25] It appears that these were apocryphal – the start of a prolonged propaganda war – and that the casualties who fell into enemy hands were well treated by the standards of the time. The two sides agreed to respect each other's captured wounded. British prisoners were treated by surgeons with loyalist sympathies and the Americans dressed by British surgeons thus sparing their hard-pressed doctors and preserving vital medical supplies.[26] Not all were grateful for this enlightened approach. In Menotomy, an American doctor from Brookline attempted to reach a wounded British soldier who had crawled into a barn. When the doctor offered to dress his leg, the regular fired on him, fortunately missing. The wounded man was quickly dispatched.[27]

There remained the task of burying the dead. Major General William Heath, now in charge of the rebel army, ordered out a company to locate the wounded and to dig graves.[28] Many of the bodies, mostly British, lay naked on or around the road.[29] The American dead were often buried in their local church. At Danvers, the fallen Danvers men were interred at the Old South Church. Men lined the route of the funeral, and three volleys were fired over the grave.

The men forming the escort at the Danvers funeral – soldiers from Newburyport, Salisbury and Amesbury – were on their way to Boston.[30] British forces under General Thomas Gage were now besieged in the city by an American army formed along a ten-mile crescent from Roxbury to Chelsea.[31] As spring merged into early summer, both sides attempted to optimise their medical provision, anticipating sickness and a further battle. The British appointed five men to lead their medical department, the 'Hospital at Boston'. Jonathan Mallet, who attended Jeremy Lister, was confirmed as purveyor. He had previously served as a staff surgeon in Louisiana in the Seven Years War. Michael Morris, who was a veteran of the Portuguese Campaign of the Seven Years War, was appointed as physician. Robert Roberts, previously a surgeon in the 3rd Dragoon Guards, was an apothecary. John Samuel Charlton, recently surgeon in the 17th Foot, was promoted to staff surgeon to the hospital. We have little information for the final appointee, Alexander Grant, who was also raised to staff surgeon.[32] A general hospital was opened in the city in mid-May. This was in an old factory (the Manufactory House) on Long Acre opposite the current Park Street Church. Auxiliary general hospitals were later opened at the Workhouse and the Almshouse and eventually there was a general hospital in Charleston. This provision was supplemented by regimental hospitals and private houses.[33]

It has been estimated that 140 Americans served as either hospital or regimental surgeons and mates at the Siege of Boston.[34] The earliest of these were with the 4–5,000 strong Massachusetts militia regiments. Each unit had a surgeon and a surgeon's mate. The Connecticut regiments, raised a little later, had two mates each.[35] Before the Battle of Bunker Hill, these were largely unofficial attachments, few or perhaps none having been examined or properly commissioned. As early as May, the Provincial Congress, mindful of the uneducated nature of many of these men, ordered the formation of a committee 'to examine the surgeons of the army'. If they were judged to be qualified to serve then their appointment was by the colonel of the regiment.[36] The first substantial American general hospital of the Revolution was opened in Cambridge, located in private houses. By the end of June, there were four general hospitals for the Massachusetts Army at Cambridge, Menotomy, Roxbury and Watertown. Two specialist smallpox hospitals were also opened. As has been discussed, the relative role of general and regimental hospitals was a subject keenly debated in the eighteenth century. At Boston, the American armies relied principally on the general facilities spurred by their convenience, more reliable supplies, and the perceived superiority of the staff. Nevertheless, the regimental hospitals played a vital part and the role of the private houses of sympathetic local citizens should not be underestimated.[37]

The British had to import hospital equipment from England. More than 5,000 palliasses, 11,250 blankets, 8,500 sheets, 2,500 coverlets, bed rugs and ward utensils of all descriptions had arrived in Boston.[38] They controlled the drug supplies in the city which caused problems for their enemy as the limited amounts in the neighbouring small towns were soon exhausted. In June, the Americans were forced to initiate another committee 'to take into consideration a complaint that the surgeons in the army are not properly furnished with medicines'. There were not enough medicine chests for all the regiments and a dearth of hospital supplies.[39]

Most of the patriot troops besieging Boston were housed in hastily improvised shelters. These were constructed from anything available including turf, sail cloth and pieces of iron. Clothes and blankets were scarce.[40] The soldiers were in rags and filthy. A visitor noted that they 'let their linen etc. rot upon their backs [rather] than to be at the trouble of cleaning 'em themselves'. A lieutenant wrote to his wife for a new shirt as it was hot and 'shirts Durttey verry fast'.[41] Inside the city the British garrison was better clothed and was accommodated in tents, barracks, and private homes. There was, however, the threat of food shortages, especially fresh provisions. Rebels had cut off supplies from the surrounding country. Children already had the pinched look of malnutrition.[42]

Both sides had some knowledge of the tenets of military hygiene. The senior military officers of the Massachusetts Army made attempts to keep the camps clean, ordering regular inspections of the men and the washing of barracks and private houses. The Provincial Congress was concerned, informing Washington that 'The youth of the Army are not possessed of the absolute necessity of cleanliness'.[43] The British had a greater tradition of such measures, and their soldiers could be more closely supervised. General orders gave explicit advice.

> 'The greatest attention and care must be taken to keep the Camp and Environs Clean and free from putrefaction, the different Corps having prepar'd Necessary Houses [toilets], the Quarter Masters will have them Cover'd with fresh Earth every Morning.'

It was forbidden for the men to evacuate their bowels elsewhere. Sea bathing was strongly recommended, and little was left to chance; 'Attention must be had the Men do not Continue long in the Water (nor those who are unacquainted with Swimming risk any Accident happening by going beyond their Depth).'[44]

A British officer writing home in January 1775 described the army as very healthy but a few weeks later he acknowledged the presence of smallpox and some attempts at inoculation. Three soldiers were dying from the disease each day.[45] Lieutenant John Barker of the King's Own Regiment agreed that the town was 'very sickly' due to the mildness of the weather.[46] Frederick Mackenzie recorded that on 23 April, forty-eight men of his regiment were sick out of a total of 303, a rate of 16 per cent.[47] Cooperative measures taken by Gage and the local authorities kept smallpox under some control. The American army was relatively healthy, sick rates in the spring and early summer were probably less than 10 per cent. This was low by the standards of the time. The presence of smallpox in Boston was, however, an existential threat to a patriot army with little previous exposure and low levels of immunity.[48]

Fear of the disease was immediately overshadowed by the first great battle of the Revolution fought on 17 June. The British could claim victory at Bunker Hill, but they suffered very heavy casualties; 226 men were killed and 828 wounded.[49] Officer losses were disproportionately high. Sergeant Roger Lamb believed them to have been singled out by American marksmen and an account by a Connecticut officer confirms this; 'a choice party of our best shots under cover were appointed to fire at none but the Reddest coats'.[50] The total losses represented 42 per cent of the attacking force and 16 per cent of the entire British garrison in Boston.[51] The equivalent American casualty figure for the forces engaged was 32 per cent. The 453 casualties were made up of 139 killed, 278 wounded and thirty-six missing.[52] American senior officers also paid a heavy price. Joseph Warren was hit by a ball below the left eye and died instantly.[53]

In this carnage, the first medical priority was to administer first aid and remove the more seriously wounded from the field. The British had no formal system for battlefield evacuation and at Bunker Hill many of their wounded lay too close to the rebel defences to be easily collected.[54] Any medical help was thus ad hoc and heavily reliant on comrades. Surgical help was a distant prospect. When Major Williams of the 52nd was badly wounded atop Breed's Hill, Captain Francis Lord Rawdon asked Ensign Martin Hunter to find a surgeon. But Hunter was not keen.

> '[I] had seen enough to know that I was much safer under the works that I could be at a few yards from it, as the enemy could not depress their guns sufficiently to do any execution to those that were close under, and to have gone to the rear to look for a surgeon would have been almost certain death.'

Hunter had just witnessed the fate of four soldiers carrying off the wounded Captain George Harris. Three were wounded in the act, one later dying. Harris was left under some trees out of reach of the American fire.[55]

A general order of 19 June suggests that some British casualties were still being brought in forty-eight hours after the battle.[56] However, the great bulk of the wounded were transferred to Boston on the evening after the battle. An anonymous officer describes spending the night carrying wounded and dead fellow officers.[57] Boats, their bottoms slippery with blood, ferried the injured men from the Charleston Peninsula to the main town. This transfer probably continued for much of the next day, all means of improvised transport being used. First Lieutenant of Marines John Clarke saw coaches, chariots, single-horse chaises and even wheelbarrows. The citizens of the city also witnessed the 'melancholic scene' of several carriages full of dead and dying officers.[58] They were taken to the general hospitals at the Manufactory House, the Almshouse and the Workhouse. The general hospital at Charleston, intended for the more lightly wounded and the sick, was not opened until eleven days after the fighting. Many of the officers were cared for in private homes.[59] Isaac Lothrop, a member of the Provincial Congress, claimed that there were not enough army surgeons to dress the wounded and that many died in the streets.[60]

According to Clarke, the British army surgeons were assisted by Boston's physicians, surgeons and apothecaries.[61] This was sorely needed as the army's hospital staff was limited to two surgeons, eight hospital mates, one purveyor and two apothecaries.[62] On 19 June, most of the surgeons still on the Charleston Peninsula, where there were presumably some dressing stations and perhaps a field hospital, were asked to return to Boston; 'the Exigence arising from the state of the sick and wounded in the General Hospital in Consequence of the Action of the 17th makes this Arrangement Necessary'.[63] Later general orders directed the provision of linen and the sending of 'careful sober women' to the hospitals where the patients were 'greatly suffering for want of attention'.[64] When 170 of the survivors were eventually evacuated to England, they provided 'a most shocking spectacle' at Plymouth, skeletons with missing arms and legs.[65]

If the relatively well-established British army medical service with its previous experience of eighteenth-century wars was so pressed then it is understandable that the embryonic American medical provision was overwhelmed. There were around thirty American doctors at the battle but no proper leadership. Many of the regimental and hospital surgeons and mates still served in a temporary capacity. All arrangements were improvised. It was the hottest day of the summer and the wounded begged for help and water. Soldiers' blankets were combined with muskets and poles to make crude stretchers and the injured men were first moved to the west side of

Bunker Hill. They were hastily dressed and then sent on to nearby barracks and private houses, some of the latter vacated by loyalists. The more seriously wounded eventually reached Cambridge, Menotomy and Watertown. Here, they were managed in tents, barracks, private homes, regimental hospitals, and the only extant general hospital.[66] New general hospitals were soon opened as previously described.

That the British hospitals were inadequate is clear from the testimony of Richard Hope, surgeon to the 52nd Regiment. He had a lucky escape, as an American musket ball was deflected by a large bunch of keys in his pocket. This did not improve his mood.

> 'We had about thirty killed on the spot of our private men, and eighty wounded, a fourth part of whom will die; forty seven of the worst cases with the whole sick of the Regiment are for want of room in the general Hospital forced on me; this is quite unprecedented to oblige a regimental Surgeon to bear the charge in time of war of wounded soldiers, and this injustice will be above forty pounds out of my pocket, a noble recompense for nineteen years service; the fatigue is so great I have not had five hours rest any night since the action, so that thro' weakness of body, weariness of mind, and being half starved I am brought low enough.'[67]

Many of the British had multiple injuries. John Randon wrote to his wife that he had received two gunshot wounds, one in the chest and one in the groin; 'The surgeons inform me that three hours will be the utmost I can survive'.[68] Captain Charles Stuart asserted that among his stricken light infantry and grenadier comrades, few had less than three or four wounds.[69]

American soldiers also received horrific injuries although in smaller numbers. Men who carried the wounded away from the field in boats were forced to bail the blood out of them.[70] Ebenezer Bridge had his head and neck sliced by a sword while Amos Farnsworth received a gunshot wound to his elbow; 'Another bawl struck my Back taking a piece of Skin as big as a Penny but I got to Cambridge that night'.[71] Americans suffered non-fatal wounds in the foot, leg, knee, thigh, groin, chest, arm, hand, neck and cheek.[72]

The surgeons of both sides confronted a grim and relentless task. British Staff Surgeon Alexander Grant, writing six days after the battle, believed the enemy to have been either short of ammunition or especially malicious.

'I have scarce time to eat my meals, therefore you must expect but a few lines. I have been up two nights, assisted with four mates, dressing our men of the wounds received the last engagement; many of the wounded are daily dying, and many must have both legs amputated. The provincials had either exhausted their ball, or they were determined that every wound should prove mortal; their musquets were charged with old nails and angular pieces of iron.'

He attributed the large number of leg wounds to an (unlikely) plan to disable British soldiers thus rendering them an extra burden to the army in Boston. Private Thomas Sullivan of the 49th supposed some of the purulent wounds to be caused by the enemy poisoning the balls.[73]

The best American account of surgery after the battle has been left by 36-year-old Dr Hall Jackson. A committed patriot, he rode for thirteen hours from Portsmouth to reach Cambridge where he offered his help:

'to describe the pitiful and miserable condition of our poor wound[ed] Brethren would be impossible, many tho' 48 hours was elapsed, had never had the least application apply'd, many lay bleeding & not a person to assist them... [Of the surgeons who were there], not one of these were possessed of even a needle, or any other proper Instruments, had they been ever so well equipped, the matter would not have been much mended. I amputated several limbs and extracted many balls the first night, the next day I was hurried to all quarters Dr. Church having got notice of my being at Mistick, [and he] the best Surgeon on the Continent being obliged to supply poor [Joseph] Warren's place at the Congress forced the principal [part] of the wounded on me, I went on with this fatigue 15 days, when a violent inflammation in my eyes forced me to return to Portsmo'.'

Remarkably, Hall lost only two of his patients, one of them an amputee.[74] He well represents the typical surgery performed although there were some more targeted procedures. George Harris, whose removal from the field proved so costly to British soldiers, had his head wound successfully managed by the ancient operation of trepanning, the making of a hole in the skull; 'before the callous was formed, they indulged me with the gratification of a singular curiosity – fixing looking-glasses so to give me a sight of my own brain'.[75]

The less fortunate were buried as quickly as possible. The night after the battle, Gage sent twenty barrels of quicklime to Charleston and the corpses were deposited in a damp hollow between the Breed's and Bunker hills. Officers generally received a more dignified funeral in Boston churchyards.[76]

Both sides had taken prisoners. At Cambridge, British navy surgeons were allowed to administer to wounded British captives.[77] The American wounded prisoners of war in Boston were apparently well accommodated but their care was probably haphazard at best and only a third were still alive in September. None of the amputation cases survived. A local physician and ex-British Army surgeon, Miles Whitworth, was later blamed for their suboptimal treatment although he was probably a scapegoat.[78]

In the period after Bunker Hill, it became clear to the American authorities and senior military officers that there was a leadership vacuum in the army's medical provision. On assuming command, Washington inspected the hospitals. He was not impressed, writing to Congress on 21 July complaining of the lack of organisation (see Chapter 3).[79]

The appointment of Dr Benjamin Church as the first British-style director general should have been part of the solution but, as has been explained, it was just the start of the dissent and discontinuity which afflicted the top of the American hospital department for much of the War. Congress intended that Church should provide direction for the staff, complete returns and take over the duty of the commissariat. Instructions were given for the further development of general and regimental hospitals and for the placement of flying hospitals near combat zones. Church was soon removed on the charge of treason and was replaced by the energetic and able John Morgan on 5 October.[80]

At the beginning of July, directives had been issued for the method of transfer of sick men to the American general hospitals. When a soldier was ill or wounded, he was to be examined by his regimental surgeon and, if his condition was thought to be serious, he was to be sent to the general hospital with a certificate.[81] This may seem straightforward but at this time there was much friction between the regimental surgeons and the directorship of the medical department and also controversy as to the respective roles of the general and regimental hospitals. General John Sullivan was responsible for the army's defences early in the siege. He weighed in on the side of his regimental surgeons.

> 'This [sending the troops to the general hospital in the rear lines at Cambridge] filled them with such fearful apprehensions that more

than half of them refused to go, Declaring they would rather Die where they were, and under the care of those Physicians they were acquainted with, than be removed from their friends under the care of Physicians they never saw. I found it vain to attempt Reasoning them out of those Sentiments.'

He accused Church of ignoring the regimental surgeons and of starving them of medicines and dressings.[82]

Many of the doctors in the general hospitals had no previous hospital experience or medical training beyond an apprenticeship.[83] The facilities were crowded. Nevertheless, Morgan defended them in October, and when Surgeon James Thacher visited them in November, he was gratified to observe that 'the brave men while in the service of their country, receive in sickness all the kind attentions from physicians and nurses, which their circumstances require'.[84] Most of the deficiencies and neglect were probably in the regimental hospitals which continued to be supported by the regiments' colonels. The status of these hospitals and the relationship of their surgeons to the general hospitals were to remain vexatious issues.[85]

Excerpts from the British general orders give some clue to the steps taken to optimise the hospital provision within Boston. In late June and early July, women were ordered to the hospitals to serve as cleaners and nurses. Any woman who refused to be a nurse was to be struck off the provisions list. Sick men were only to be sent to the general hospital if they had a written order from a military officer or their regimental surgeon. In September, a house in Charleston was adapted to be a convalescent hospital.[86] These directives suggest real attempts at organisation and indeed the secretary at war wrote to Gage in March 1776; 'I am glad to find you are so well satisfied with the care and attention of the gentlemen in the medical department'.[87]

Expectations were low. Correspondence from the Boston garrison suggests that the improvised British hospitals were often squalid. A letter from an anonymous officer written in August was later published in the *Morning Chronicle and Daily Advertiser*.

'Our distresses accumulate every day; our barracks are all hospitals and so offensive is the stench of the wounds that the very air is infected with the smell.'[88]

Another officer agreed; 'Could you view our hospitals, and see how fast we drop off, your heart would bleed within you'. He claimed that as many thirty bodies a day were thrown into a trench 'like those of so many dogs'.[89]

The unsanitary conditions in the British general hospitals reflected the impoverished state of the besieged army. The soldiers were forced to live on a diet of salt beef and salt pork which was as hard as wood.[90] Frying the pork was forbidden in general orders as it was thought to be especially injurious to health.[91] The spruce beer caused diarrheoa.[92] Although the men were well clothed, they were not moved out of tents into warmer winter quarters until mid-December.[93] Outside the city, the American forces were short of clothes, blankets and fuel. Major General Artemas Ward complained to the Massachusetts Provincial Congress that his soldiers were 'almost naked'.[94] Only in October was there a sustained effort to build wooden accommodation. These barracks were too small and full of smoke due to the lack of chimneys.[95] Under such conditions, both armies were vulnerable to disease. British soldiers were soon calling Boston 'the graveyard of England and the slaughter-house of America'.[96]

The most feared disease was smallpox. In November, it broke out in the city with renewed virulence despite quarantine measures. Major General William Howe, who had replaced Gage, was forced to adopt the policy of inoculating all soldiers who had not previously had the disorder. It is clear from his orders that this was strongly recommended but not mandatory. Men who accepted the inoculations were to be put in houses by themselves and kept apart from those who refused. The troops of a European army such as the British would have had widespread exposure to the virus in childhood. The number susceptible was thus small and the risk of inoculation to individuals and to the wider army was relatively low. To facilitate this approach, a floating smallpox hospital was opened, and inoculation was extended to the residents of Boston.[97]

Howe's inoculation strategy was successful. The British general also ejected several locals from the city. There was now a real danger of the spread of the disease into the much more vulnerable American forces outside. Washington shared his 'dreadful apprehensions' with the Congress. It is possible that the fear of smallpox was a factor in his decision to besiege rather than attack the city. At the end of November, Washington reinforced the American quarantine, excluding any refugees from the Continental Army's camp. Letters coming out of the city were dipped in vinegar. Smallpox remained a constant threat through the winter. A guarded smallpox hospital was established distant from the lines. These precautions worked and the disease was kept in check for the duration of the siege.[98]

British eyewitness accounts confirm the presence of dysentery in Boston in the summer of 1775. There are references to the 'bloody flux' which caused much suffering and some deaths. It was usually blamed on Boston's water supply or the consumption of spruce beer.[99] One British officer noted that the disease 'runs us off our legs in a few days, and has made the remains of our famished army look like so many regiments of skeletons'.[100] In September, Gage complained that the hospitals had been 'crowded for some time by Dissentry'.[101] Unsurprisingly, the affliction also made inroads into the American ranks. Isaac Bangs was entirely debilitated, 'the Bloody Flux raged so hard upon me & nothing suitable for my Diet to be bought, it was thought best for me to go into the Country.'[102] The epidemic extended to the civilian population of East Massachusetts leading to some eccentric 'cures' being published in local newspapers.[103]

The shortage of fresh provisions in Boston made an outbreak of scurvy inevitable. Together with dysentery, this was a major cause of indisposition in the British garrison. In December 1775, Captain William Evelyn believed that they had escaped lightly, 'we are in tolerable good health and spirits, and not yet so overrun with the scurvy as you would expect of people who live upon salt pork, without roots or vegetables of any kind'.[104] By January 1776 this paltry diet was becoming more problematic, Lieutenant William Fielding declaring that many of the soldiers were severely affected by the disorder.[105] The authorities attempted to ward it off by the increased issue of antiscorbutics such as spruce beer and 'Sour Crout'.[106]

Other diseases affecting both armies were respiratory infections, colds, and rheumatic disorders. These were more debilitating than life-threatening. In Boston, there was an ample supply of alcohol and drunkenness was commonplace. The alcohol was often of very low quality and even poisonous. Two soldiers died after drinking cheap New England rum.[107] New cider caused diarrhoea in the American troops and Washington forbade the drinking of it.[108]

The sick rate in the British Army peaked at twenty-three per cent in November 1775, more than 1,700 men. A few of these were still recovering from wounds but the vast majority were victims of disease. By March of the following year the rate had fallen dramatically to only eight per cent. This was probably due to a combination of increased immunity to dysentery, the use of antiscorbutics, and the inoculation programme against smallpox.[109] In the Continental Army, the average sick rate between July 1775 and March 1776 was 12 per cent, the highest level of 17 per cent occurring between August and September.[110] This equates to an average daily sick list of around 2,000, allowing for an average troop strength of 17,400 for the duration of the siege.[111] It was normal for armies of this period to have a sick rate of 12 per cent in the autumn so if one considers the poor hygienic state of the soldiers and the primitive nature of the medical services, the American sick rates are surprisingly low. The reason for this was very likely multifactorial, a cumulative effect of the underlying tough constitution of the provincials, limited combat and long marches, the proximity of supplies, and the personal interest Washington had shown in the wellbeing of those under his command. Smallpox had been limited by quarantine, dysentery was weakening but rarely fatal, and typhus had not made a significant appearance.[112]

The British have been accused of waging biological warfare at the siege of Boston. What was Howe's motivation for sending refugees out of the city? Was it simply to safeguard the health of his soldiers and the citizenry or was it a sinister plot to introduce smallpox into the enemy camp? Washington was initially disbelieving of the reports of such a 'diabolical scheme', but he eventually became suspicious and then convinced. On 11 December 1775, he wrote:

'The information I received that the enemy intend Spreading the Small pox amongst us, I coud not Suppose them Capable of — I must now give Some Credit to it, as it has made its appearance on Severall of those who Last Came out of Boston.'[113]

There were allegations that a Boston doctor had intentionally planted recently inoculated persons among the refugees. One refugee claimed that he had been forcibly expelled from the city with disease pustules on his legs. The accusations fell away in early 1776 only to resurface when the city was evacuated in March. The case against Howe is inconclusive. It may be that his discharge of people from the city was self-serving but not a pre-meditated attempt to induce an epidemic of smallpox.[114]

At the outset of March, Washington planned to seize and fortify the strategically vital Dorchester Heights, an area of high ground beyond Boston

Neck. A battle was expected. Surgeon Thacher saw the military and medical preparations:

> 'Several regiments of militia have arrived from the country; and orders have been received for surgeons and mates to prepare lint and bandages, to the amount of two thousand, for fractured limbs and other gunshot wounds. It is, however, to be hoped that not one-quarter of the number will be required, whatever may be the nature of the occasion.'[115]

Washington ordered the surgeons of the Cambridge general hospital and the regimental surgeons of the centre and left wings of the army to assemble at Brown's Tavern not far from Concord. Here, Morgan was to give instructions as to their posting on the field and the collection and evacuation of the wounded. The director general also advertised in local newspapers for nurses and orderlies for the hospitals. He selected soldiers to act as stretcher-bearers.[116] The regimental hospitals were to be emptied and the sick and wounded transferred to the college buildings at Cambridge. Barracks on Prospect Hill were to receive the wounded from the expected engagement.[117]

This laudable planning could not disguise troubling deficiencies. Surgical supplies were critically low. Surgeons of twenty-four of the twenty-six regiments had only the following available: six cases of amputation instruments, one in bad condition, twenty-one cases of pocket instruments, two cases of lancets, twelve cases of crooked needles, two cases of knives, 859 bandages, twelve pounds of lint, and twenty-four tourniquets. Medicines and sheets were also hard to find. The hospitals were a little better off.[118]

Fortunately, the Americans caught their torpid foe by surprise and Howe aborted a counterattack, limiting the British reprisal to an intense but short-lived cannonade of the new Dorchester fortifications. Among the American wounded at Roxbury was a young lieutenant, hit by a cannon ball in the thigh, who needed amputation. 'He did not bleed to excess yet his pain was so exquisite, occasioned by the bone being shivered to pieces quite to his hip joint, that he died about 9 o'clock the next morning'.[119] Injuries to major joints were often fatal.

The British occupation of Boston was now untenable, and orders were given for the abandonment of the place by the 9,000-strong army and some of its followers. The initial move would be to the British base at Halifax, a two-week voyage to the north-east.[120] General orders of 10 March stipulated that the commanders of corps were to have all their sick, convalescents and women on board by six o'clock in the evening. The transports, overcrowded with soldiers and loyalists, finally departed a week later.[121]

In mid-April, there were eighty-nine British sick in a Halifax garrison of 1,113 men, a rate of only 8 per cent. At least some of these men were affected by smallpox. Howe's orders refer to hospital ships and also to a hospital on St George's Island where the smallpox cases were sent.[122]

Washington triumphantly rode into Boston. He remained suspicious of enemy schemes to infect his army. The first thousand Continental troops to enter the city were smallpox survivors who were instructed to search for evidence of the disease.[123] There were even insinuations that the British had poisoned the city's drug supplies. The Americans had taken over the British general hospitals and had inherited significant hospital stores which the fleeing army was unable to carry away. On 15 April, the *Boston Gazette* reported that, 'it is absolutely fact that the Doctors of the diabolical ministerial butcher when they evacuated Boston, intermixed and left 26 weight of Arsenick with the medicines which they left in the Alms House'. Dr John Warren later swore under oath that he had visited the medicines storeroom of the hospital and discovered about twelve to fourteen pounds of arsenic mixed in with the drugs. On Washington's orders, Morgan confiscated the drug supplies of two Tory physicians in the city.[124]

Washington had distanced his enemy, but the smallpox virus was still close. On 21 March, he again communicated his concern to the Massachusetts legislature. Two weeks later, he headed towards New York leaving only two regiments behind. His men had been spared the ravages of a smallpox epidemic. That Washington's fears were well-founded is illustrated by the spread of the disease in Boston after the departure of the two armies. By May, James Thacher was being advised by his friends to resort to inoculation. This was against general orders, but Morgan was also a supporter of the procedure and, in early June, the authorities lifted the ban. By late 1776, 5,000 Bostonians had been inoculated. The combination of large-scale inoculation and quarantine was effective and in September there were only a handful of cases in the city.[125]

The move of the Continental Army south to the defence of New York left Morgan with a major logistical challenge. If we are to believe his own words, the transfer of medical resources was remarkably slick.

'When the troops marched from Cambridge for New York, all the sick were left behind in the General hospital, amounting to upwards of 300 men. In less than six weeks, during which time but few died, I was able to discharge the hospital of every man, to settle and pay every account, insomuch as never to have had any demands from that quarter.'[126]

Economy was foremost in the director general's mind, a characteristic he shared with his commander-in-chief. Thousands of pounds worth of medicines, furnishings and hospital stores were to be sent on to New York 'with little or no expense to the public'. Most of these supplies had been abandoned by the British.[127]

The American medical department in New York would commence its role with better organisation and resources than was the case at the start of the siege of Boston. With respect to smallpox, Washington's soldiers had dodged a bullet. An American army to the north had been less fortunate.

Chapter 5

The American Invasion of Canada

May 1775–September 1776

T[hursday] 28 and 29. Very plesent / Sum of our Company dieth with
ye small pox / a very brisk cannading both sides.
Journal of Private Jeremiah Greenman, Quebec, December 1775

The aftershocks of events at Lexington and Concord were felt 300 miles away. Canada was a country of 100,000 people, mostly French-Canadian peasants with a resentful allegiance to their new ruler, the British Crown.[1] It was inevitable that it would be drawn into the conflict. The British valued it as a strategic North American base and a source of manpower. The Americans were convinced that the country was a natural part of a united North America.[2] After rebel forces seized the British posts of Ticonderoga and Crown Point in May 1775, Major General Philip Schuyler was ordered to attack Canada. He informed Washington that he was determined 'to Do it' but he was soon laid low by a 'bilious fever', a 'violent flux' and a 'barbaric complication of disorders' – perhaps an omen for the American expedition – and his command devolved to Richard Montgomery, a former British general.[3]

In describing the medical aspects of the American invasion of Canada it is convenient to divide the campaign into four parts. Firstly, Montgomery's advance on Quebec via Montreal; secondly, Benedict Arnold's epic march through the wilds of Maine; thirdly, the joining of the two forces and the unsuccessful assault on Quebec and death of Montgomery on the last day of 1775; finally, the tortured American retreat under the command of Brigadier General John Sullivan which reached Crown Point in July 1776.

To defend the vastness of Canada, the British commander Guy Carleton had only 800 seasoned troops. The Canadians had not rushed to his side. He first concentrated most of this paltry force in Montreal although the city was soon to be abandoned in the face of Montgomery's inexorable progress towards Quebec.[4] The British medical resources were equally sparse. At Montreal, the staff was made up of three surgeons, two apothecaries, a purveyor, twenty mates and five temporary mates enlisted locally. General hospitals were sited at Montreal, Quebec and later at Trois-Rivières with smaller facilities at St Johns south of Montreal, Oswego on Lake Ontario, and at Sorel on the St Lawrence River.[5] The senior medical officers were Robert Knox, inspector of hospitals at Montreal, and Hugh Alexander Kennedy, inspector of hospitals at Quebec. Knox had been appointed an army physician in Germany in 1760 and Kennedy at Havana in 1762 so the department had experienced leadership.[6] We have little information as to its quality at this time but the failure to provide Quebec with any substantial medical supplies for more than ten years suggests complacency.[7]

While the British medical department in Canada was small, the American medical planning for the invasion was wholly inadequate. The authorities, preoccupied by the siege of Boston, did not rise to the considerable challenge of providing proper medical care to an army about to enter a wilderness. Schuyler expressed his concerns in a letter to the Continental Congress written at Ticonderoga on 6 August 1775:

> 'Out of about five hundred men that are here, near a hundred are sick, and I have not any kind of hospital stores, although I had not forgot to order them, immediately after my appointment. The little wine I had for my own table, I have delivered to the Regimental Surgeons. That being expended, I can no longer bear the distress of the sick, and impelled by a feeling of humanity, I shall take the liberty immediately to order a physician from Albany, (if one can be got there, as I believe there may), to join me, with such stores as are indispensably necessary. If Congress will approve of this measure, they will please to signify what allowance of pay shall be made. If not, I shall discharge the person whoever he be [Stringer], paying him for the services he may have performed.'[8]

The general and his reluctant newly appointed medical director, Samuel Stringer, were forced to improvise, recruiting surgeons and mates, adapting barracks and houses at Fort George and Albany for hospitals, and scavenging for drugs and equipment. Some units still lacked regimental surgeons.[9] Congress, anticipating a quick victory, authorised a staff of only two surgeons and two mates.[10] Stringer's role was confirmed in September. His difficulties were exacerbated by a failure to define his relationship to John Morgan, the director general. This led to friction between the two men and was an early example of the confused leadership that was to plague the American medical department.[11]

Montgomery's Northern Army captured the British advance posts of St Johns and Chambly and Montreal capitulated on 14 November. However, his original strength of 2,000 men was reduced to 800 by a combination of sickness, desertion and expiring enlistments.[12] There were only the regimental surgeons and mates for medical support and no formal arrangements were made for opening hospitals along the St Lawrence or for inoculating the troops.[13]

Arnold departed Cambridge in mid-September 1775 with just over 1,000 men. His route to Quebec was through the uncharted, freezing and flooded Appalachian Highlands. The medical provision for this heroic undertaking was limited. There were no surgeons or surgeon's mates available from the hospitals at Cambridge or Roxbury. Isaac Senter was the regimental surgeon to the New England detachment. He was 22 years old and had not completed his apprenticeship. He had help from a surgeon's mate (Green) and two assistants (Barr and Jackson) but Green soon developed dysentery and was left behind. There was possibly a physician (Coates) with the Pennsylvania contingent and Ensign Matthew Irvine of Morgan's Rifle Company and Captain Henry Dearbon of the New Hampshire Company were both doctors who had left the scalpel for the sword.[14]

The focus was on survival rather than elaborate medical arrangements. Senter describes a blockhouse being built for the sick at the second portage of the Great Carrying Place; the soldiers christened it 'Arnold's Hospital'. Not far from this, Irvine, ill with dysentery and rheumatism, was left with four men of his company in a small bush hut constructed by the riflemen. Both Irvine and Green refused medication.[15] That it was not possible to carry the sick for any significant distance is clear from Private Jeremiah Greenman's journal entry two weeks later:

'T[uesday] 31. [October] Set out this morn very early / left 5 sick men in the woods that was not abel to march / left two men with them / but what litel provision they had did not last them / we gave out of our little / every man gave sum but the men that was left was obliged to leave them to the mercy of wild beast.'[16]

Arnold's men were exposed to conditions that were extreme even in the context of the War. Senter documents the suffering in his journal:

'Monday 30 October… We wandered through hideous swamps and mountainous precipices, with the conjoint addition of cold, wet and hunger, not to mention our fatigue – with the terrible apprehension of famishing in this desert.'[17]

The boiled bare jawbone of a pig had been 'sumptuous eating'.[18] Greenman survived by consuming 'the head of a Squirl with a parsol of Candill wicks boyled up to gether wich made very fine Supe without Salt'.[19] Boats were wrecked in the rivers and the remaining supplies spilt. Senter lost his medical box and surgical instruments and had only his lancet in his pocket.[20]

In mid-October, Senter refers to cases of diarrhoea and to a 'very formidable' number of sick in the temporary blockhouse hospital but he makes few references to specific diseases after this.[21] More than 600 men reached Quebec. Of these, 120 were unfit for duty with dysentery, diarrhoea, or rheumatism.[22] The losses were surprisingly low considering the appalling hardships endured. The men were hardy and well led and the constant movement protected against camp diseases such as typhus. Arnold wrote to Montgomery that he had advanced 320 miles 'through morasses, thick woods, and over mountains'. It was, he informed another correspondent, a march 'not to be paralleled in history'.[23]

Arnold's force was too weak and too late for a surprise assault on Quebec. At the start of December, Montgomery's army joined him outside the fortress walls. An American general hospital was established in a stone convent upon the St Charles River at the far end of the suburbs of St Roch. Senter was placed in charge, and he comments that the building was fit for purpose with a fine ward large enough for fifty patients and heated by a fireplace and stoves. The British batteries, only half a mile away, spared the hospital but Senter had to face some sniping from the walls when he visited.[24]

Senter was later to become an eminent member of his profession and he appears to have been a conscientious doctor but the entrusting of the general hospital to a young inexperienced regimental surgeon reflects a shortage of

Portrait of George Washington by William Williams (1794) showing smallpox scars on the cheeks and nose.

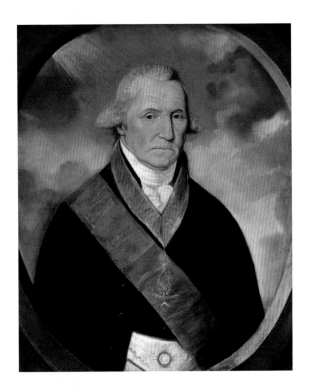

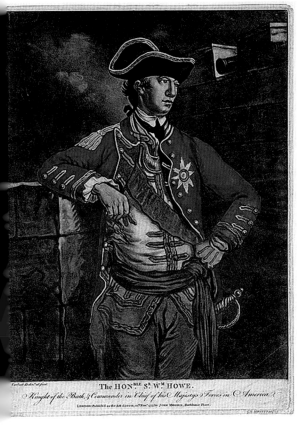

The HON.^{BLE} S.^T W.^M HOWE.
Knight of the Bath, & Commander in Chief of his Majesty's Forces in America.
LONDON, Published as the Act directs, 10.th Novr 1777 by JOHN MORRIS, Rathbone Place.

Major General William Howe.

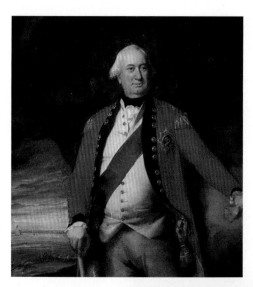

Charles Earl Cornwallis.

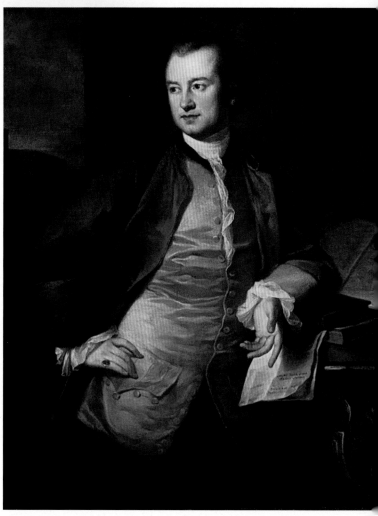

John Morgan.

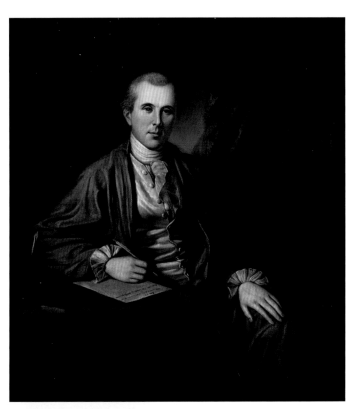

Benjamin Rush.

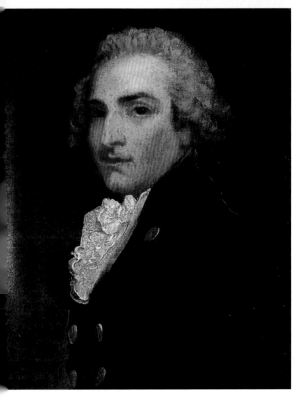

Robert Jackson.

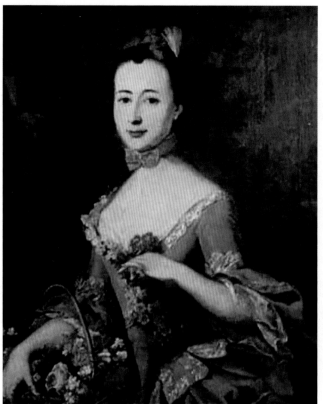

Left: *Baroness von Riedesel.*

Below: *Satirist James Gillray's 1802 caricature of smallpox vaccination ('the New Inoculation!').*

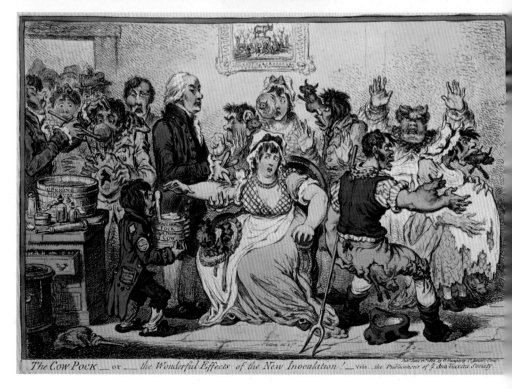

The Cow-Pock — or — the Wonderful Effects of the New Inoculation! _ Vide _ the Publications of ye Anti-Vaccine Society.

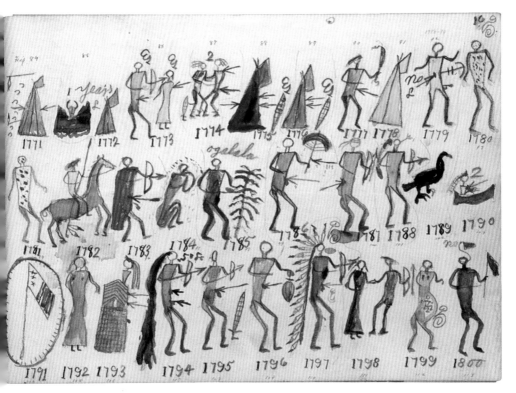

Animal hide drawing by Battiste Good showing events in the history of the Lakota people. Smallpox epidemics occurred in 1779–80 and 1780–81 (Manuscript 2372, NAA INV 08746804, Department of Anthropology, Smithsonian Institution).

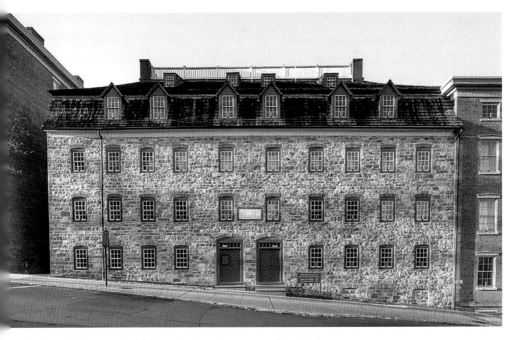

Brethren's House at Bethlehem. An American general hospital.

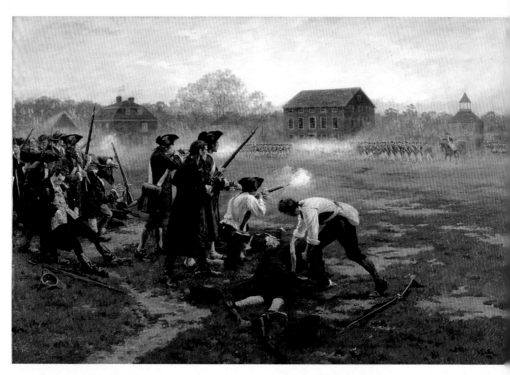

Above: *The Battle
of Lexington.*

Left: *The Battle
of Bunker Hill.*

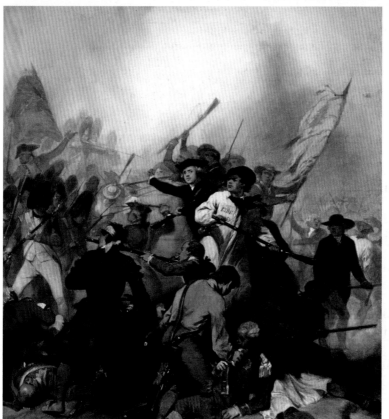

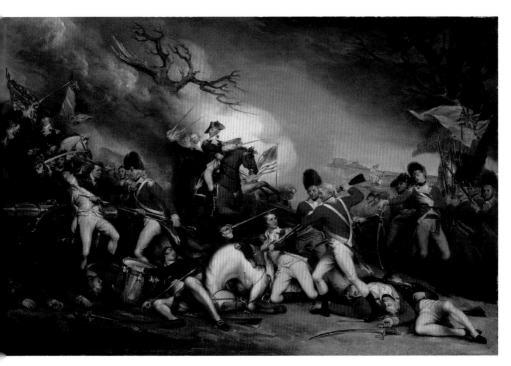

The death of General Hugh Mercer in the Battle of Princeton. The mortally wounded Mercer rests against his horse. Washington enters the scene accompanied by Benjamin Rush (Colonel John Cadwalader between them).

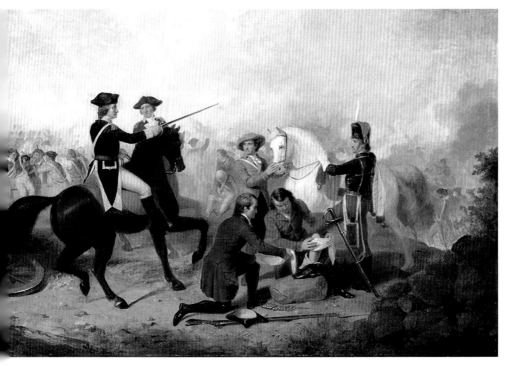

John Cochran bandages the wound of the Marquis de Lafayette at the Battle of Brandywine.

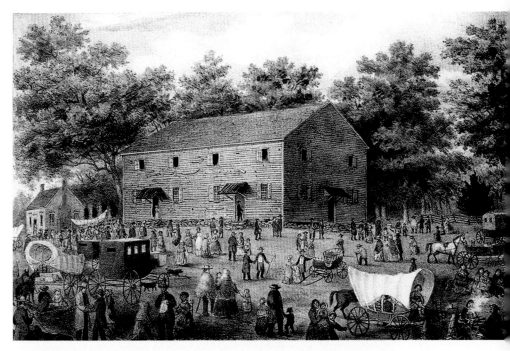

The Quaker New Garden Meeting House at Guilford Courthouse. Watercolour of 1869.

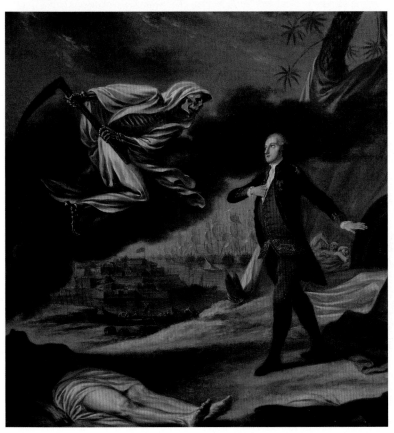

Allegorical portrait of a French naval officer of the American Revolutionary period. Thomas François Lenormand de Victot was fatally wounded at the Battle of the Saints in 1782.

senior medical staff with the American forces. Sergeant John Pierce, one of Arnold's men, was ill with jaundice. His diary entry for 13 December suggests a medical service under duress and lacking expertise:

> 'I thot several times I should be extremely Glad to be at Home where I could be better taken Care of for in this Country they have no herbs for the Sick that we Could find and but very few Druggs and our Surgeons and Physicians Lost all their Drugs and Instruments on our march thr,o the wilds of Canady and if they had not they were a Poor Set of men indeed.'

A few rebels had been injured by British cannon fire and Pierce says there were about twenty sick and wounded in the hospital at this time.[25]

Inside Quebec, the British garrison was also afflicted by the extreme cold. Militia captain Thomas Ainslie complained that the soldiers' senses were benumbed and that after ten minutes exposure to the air they could not handle their weapons. One night was 'inconceivably cold'. It was 'employment enough to preserve one's nose'. The garrison was relatively healthy, but Ainslie admitted that smallpox had been present for some time.[26]

Senter reported that there were only a few American sick at the start of December. There were respiratory ailments and cases of dysentery.[27] On the 6th, Caleb Haskell of Captain Samuel Ward's Rhode Island Company recorded in his diary that, 'The smallpox is all around us and there is a great danger of its spreading in the army'.[28] This suggests that this was not an entirely new occurrence, but it is the first mention of smallpox in contemporary accounts. A week or so later, Jeremiah Greenman describes the disorder as being 'very plenty'.[29] Senter makes no mention of it until the 17th; 'From this to the 23rd no occurrence of consequence, except the smallpox broke out in the army'. Five men were admitted to the hospital with the diagnosis.[30] The casual nature of Senter's allusion to the outbreak of smallpox perhaps reveals his own inexperience and a failure to recognise the potentially catastrophic nature of an epidemic. Some action was taken. Victims were removed to quarters three miles from camp and later a small smallpox hospital was opened. However, preventative measures were not pursued with the vigour that had been displayed at Boston.[31]

In this leadership vacuum, soldiers sought help from local quacks or inoculated themselves. Seventeen-year-old John Joseph Henry, a rifleman in

Arnold's detachment, saw men self-inoculating by inserting pins or needles under their finger nails 'either to obtain avoidance of duty or to get over that disease in an easy and speedy way'.[32] Senter had himself inoculated on Christmas Day.[33] Quarantine was poorly enforced, smallpox cases spilling over into local houses and at least some soldiers refusing to go to the new smallpox hospital.[34] Montgomery's pockmarked face signified his own immunity but he had no equivalent protection for his army. It is unclear why he and Arnold did not immediately institute a formal inoculation policy. They were presumably distracted by military matters, and they lacked experienced medical advice.

Ainslie relished the news that smallpox had taken hold in his enemy, 'tis a deadly infection in Yankee veins'. On the day before the assault on Quebec, he describes the disease as 'raging' among the rebels.[35] Such sentiments raise the question as to whether Carleton, in command in the city, deliberately introduced smallpox into his opponent's ranks. American soldiers on the scene had little doubt of British guilt. Henry thought the disease to have arrived by means of 'the indecorous, yet fascinating arts of the enemy'.[36] Haskell alleged that men and women were covertly sent out from the city, implying that they may have carried smallpox.[37]

At a later American inquest into the failure of the expedition, Thomas Jefferson concluded that the charges of biological warfare were credible.[38] As at Boston, this was possible but there is no proof. Historian Elizabeth Fenn, who has made the most detailed study, points out that it is quite likely that the disease was contracted by American troops mingling with the locals outside Quebec. Carleton's humane treatment of American smallpox victims after the siege also undermines the argument that he deliberately spread the infection.[39]

John Pierce, a surveyor and engineer with Arnold, gives a very human account of the futile attack on Quebec:

> 'General Montgomery marched to the walls his Ladder being in the rear he raised what there was and Indevered to mount one himself and was Shot with a musquet Ball Dead in the Spot – and orders being immediately Given out to retreat the whole retreated immediately and Arnold was in the Lower town fighting it out – I had a fair view of the whole. The bells were all Set on ringing Cannon playing bombs flying small armes Constantly going Drums beating men Groaning with their wounds Women and Children Screaming and Crying a terrible Scene to behold. Col.

Arnold was wounded in his Leg Maj^r Ogden was wounded in his Shoulder Capt. Morgan in his Thys we heard Capt. Hubbard was wounded in his ancle.[40]

The Americans had been, in Carleton's words, 'repulsed with slaughter'. They suffered 461 casualties including thirty killed, forty-two wounded and 389 captured. The British had only five dead and forty-one wounded.[41]

The American hospital, now in effect a field hospital, had been readied for the action. Horses and wagons had been secured from local villages for the carriage of the wounded.[42] All movements were impeded by the winter weather, the snow up to six feet deep. According to Senter, wounded men came 'tumbling in' within an hour of the start of the fighting. The hospital's grand ward was soon full. Once the British had captured the horses and carriages, only the more slightly wounded were able to make their way back.[43] The convent's nuns gave valuable help in the care of the wounded rebels, applying bandages and praying for those beyond medical help.[44]

A musket ball entered Arnold's left leg causing bleeding and rendering him very weak. Despite this, he says that he walked a mile to the hospital, 'being obliged to drag one leg after me'.[45] It is surprising that a wounded senior officer was left so isolated. Senter recalls that Arnold was carried in by two soldiers. The young surgeon gave him his immediate attention:

> 'The ball had probably come in contact with cannon, rock, stone or the like, ere [before] it entered the leg which had cleft off nigh a third. The other two-thirds entered the outer side of the leg, about midway, and in an oblique course passed between the tibia and fibula, lodged in the gastroennemea muscle [gastrocnemius muscle which forms the calf] at the rise of the tendon Achilles, where upon examination I easily discovered and extracted it.[46]

Arnold was lucky to avoid a more serious injury to a joint, the bones or nerves. Within a month, the wound had entirely healed, and he was able to hobble about.[47] Not all were so fortunate. The captured rebels in Quebec morosely watched wagons loaded with the fatalities making their way to the 'dead house'. Here, the bodies 'were heaped up in monstrous piles... their limbs distorted in various directions, such as would ensue in the moment of death'.[48]

A British attack on the hospital had been feared. Arnold loaded his pistols and kept his sword on his bed. He ordered his wounded men to have a gun by their side. In the event, the Redcoats stayed away, and the city was blockaded, both sides waiting for reinforcements. The fate of the American prisoners was mixed, reflecting the importance of rank in access to good accommodation and medical treatment. There is evidence of humanity on the British side. John Pierce heard that his comrades were being well looked after and had been offered inoculation.[49] Captain Henry Dearbon was lodged in a private house and was soon inoculated by a Dr Bullen, an expert practitioner.[50] For the ordinary men much more was left to chance. Eyewitnesses testify that conditions in the hospital at the *Hôtel-Dieu* were generally good.[51] In the prison, there was overcrowding, and the shortage of water forced men with fevers to drink their own urine.[52] It was not coincidental that of the twelve prisoners who died of their wounds, none were officers.[53]

The close confinement of the captured men facilitated contagion and in mid-January Greenman reported that smallpox was rife.[54] Soldiers with persisting sores were discharged from the hospital back to the prison. Nineteen-year-old Private Simon Fobes witnessed the inevitable consequences; 'Of course, all who had not had it took the disease, and there we were, without doctor, medicine, or any preparation for such a dangerous disease'. He survived and later estimated that over the winter about one-twelfth of the prisoners died of smallpox.[55] Another prisoner, Private Abner Stocking, believed it to be one-ninth.[56]

There were also several cases of diarrhoea, and, in April 1776, scurvy made its appearance among the captives. Rifleman Henry developed the disorder, and he says that it was soon widespread:

> 'their limbs contracted, as one of mine is now: large blue and even black blotches appeared on their bodies and limbs – the gums became black – the morbid flesh fell away – the teeth loosened, and in several instances fell out. Our men were now really depressed.'

The victims received sympathetic attention from British doctors, notably from Adam Mabane, a staff surgeon in the garrison. The affliction only started to resolve when the weather improved, and their diet included vegetables.[57]

Outside the walls, the American medical services were compromised by a lack of supplies. On 2 January, the quarter master general wrote in desperation to General David Wooster, 'I hope you will not forget to remind Congress of the necessity of furnishing a suitable [medical] chest for the Army... a thing much neglected in this campaign'.[58] Wooster, in temporary command of the siege, pleaded with Congress in late April for more surgeons and medicines.[59] Congress soon replaced Wooster with General John Thomas, a Massachusetts physician who had a particular fear of smallpox. On arrival at Quebec in May, Thomas discovered that his paper army of 1,900 troops had been reduced to only 500 men fit for combat, the rest being invalids 'chiefly with the smallpox'.[60]

The disease was becoming more virulent. Two hundred men were officially inoculated and there was much secretive self-inoculation despite an order forbidding the practice.[61] Josiah Sabin, one of Seth Warner's Green Mountain Boys, contracted smallpox.

'He [Sabin] inoculated himself; got the infection from the hospital. He also inoculated many of the soldiers, but as this was against orders, they were sent into his room blindfolded, were inoculated, and sent out in the same condition.'[62]

Sabin claims that this subterfuge saved many lives, and he was probably correct. Very few of the New England recruits had ever had the disorder and they were especially vulnerable.[63] Quarantine measures proved inadequate. Arnold feared 'the entire ruin of the Army'.[64]

In contrast, the British garrison remained healthy. There were some 'slight fevers and diarrhoeas' and only a few men in the general hospital.[65] Thomas Ainslie suspected that some were exaggerating their symptoms.

'It is proposed to raise a company of Invalids in Town. Some people from real ailments, have been incapable of doing garrison duty, but there are many shameless beings within the walls, who under pretence of bad health, skulk from their duty & sleep soundly at home, while their fellow Citizens watch exposed to the rigours of a Canadian Winter.'[66]

If this was a sign of poor morale, the situation was entirely transformed by the arrival of a British fleet carrying reinforcements. On 6 May, Redcoats emerged from the city's gates on to the Plains of Abraham and the American forces fled upriver.[67] It was a chaotic retreat. Senter describes it as 'helter-skelter'.[68] The American general hospital and most of the sick were soon in British hands. Ainslie witnessed the panic:

> 'To lighten the boats they inhumanely threw out many of their sick men upon the beach, some of them expired before our parties cou'd get to their relief, those objects of compassion whom we found alive were sent to the General Hospital.'[69]

Carleton had given the order to send out search parties. In the following days, the British rescued between 200 and 500 men, almost all infected by smallpox.[70]

Thomas ordered Senter to Montreal to open a hospital for the reception of the sick. He commandeered a large house belonging to the East India Company which could accommodate 600.[71] This suggests a semblance of medical organisation, but Senter was too often acting alone. Congress had failed the medical department. On the long retreat to Crown Point, 'shortages, sickness, inexperience and confusion engulfed the regimental surgeons of the army'.[72] Sick men lay in the bottom of leaking boats. Stringer wrote to Washington in mid-May asking for help; the surgeons had no medicines or instruments. He informed Schuyler that the situation was hopeless and threatened to resign, 'if I had seen the irregularity of our affairs, I would not have entered the service'.[73] He eventually received permission to hire a larger medical staff and Dr Jonathan Potts, a well-trained physician, was sent north to support the hospital at Fort George.[74]

The British service was comparatively well organised and advantaged by military ascendency. Kennedy accompanied Carleton as chief medical officer. Because of the extended line of communications, a flying hospital was established to link the regimental facilities and the base general hospitals. It was first at St Johns and then was moved forward behind the advancing troops.[75]

In Arnold's words the retreating rebel army was now a 'rabble'.[76] The American cause was not helped by further military misadventures at 'The Cedars', forty miles north of Montreal, and at Trois-Rivières. Thomas died of smallpox on 2 June. His scarred and rapidly decomposing body was buried immediately.[77] He was replaced three days later by John Sullivan, but no general could outrun the virus.

In early June, 1,000 out of 1,500 Continental soldiers at Montreal had smallpox. Along twenty miles of the Richelieu River, there were more than

3,000 American sick and more than 1,000 of these had the disease. Attempts at inoculation did not stop its spread and the army that arrived at the Ile au Noix ten miles north of the New York border had been effectively destroyed. Dysentery and malaria were now also making inroads.[78] Lewis Beebe, a surgeon's mate from Massachusetts, was ordered to the small island:

'sailed in a bateau [to Ile au Noix] and arrived there about 3 P.M. was struck with amazement upon my arrival to see the vast crowds of poor distressed Creatures. Language cannot describe, nor imagination paint, the scenes of misery and distress the Soldiery endure. Scarcely a tent upon this Isle but which contains one or more in distress and continually groaning, & calling for relief, but in vain! Requests of this Nature are as little regarded as the singing of Crickets in a Summer evening. The most shocking of all spectacles was to see a large barn Crowded full of men with this disorder [smallpox], many of whom could not See, Speak, or walk – one nay two had large maggots, an inch long, Crawl out of their ears, were on almost every part of the body. No mortal will ever believe what these suffered unless they were eye witnesses.'[79]

To their credit, Arnold and other senior officers made well-meaning attempts to promote military hygiene, ordering the latrines to be kept apart from the encampment.[80]

For the final stage of the retreat to Crown Point, the sick were packed into open boats. After a five-day voyage of 100 miles, lashed by heavy rain, 3,000 men were dragged ashore.[81] Bostonian John Adams, a member of the Continental Congress and a future United States president, wrote to his wife on 7 July:

'Our Army at Crown Point is an object of Wretchedness, enough to fill a Humane mind with Horror; Disgraced, defeated, discontented, dispirited, diseased, naked, undisciplined, eaten up with Vermin – no Clothes, Beds, Blankets, no medicines, no Victuals but Salt Pork and flour.'[82]

Desperate men attempted to inoculate themselves with dried scabs.[83]

Compared with this medical catastrophe, the pursuing British forces escaped lightly. Kennedy gave dietary advice to prevent outbreaks of scurvy.[84]

There were numerous cases of dysentery and malaria, but the mortality was low. Orders were given at Montreal to inoculate all men who had not had smallpox. This precaution resulted from American cases of the disease being left in the hospital there. The summer heat debilitated some of the troops but all were able to rejoin the march.[85]

Carleton failed to catch the Americans and he was short of boats. The rebel army, now under the command of General Horatio Gates, gained respite at Crown Point and Ticonderoga while the British remained at St Johns. The invasion of Canada had been a dismal failure. American casualties were estimated to be 40 per cent. More than 5,000 men had perished, been captured or were unfit for service.[86]

When Jonathan Potts arrived at the small stone fortress at Fort George in early July 1776, he little anticipated that he was to oversee the largest military hospital of the War. A hospital return for 12–26 July showed 1,497 men admitted, 439 discharged, fifty-one dead, three deserted and 1,004 remaining. At the end of the month, Potts noted that 1,500 had been admitted and 300 discharged but he admitted that all figures were approximate as he was so overworked. He appealed to Director General Morgan:

> 'Without clothing, without comforts, or a shelter sufficient to screen them from the weather, I assume your known humanity will be effected when I tell you upwards of one thousand sick... labor under the various disorders of dysentery, bilious putrid fevers, and the effects of confluent smallpox; to attend the large number we have four seniors and four mates.'[87]

Medicines were running out and there were no bandages or lint. Morgan and Stringer continued to dispute their relative seniority. The director general was also distracted by the likelihood of a British attack on New York and Congress remained lethargic.[88] Surgeon Samuel Meyrick bemoaned the medical mismanagement, 'it is enough to move the heart of a stone to be in the situation of a Physician under the present circumstances.'[89]

Smallpox remained the greatest fear of the army. It terrified the men more than the enemy and was the cause of large-scale desertions.[90] However, as recorded by Potts, it was not the only affliction. At Ticonderoga, Beebe reported 'dysentery, jaundice, putrid, intermitting, and bilious fevers'. Half his regiment, perhaps half the Continental Army, was unfit for duty.[91] Samuel

Kennedy, surgeon to the 4th Pennsylvania Regiment, produced a similar list of disorders.[92] It is likely that these doctors were describing a lethal combination of dysentery, malaria, and typhus. Men burned brush piles in the mornings and evenings in a vain attempt to purify the air.[93]

Fortunately, Gates was a proactive officer, and he took practical steps to try to improve the state of his men. Sanitary regulations were enforced. These pertained to clothing, water supplies, soap, and the use of latrines. He also asked his surgeons for advice. They were quick to point out the lack of medicines and equipment. The situation was best summarised by an army officer from the artillery companies which had no surgeon to reply to Gates. His scribbled note read 'Medicines and surgeons none. Instruments none. Assistance none'.[94]

Military hygiene initiatives were allied to better quarantine enforcement and a more controlled inoculation regimen. New recruits were screened, self-inoculation was forbidden, and soldiers were given certificates confirming official inoculation.[95] By early September, this led to improvement in the health of the troops and particularly a fall in the number of smallpox cases. Gates' assertion to Washington that the disease was eradicated may have been an exaggeration, but other diseases were now more problematic.[96] Lewis Beebe reports dysentery still 'raging' at the start of October.[97] At this time, there were 4,000 sick out of a total strength of 14,500.[98]

Thomas Dickson Reide had arrived at Quebec from England with the British reinforcements. His predilection for collecting data makes him the best single source for the diseases afflicting Carleton's army. In early July 1776, he accompanied four companies of his regiment to the village of Lachine, on the St Lawrence River a few miles from Montreal. In the following two months, there was a little malaria and dysentery, but the sick list never exceeded twenty-five men. When the troops advanced to St Johns in mid-September, they encountered heavy rain and swampy ground. Within a few days, there were more than a hundred men sick with 'fluxes and fevers'. The army's overall sick rate was more than 12 per cent compared with 7 per cent two months earlier. Reide himself was weakened by malaria but there were few deaths.[99]

There was a British forward camp at the notorious Ile au Noix. Dysentery had replaced smallpox as the chief ailment and here there was significant mortality. A British cemetery soon opened next to the rebel graves. German surgeon Julius Wasmus echoed his American peers; 'The misery of this island is indescribable'.[100] When hostilities resumed in the autumn of 1776, the British sick were sent to a temporary hospital at St Johns.[101]

Events far to the south in Virginia were a reminder that not all British-led forces had higher levels of immunity against smallpox. At the end of 1775, the colony's Royal governor, John Murray, Earl of Dunmore, promised refugee African American slaves their freedom if they joined the British cause. Eight hundred to 1,000 of Virginia's black population joined the Ethiopian Regiment. In early 1776, smallpox appeared in Dunmore's fleet in the Chesapeake, and it subsequently savaged the black and white army on shore, first at Tucker's Point near Norfolk and then to the north at Gwynne's Island. Some inoculation was undertaken although the extent of this is not clear. It had little impact on the number of disease deaths, perhaps because the smallpox epidemic was compounded by other disorders including typhus.

It was obvious that the black troops were more vulnerable to smallpox than their white comrades. An escaped American prisoner confirmed that it was the black ranks that were most depleted. The Ethiopian Regiment was continuing to recruit but it was soon reduced to a few hundred men rather than the 2,000 that Dunmore would have had, 'had it not been for this horrid disorder'. Five hundred men had been lost on Gwynne's Island alone. Virginian troops later found the place to have been evacuated, a few smallpox sufferers still hanging on to life. Others had been consumed by the flames that had torn through the brush huts. Dunmore was eventually to sail for England leaving the seeds of the disease among the Virginian patriot soldiers and the civilian population.[102]

Chapter 6

The New York Campaign

June 1776–November 1776

I have the canopy of heaven for my hospital and the ground for my hammock.

Private Joseph Plumb Martin, October 1776

New York was of great strategic significance. Washington described it as being of 'infinite importance'. If they lost it to the British, the rebels in the northern and southern colonies would be divided. In the years leading up to the Revolution, the city had flourished, benefitting from open trade with Britain and clandestine deals with France. Visitors commented on the 4,000 wooden and brick buildings, comparing them with the best of British and Dutch architecture. They were interconnected by cobbled lanes and tree-lined walkways.[1]

The rapid transformation of this increasingly sophisticated metropolis into a garrison town put intolerable strain on what was a relatively new infrastructure. American troops poured into the suffocating streets, many working on the new fortifications. In the early summer of 1776, the city was hot and obviously unhealthy. Sparkling ponds and springs had mutated into stagnant pools and the thoroughfares exuded a horrible smell. The unsanitary habits of the American troops hardly helped. They dumped refuse in the streets and relieved themselves into the ditches of the fortifications. The same water was used for washing, cooking, and drinking. Senior officers, notably Washington and General Nathanael Greene, issued orders that the men should clean their encampments, dig latrines, bury offal, and seek fresh sources of water.[2]

By late June, Washington had approximately 19,000 soldiers around Manhattan; this number would swell to 28,000 by August. William Howe's British army was ultimately to be 32,000 strong. It was escorted by a fleet commanded by his brother, Richard Howe, and was first sighted off Long Island on 29 June. It appeared a 'forest of masts'. General Howe put men ashore on Staten Island at the start of July but there was to be no fighting for another two months while he considered his options, gathered intelligence, and waited for more supplies and reinforcements.[3]

In New York, medical preparations were being made for the coming campaign. These were compromised by discord in the department. The director general, John Morgan, was supported by his hospital medical staff but he had a poor relationship with the regimental surgeons and there was still uncertainty regarding the relative roles of the general and regimental hospitals (see Chapter 3). Morgan was not helped much by the military authorities. He was refused masons and carpenters to work on hospital buildings and soldiers sent to help soon drifted away.[4]

Battling against indifference, Morgan worked hard to ready the city for what one of his doctors referred to as 'the horrible effects of a general action'.[5] The general hospitals in Manhattan were at King's College, at the newly rebuilt City Hospital, at the workhouse, and at the city barracks. Vacated loyalist homes and country seats outside the city were appropriated despite resistance. King's College was the primary unit. There was also a general hospital on Long Island under the supervision of Dr John Warren. Morgan gave Warren detailed instructions for its management. It was to be staffed by a combination of hospital mates and surgeon's mates from Nathanael Greene's brigade. A smallpox hospital on Montresor's Island had admitted only a few patients.[6]

Advertisements were placed in New York newspapers for nurses for the hospitals.[7] Wider local help was sought, the city's inhabitants contributing 2,000 sheets and hundreds of shirts.[8] Drug supplies were an ongoing headache for Morgan despite the transfer of medicines from Boston. Many of the New York druggists were loyalists and their stocks disappeared when needed for Washington's army. Congress agreed to the procurement of more medicines but not before the director general had been forced to place an advertisement in the *New York Gazette* of 29 July:

> 'WANTED immediately... a large quantity of dry herbs, for baths, fomentations, &c. &c. particularly baum hyssop, wormwood and mallows, for which a good price will be given.'[9]

Morgan's instructions for hospital management were detailed and included measures to optimise bedding and ensure cleanliness.[10] The hospitals in New York were of reasonable quality. Hospital Mate Solomon Drowne worked at the King's College facility, which, he says, was in an elegant building; 'its situation pleasant and salubrious... We have things in pretty good readiness'.[11]

Morgan judged himself to be 'well off' in the general hospitals despite the niggling shortages. However, he despaired of the regimental surgeons who lacked the most basic equipment and who, at least in some cases, seemed not to care. He sent them some of the hospital stores including bandages, sheets, lint, and tourniquets. He could spare no surgical instruments and was unable to solve the problem.[12]

There were still regimental hospitals in use, but they were poorly regulated. Around this period, Morgan visited one serving the men of General John Fellow's Massachusetts Brigade.

> 'On looking into the rooms, they were found to be filled with sick, and the surgeons who had their care, panting for breath, in the midst of them. It was amidst the sultry heat of summer. In vain I represented to him [the regimental surgeon] the danger of engendering a putrid, malignant fever [typhus], from crowding so many sick in confined rooms in that hot season. He had near a hundred sick in the house.'

Morgan advised that some of the patients should be moved to a general hospital. He had previously ordered that regimental surgeons should not care for more than thirty to forty sick. His advice was ignored, underlining his lack of authority and the indiscipline of the wider medical department. The regimental surgeon soon died from infection.[13]

The British medical arrangements for the New York campaign were along traditional lines with a hospital staff and the regimental contingent. Jonathan Mallet had been appointed as chief surgeon to North America and Michael Morris was the inspector of regimental infirmaries.[14] Among the fleet were several hospital ships designed to care for the sick and to allow evacuation of the wounded for surgical treatment.[15]

The American army that had arrived in New York was healthy, but the unhygienic state of the city soon led to the eruption of infectious disorders including dysentery, typhus (or typhoid), scabies, smallpox, and venereal complaints.[16] The sick rate climbed inexorably. In the third week of June, 2,600 were ill out of a force of 18,000. By 7 August, there were 6,500 sick out of 17,000.[17] Approximately a third of Washington's army was incapacitated before any clash of arms.

Dysentery was not a cause of great mortality, but it debilitated large numbers of men. Lieutenant Isaac Bangs of the 2nd Massachusetts wrote in his journal for July that almost his whole regiment was struck down with the 'camp distemper' or 'bloody flux'.[18] Surgeon Ebenezer Beardsley of the 22nd Continental Regiment later left a detailed account of the disease. In the middle of May, his previously healthy regiment was 'taken down with the dysentery in the space of a week'. Unlike other units, the men had not been moved to tents but had remained in their quarters on Smith Street. Soon, a hundred soldiers were ill, and Beardsley admits that he was perplexed as to the cause. He eventually deduced that the disorder originated from the 'confined and putrid atmosphere in which these unfortunate men lived'. The surgeon's successful request that his patients be removed to more capacious accommodation led to an obvious reduction in the number of cases. Only two men died.[19]

Skin disorders were also not associated with many deaths, but they caused much suffering and incapacity. Lieutenant Bangs complained of boils breaking out all over his body.[20] Bangs is a good witness of military life in New York. The 'Holy Ground' near Saint Paul's Church was a favoured haunt of prostitutes:

> 'The whole of my aim in visiting this Place at first was out of Curiosity... it seems Strange that any Man can so divest himself of Manhood as to desire an intimate Connexion with these worse than brutal Creatures, yet it is not more strange than true that many of our Officers & Soldiers have been so imprudent as to follow them, notwithstanding the salutary advice of their Friends, till the Fatal Disorder seized them & convinced them of their Error.'

Forty men from one regiment contracted syphilis or gonorrhoea.[21] Many were presumably seeking a transitory escape from an alien and threatening environment. Samuel Kennedy, surgeon to the 4th Pennsylvanian Battalion, wrote to his wife that he found their separation intolerable; 'sometimes I feel almost ready to resign'.[22]

Squalid conditions were also common at sea. A British Guards officer summed up life aboard the transports; 'There was continued destruction in the foretops, the pox above-board, the plague between decks, hell in the forecastle, the devil at the helm'.[23] There were well-meaning efforts to improve the lot of soldiers and sailors afloat. British physician William Rowley had just published his *Medical Advice for the use of the army and navy in the present American expedition.* This contained common-sense instruction relating to diet, water supplies and ventilation. The sick were to be kept away from the lower parts of the ship where the air was 'dangerously fetid' due to filth thrown down by the crew.[24] Between 1775 and 1783, about 8 per cent of the British soldiers shipped to North America died in the Atlantic.[25]

The British troops arriving at New York in the summer of 1776 were quite healthy, the most prevalent disorders being a variety of fevers and sore throats.[26] The Hessian regiments had travelled further and there is anecdotal evidence of disease, particularly scurvy and diarrhoea. An anonymous German solder with the First Hessian Division complained that the tedious voyage had caused sickness despite prophylactic measures such as disinfection and pumping in clean air. The soldiers drank seawater and chewed tobacco in vain attempts to prevent scurvy, a disorder which 'reigned supreme'.[27] The Von Ditfurth Regiment, which arrived at Staten Island on 15 August, had embarked at Marburg in February. Only thirty-eight men out of more than 600 were sick, fewer than later in the year. This suggests that the newly arriving German troops were variably affected by illness.[28]

At the Battle of Long Island on 27 August, Washington was outmanoeuvred by Howe, British forces attacking the American flank and rear. The Continental Army was forced to fall back on Manhattan. The American losses totalled 1,100 compared to only around 400 for the British.[29] A few weeks prior to the fighting, Morgan had issued detailed instructions to his regimental surgeons 'in case of action'. On the field, they were expected to attend their own corps to dress the wounded. Their post was to be a few hundred yards behind the line, ideally under cover. It was expected that casualties would initially be taken to the Long Island general hospital or evacuated to facilities in the city.[30] Morgan had appealed to the New York Convention for extra buildings for the wounded.[31] There was still a need to improvise. Surgeons were asked to use their razors where surgical instruments were lacking.[32]

The scale of the American defeat undermined these preparations. Once battle was joined, the American surgeons were quickly caught up in the retreat and several were captured.[33] Sixty-five-year-old Bodo Otto, surgeon of the Battalion of the Flying Corps Troops of Berkshire County, escaped this indignity but lost all his medicines and instruments in the chaos.[34]

The patients in Warren's Long Island hospital were hastily evacuated. Washington ordered that the remaining wounded be removed to New York City on 29 August. Several hundred were shipped across from Long Island, arriving at various wharfs. Perhaps a fifth of these were seriously wounded, many having fallen into enemy hands. Drenched by heavy rain, they were carried to the general hospitals. Morgan dressed and operated on the men admitted to King's College.[35]

The best account of the British medical provision for the battle is that of Staff Surgeon Thompson Forster. He accompanied James Grant's division together with three surgeon's mates and two servants who carried the bandages and surgical instruments. They set up a dressing station behind the main body of the attacking brigade. This was on a 'considerable eminence' which would have made it easily identifiable to the wounded but also a target for enemy artillery. Forster was soon forced to move, fully admitting his apprehension. 'That time which was taken up making the disposition for the attack was dreadful to me beyond description'. He arranged for the casualties to be carried to a neighbouring barn and dispatched one of the mates to attend to wounded prisoners.

> 'Hurt as I was at seeing so many or our brave soldiers wounded, I yet must acknowledge I felt a secret pleasure in being instrumental in their relief as well as a conscious dignity at being appointed to such a department where I was of real use to my King and Country!'[36]

Most of the British wounded were sent back to hospital ships off Long Island while the more serious cases were operated on and held onshore until they were recovered enough to move. It was judged too risky to open a proper hospital on land 'lest they should be surprised by the Rebels'. In the days after the action, Forster was posted to a flying hospital. He was joined by two other surgeons and six mates. Located near headquarters, individual surgeons were sent on horseback to tend the wounded.[37]

Washington was forced to abandon New York on 14 September. The commander rode back to his new headquarters, a Georgian mansion south of King's Bridge.[38] Morgan faced the daunting task of evacuating the sick and wounded. He quickly identified possible sanctuaries at Hoboken, Weehawken, and Newark.[39] The director general tried to be everywhere, but the medical department was close to disintegration. Many doctors and nurses had either been captured or had fled, the wagons had been impressed by the militia, the boats were late in arriving, and the citizens of Newark were resisting the opening of a hospital for soldiers with infectious diseases.[40] Morgan was soon in personal charge of upwards of a thousand ill and wounded soldiers. He left instructions to Warren and to several hospital staff to follow the sick.[41] On the 18th, Washington had to order regimental surgeons to care for their own patients 'until the General Hospital can be established on a proper footing'.[42]

The Continental Army was defeated and miserable. Food remained scarce. Men slept in the open on cold wet ground. Many had no blankets. Service, according to one soldier, was reduced to 'hard duty and nakedness'.[43] In such conditions, diseases were bound to proliferate. Surgeon James Tilton later described the American encampment at King's Bridge:

> 'our raw and undisciplined condition at that time, subjected the soldiers to great irregularity. Besides a great loss and want of clothes, the camp became excessively filthy. All manner of excrementitious matter was scattered indiscriminately through the camp insomuch, that you were offended by a disagreeable smell, almost everywhere within the lines. A putrid diarrhoea was the consequence. The camp disease [dysentery], as it was called, became proverbial. Many died, melting as it were and running off by the bowels. Medicine answered little or no purpose.'

Tilton noted that the army's health was always worse when it was static.[44] He infers that not much treatment was given. Many doctors were themselves ill. A single surgeon's mate was responsible for five Connecticut regiments. A chaplain perished from dysentery only attended by 'an unskilful quack of a surgeon's mate'.[45] Sick rates remained stubbornly high. In the middle of September, there were 8,500 sick, more than a third of the American army.[46] The British were not entirely spared the toll of disease but Royal Marines Captain John Bowater's declaration that the fleet and army were 'both very healthy', and in 'exceedingly high sperrits' reveals the contrast between the two adversaries.[47]

On 15 September, the British attacked at Kip's Bay in the first of several probing manoeuvres which drove Washington's beleaguered force northwards into Westchester County. The thin line of American musketeers guarding the Bay broke and fled. Thompson Forster was with the British troops, and he set up his first aid post in the captured American camp. There were, he says, American wounded everywhere. With the help of his colleague, Staff Surgeon Richard Proctor, he turned a cow house into a temporary field hospital. Having done their work, the two doctors spent a 'jolly evening' in a barn.[48]

This was a bloodless action for the British, but this was not the case at Harlem Heights the following day. Here, Washington's forces had adopted a strong position and they forced a British withdrawal after hard fighting that eventually engaged 3,000 men on each side. It was a morale boost for the rebels. American casualties were around 100 and the British losses exceeded 170.[49]

Thompson Forster learned a harsh lesson. He dressed the wounded in barns and stables and then, on the following day, commandeered three nearby houses; 'I had nurses, stewards, orderly men, and in short as complete an Hospital as if I had been a month about it – I thought I should gain great credit'. The buildings were soon targeted by two American six-pounders and had to be abandoned amid scornful laughter from the doctor's own comrades. It was risky to set up dressing stations and field hospitals so close to the action. Forster, who had to flee his hospital in the middle of the night clothed only in a shirt, conceded that it was his own fault.[50]

The was no proper American hospital at Harlem Heights and the wounded were opportunistically removed to local taverns such as the Blue Bell and the Cross Keys, the latter on the King's Bridge Road.[51] Major Charles Gilman, an American doctor serving as a military officer, was wounded in the back of the hand. The injury became infected and stubbornly refused to heal until he accidentally spilled rum on it; 'in two days... I removed the cover and the wound was healing'. Thereafter, all wounds were soaked in rum.[52]

Howe's landing of 4,000 men at Frog's Neck on 18 October was strategically sound but poorly executed. It was a bad landing point, and the British force was hemmed in to the marshes by Pennsylvania riflemen who controlled the only bridge.[53] Forster was on the misnamed hospital ship *Peace and Plenty*. He went ashore and attended to General Charles Cornwallis who had been stunned by a shell blast. Fortunately, the Earl recovered quickly and was spared a bleeding.[54]

Realising that Frog's Neck was a dead end, Howe moved his forces to Pell's Point where British progress was hotly contested by Colonel John Glover's brigade. The rebels eventually withdrew but only after inflicting more casualties than they suffered.[55] Forster landed with the troops but soon returned to the hospital ship. Among the British wounded was Captain William Glanville Evelyn. He received three bullet wounds while vaulting a stone wall. The first grazed his left arm, the second entered his upper thigh, and the third shattered his right leg above the knee. He was offered amputation, but the young officer would not consent to the operation, and he died three weeks later in New York.[56] Refusals of amputations during the War are anecdotal but appear to have been common and not always associated with an unhappy outcome.

The more major but inconclusive Battle of White Plains was fought on 28 October. There were approximately 150 killed and wounded on each side.[57] Again, Forster is a reliable witness. The British wounded were collected in carts, and many were transferred offshore for dressing and surgery. Both the *Peace and Plenty* and another ship were filled for the return to New York.[58]

On the American side, there was a constant need for improvisation, but Morgan's prodigious efforts ensured the presence of a basic medical service. Orders earlier in the month stipulated that a 'stout able bodied man' from each company was to be appointed to help the musicians and camp colourmen in assisting the wounded.[59] There were few regimental surgeons at White Plains, many of them absent from their units. Morgan was forced to rely on the hospital surgeons and mates to assist him on the battlefield. The wounded were evacuated to a general hospital at North Castle.[60] The director general later justified his actions to Washington:

> 'While we were getting in readiness, a firing of cannon was heard anew... On learning it was at the White Plains, every surgeon of the hospital then present set out with me, immediately for the Plains, several mates following with a wagon, to bring the instruments and dressings. We fixed [located] near lines, and I never stirred from thence till the enemy retreated, which was about a week later.'[61]

Morgan spent a few hours at North Castle giving directions and assisting with the wounded in the hospital. He left a hospital surgeon and a few mates at White Plains in case of a renewed British attack. He admitted that the hospital surgeons had been 'overwhelmed' by the number of sick and wounded and lamented that they could not be both with the troops in the field and in the hospital at the same time.[62]

Fort Washington was captured on 16 November, all its stores and 2,700 prisoners falling into British hands.[63] Forster describes the incessant British cannonade and the impatience of the besiegers, eager to use their 'grinning bayonets'. Stuffing his pockets with bandages, the surgeon made his way to the front where he came upon the British wounded, including his friend, Captain Dering of the 15th Foot:

> '[He] squeezed me by the hand but could not speak. I beckoned to my servant to bring me some Lint to dress a large wound in his Chest by a three pound Ball – I was so much shock'd myself that I could not speak – I kneeled down to apply the Lint to my dying Friend – I was tying a Bandage round his Body – the young lad who had carried my Bandages was standing by me much distressed at the Scene, looking down at the Captain with that compassionate Countenance which shewed a good heart – a three Pound Shot knocked him dead at my feet, the Captain at this instant was insensible. I layed still on the Ground for some minutes not knowing what to do.'[64]

Forster recovered enough to make his way to the rear. He was not the only doctor in danger. Pennsylvanian surgeon James McHenry, later secretary for war, was seen sitting on a rock extracting a musket ball from a wounded officer, 'exposed to all the fire of the enemy, and but a few minutes before the British charged.'[65] McHenry and his medical colleagues, Hugh Hodge and John Beatty, were taken prisoner.[66]

Among the American wounded was Ensign Jacob Barnitz, a blacksmith who was 'the most uncouth-looking man in the army'. Barnitz was shot through both legs and later stripped naked by Hessian soldiers. He was collected the next day and taken to New York where, like Captain Evelyn at Pell's Point, he refused a British surgeon's offer of removal of one of his limbs. Unlike the aristocratic British officer, Barnitz survived. The ball below his knee caused constant pain and, thirty-two years after the fall of Fort Washington, he consented to amputation of the leg above the knee.[67]

The British had seven general hospitals in New York. These were the General, the College, the Vauxhall, the Brick Meeting House, the Ranelaugh, the Poor House, and the Quaker Meeting House. These gave a total of 3,000 beds, the College being the largest facility and able to house more than 1,000 sick and wounded. There was a hospital staff of five physicians, three purveyors, eight staff surgeons, eight apothecaries, and sixty hospital mates. In addition, there were the vital subordinate clerks, stewards, storekeepers, and cooks who were often appointed from the local population. Ward orderlies were usually recruited from the regiments and soldiers' wives acted as nurses.[68]

The American medical services were under much greater strain. After the fall of forts Washington and Lee, Morgan was forced to move the sick to Newark and Hackensack. He subsequently directed the endless stream of frozen miserable men to hospitals at Perth Amboy, Elizabeth, Brunswick, Trenton, and Morristown. Because of the threat of invasion of New Jersey, patients also ended up at Fishkill and Peekskill on the Hudson and at Norwich and Stamford in Connecticut.[69]

The British were not Morgan's only enemy. An old feud had resurfaced. William Shippen had been appointed by Congress as director of hospitals for the militia's flying camp at Perth Amboy. In early October, Morgan was instructed to provide and supervise a hospital for the army posted on the east side of the Hudson River while Shippen was to do the same in the state of New Jersey. The division of responsibilities was unclear, and the two men were soon competing for staff, supplies, hospital locations, and the approval of senior military officers. Washington was later to comment to Morgan that his clash with Shippen 'was no small cause of the Calamities that befell our sick in 1776'.[70]

The medical department was being harshly judged by the men it was designed to serve. Nathanael Greene believed Morgan to be overly preoccupied with points of procedure. 'It is wholly immaterial, in my opinion, whether a Man dies in a General or Regimental Hospital'.[71] General William Heath complained that he had no proper hospital for his soldiers. Yet when Morgan offered to construct and staff a facility for 300 men, Heath failed to give the necessary orders to the quartermaster general's department.[72] There were demands for a Congressional inquiry into the hospitals and even an accusation that the doctors had killed ten times as many men as the enemy.[73]

Morgan's frustration was understandable. Commanding officers, he claimed, expected a general hospital to follow wherever they went, 'as if it were possible... an entire Hospital, properly furnished with necessary accommodation, attendants, and conveniences, although amidst Highlands, alps, or a forsaken and wasted country'.[74]

Harassed and exhausted, the director general appeared a distant figure to his critics. When, following another complaint, the Maryland authorities sent Dr John Pine to visit Morgan at the camp at White Plains, there was only an abrupt, and apparently unfeeling, response.

'he [Morgan] had nothing to say to the Maryland troops, and that it was not his business to supply the Regimental Surgeons with medicines, and that it must have been a mistake of the Convention or Council of Safety of Maryland, to send their Surgeons here without them and think they were to be supplied here.'[75]

Some military officers took matters into their own hands, removing their regimental sick away from the army into the surrounding country.[76] In November 1776, as Washington began his retreat through New Jersey, sick rates were little changed. It remained normal for a third of the rebel army to be incapacitated by wounds and disease. General Charles Lee had command of thirty regiments of New England troops. On the 24th, 5,589 were fit for duty, 1,290 were present and sick, and 1,599 absent and sick. It is not clear how many of the men 'present and sick' were fit enough to fight. General Heath's New England men were similarly afflicted.[77]

Morale was low and many were likely suffering from cold exposure and seasonal viral infections. Private Joseph Plumb Martin of Connecticut caught a 'violent cold' as did several of his comrades. The 16-year-old was ordered to the general hospital at Newark to act as a nurse.

'I had on my ward seven or eight *sick soldiers* who were (at least, soon after their arrival there) as well in health as I was. All they wanted was a cook.'

Newark was a Tory heartland and the hospital's patients were suspicious of local produce such as milk, worried that it might be poisoned.[78]

The American prisoners taken on Long Island, at Fort Washington and elsewhere were incarcerated at New York, either in jails in the city or in hulks in the harbour. Allegations of neglect were rejected by the British but there is evidence that the treatment of the American prisoners of war was inhumane even by the low standards of the time. A number of churches and other buildings had been crudely converted into prisons. In the Dutch Church, there were 3,000 inmates. Men shivered and wallowed in their own filth, clothed only in rags, and subsisting on nauseating food. The hulks were even worse, with as many as a thousand Continental soldiers confined on board. There was no medical provision.

In such conditions, there were inevitable outbreaks of smallpox and typhus and men died in large numbers. Every morning, on the hulks, the jailors' familiar cry was 'Rebels, turn out your dead'. According to the *New Hampshire Gazette*, 1,700 prisoners perished in just three days during the winter. Disease, particularly smallpox, spread to the city and wealthy New Yorkers fled their homes seeking out inoculation in the country.[79]

There were two other major theatres of operations in 1776. To the south, Henry Clinton led a British expeditionary force in an unsuccessful assault on Sullivan's Island at the mouth of the estuary leading to Charleston. This culminated in the battle of 28 June. The operation highlighted the problems of coordinating an amphibious operation, the Redcoats put ashore defeated mostly by poor intelligence and the terrain, and the Royal Navy's cannonade ineffective against determined American resistance. The British fleet came under heavy fire from the fort on the Island and the attackers suffered more than 200 casualties compared with only about forty killed and wounded among the rebel defenders.[80]

Surgeon Thompson Forster was ashore and a distant witness of the devastation on the Royal Navy ships *Bristol* and *Experiment*. Red-hot cannon balls shattered masts and caused terrible wounds.[81] An officer on the *Bristol* described a 'slaughterhouse' with 'blood and entrails lying about'.[82] Surgery was performed below deck but there was no safe place. When Captain John Morris of the *Bristol* was carried down for an above elbow amputation, the operation was interrupted by a cannon ball entering the cockpit and killing two of the medical staff. Men were still dying of their wounds in July.[83]

It is likely that the smaller number of American wounded were taken to the newly opened general hospital in Charleston.[84] The city was a notoriously unhealthy place, threatened by diseases such as malaria and, at least in the past, yellow fever. There was a seasonal element to this; 'in the spring a paradise, in the summer a hell, in the autumn a hospital'.[85] British soldiers who had landed just to the north of Sullivan's Island encountered a desolate landscape, oppressive heat and swarms of insects. 'There is nothing that grows upon this island, it being a mere sandbank, and a few bushes which harbour millions of musketoes, a greater plague than there can be in hell itself'.[86]

Despite the obvious risks, the contemporary accounts suggest that Clinton's force was not greatly affected by disease. Forster describes men being weakened by dysentery and there are references to scurvy at sea but there was no epidemic.[87] This is in marked contrast to later British campaigns in the South and the 1776 expedition was probably spared due to its relatively short duration. There may have been other factors. An officer of the 57th concluded that he and his comrades had been protected by the 'sea breeze'. Another officer attributed the army's good health to the taking of regular exercise, 'which I fancy is necessary in every climate'.[88]

A thousand miles to the north, Guy Carleton and Benedict Arnold had been building ships, determined to contest Lake Champlain. On 11 October, the two fleets came together at Valcour Island. Arnold was outgunned by the larger British vessels and had to fight a rear-guard action. He was eventually forced to beach and set fire to ships to prevent them falling into enemy hands. Only eleven of the sixteen American vessels made it to Crown Point. The largest American naval engagement of the War was a pyrrhic victory for the British, the delay in seizing control of the lake meaning that it was too late in the season to continue the campaign.[89]

Arnold's improvised navy had only a skeletal medical service. Naval Surgeon Stephen McCrea was on the schooner *Royal Savage*. He informed Jonathan Potts that the two surgeon's mates who provided for Arnold's 800-strong force were of low calibre. One had 'no practice and little theory' and the other 'neither theory or practice'.[90] The sloop *Enterprise* served as a hospital ship for the sixty or so American wounded. Jahiel Stewart, serving with Samuel Brewer's Massachusetts Regiment, is the best witness:

> 'the Cannon ball & grape shot flew verrey thick & and I believe we
> had a great many Cild [killed]... they brought the wounded aboard
> of us the Dockters cut of[f] great many legs and arm[s].'

Several men who died of their wounds were thrown overboard.[91] McCrea wrote to Potts, 'I am so hurried in getting off the wounded of our little navy that it is impossible to give you an account of our action'.[92]

The nature of Arnold's subsequent care of his wounded was disputed. A story was soon circulating in British ranks that the American general, while burning his boats, had failed to remove about thirty sick and wounded men who were on board. The key British witness supporting this account was Robert Knox, the most senior British physician in North America, who was on the British flagship the *Lady Maria*.[93] In Knox's words, 'Mr Arnold ran five ships ashore, and remained on the beach till he set fire to them, burning the wounded and sick in them'.[94]

Knox had no clear motive to make such a damaging allegation against Arnold. A later interview with a local inhabitant of Ferris Bay, the site of the incident, gives a different version of events.

> 'Lieutenant Goldsmith of Arnold's galley had been severely wounded in the thigh by a grape shot in the battle near Valcour Island, and lay wholly helpless on the deck, when orders were given to blow up the vessels. Arnold had ordered him to be removed on shore, but by some oversight he was neglected, and was on the deck of the galley when the gunner set fire to the match. He then begged to be thrown overboard, and the gunner, on returning from the galley, told him he would be dead before she blew up. He remained on deck at the explosion, and his body was seen when blown up into the air. His remains were taken up and buried on the shore of the lake. To his credit Arnold showed the greatest feeling upon the subject and threatened to run the gunner through on the spot.'[95]

This account, portraying Arnold as the hero rather than the villain, is the more believable of the two. Knox was more distant from events and could easily have misinterpreted Arnold's actions.

Chapter 7

The Battles of Trenton and Princeton

November 1776–June 1777

You would think it had been desolated with the plague and an earthquake.

Benjamin Rush at Princeton village, January 1777

Washington continued his retreat through New Jersey pursued by forces under General Charles Earl Cornwallis. In the first week of December 1776, the rebels crossed the Delaware into Pennsylvania. The American commander organised a thin defensive line, posting his troops along a 25-mile stretch of the river. The British commander, William Howe, decided to suspend the fight, ordering his men into winter quarters in New Brunswick, Princeton, Trenton, and Bordentown. Howe planned to return to New York and Cornwallis to England.

British senior officers thought their troops to be 'in perfect security'. The American army had shrunk to less than 3,000 men, many soldiers melting away at the end of their enlistments.[1] Those who remained were in a poor state. As the temperature dropped, there were disastrous shortages of tents, blankets, clothing, food, and medicines.[2] A British officer made a damning comparison of the two armies:

'The rebel Army are in so wretched a condition as to clothes and accoutrements that I believe no nation ever saw such a set of tatterdemalions. There are few coats among them but what are out at elbows; and in a whole regiment scarce a pair of breeches. Judge then how they must be pinched in a winter campaign. We that are warmly clothed and well equipped already feel it severely.'[3]

This was not cheap propaganda. Washington reported that many of his men were 'nearly naked', so poorly clad as to be unfit for service. A Pennsylvanian militiaman failed to recognise his own brother, his face covered with sores and a long beard.[4]

The American sick and wounded were dragged from place to place in open and springless wagons. Villagers who lived along the route of retreat long remembered the cries of the invalids as the vehicles jolted over the stone roads.[5] The Continental Army's doctors were forced to react to events and the hospital situation was confusing and ever-changing. There were temporary facilities at Hackensack, Perth Amboy, Fort Lee, Newark, Elizabethtown, Morristown, New Brunswick, and Trenton. More permanent hospitals were established at Easton, Allentown, Bethlehem, and Philadelphia.[6]

Wagonloads of sick had been arriving at Philadelphia since the last week of November; there were perhaps 500 invalids in the city by the end of the year. The city's hospitals were under Morgan's jurisdiction but in view of the growing number of sick the Council of Safety requested that Jonathan Potts take local control of the medical arrangements. Army hospitals were opened in the Pennsylvania Hospital, the Bettering House, the smallpox hospital on Pine Street, and in houses vacated by loyalists.[7] There was real concern that Cornwallis might occupy the city and Morgan asked faculty members of his own medical school to stand by to provide care for any patients too ill to be evacuated.[8]

Washington had asked for medical help from the Pennsylvania authorities, hoping that civilian doctors would assist his surgeons. Dignitaries cooperated with army officers in the organisation of housing and care for disabled soldiers. Patriots were importuned for vital supplies.[9] Not all the local population were willing to give help. Shippen had set up his headquarters at Bethlehem on 3 December. It was soon obvious that the 2,000 patients expected from Morristown could not all be accommodated there and that some would have to be diverted to neighbouring towns and villages. The citizens of Reading hoped that they might be spared:

> 'We have heard that a hospital is to be made at this place. Strange this, when we have no unoccupied houses in town, for many families have come hither from Philadelphia.'

Their fear was understandable. Infectious diseases were easily transmitted to the civilian population and sick rates in the rebel army were high. Shippen was prone to make optimistic reports to his seniors, but he was forced to admit that large numbers of patients not yet under his control were lodged in barns in the countryside.[10] The full impact of disease on Washington's army may be extrapolated from the experience of Smallwood's Maryland Regiment of the Continental Line. This proud unit marched through Philadelphia in June 1776, 1,100 strong. By the end of December, it could muster only sixty men. The great majority of deaths were due to disease.[11] In Potter's Field at Philadelphia, single graves were replaced by mass burials in large square pits. The gravediggers struggled to keep up.[12]

The predominant afflictions in the fall and early winter were typhus and frostbite. In the words of Surgeon James Tilton:

> 'The [American] flying camp of 1776 melted like snow, in the field; cropped like rotten sheep on their struggling rout home, where they communicated the camp infection [typhus] to their friends and neighbours, of which many died.'[13]

Another patriot surgeon bemoaned the 'universal face of despondency'.[14]

The string of defeats and the miserable retreat mortified Washington. He was determined to take the initiative, motivated in part by revenge but also by the need to restore morale. Recruitment for 1777 depended on immediate success. On Christmas Day, he made an audacious night attack on a Hessian garrison at Trenton under the command of the veteran Colonel Johann Rall. Surprising their foe, by the following morning the Americans had won a sensational victory. Roughly 500 Hessians escaped but 150 were killed or wounded and 900 taken prisoner. American artilleryman Sergeant Joseph White entered the town after the battle but did not stay long, his 'blood chill'd to see such horror and distress, blood mingling together.'[15] Astonishingly, American losses were limited to four men killed and eight wounded.[16]

As the British presence in Trenton was limited to a handful of light dragoons who promptly escaped, the German wounded were tended by their own surgeons with American help. On the evening of the battle, Washington despatched an express rider to Bethlehem directing Shippen and his surgeons to join him. As the attack was made just after midnight, there was no realistic chance of Shippen reaching the field in time and at the outset of the action there was little or no medical cover. In subsequent correspondence with Morgan, Washington complained of the lack of 'any assistance from the

Hospital Department', adding that he thought this to be 'very strange'. The details are unclear, but it seems that Shippen, who remained responsible for the medical provision of the flying camp, had not anticipated the battle.[17]

The rebels were keen that the Hessian mercenaries change their allegiance and the German wounded at Trenton were paroled under the care of their own surgeons and given hospital facilities. This cooperation is confirmed by the following note sent by an American surgeon to Jonathan Potts:

> 'The amputating instruments which you sent for use of the Hessian Surgeon were taken away yesterday by Mr. Wood, and I am told by the former that they were so bad that he could not make use of them, had they been left. There are four or five men here who must soon submit to an operation or lose their lives. I therefore beg you to send a full set.'[18]

On 29 December, Washington ordered that the American sick be moved to Newtown on the other side of the Delaware pending their evacuation to Philadelphia.[19] On the same day, Sergeant William Young of the 3rd Battalion Pennsylvania Militia came across more German casualties at Bordentown:

> 'Saw a Room full of wounded hessians, one of them with his nose shot off. All of them in a wretched condition.'[20]

When Hessian troops re-entered Trenton in early January, they found their wounded to have been well cared for. Some of these men were eventually left in the hands of Continental Army doctors. Bodo Otto cared for a young officer, Lieutenant George Saltzmann, who showed his appreciation with gifts of a German song book and a sword.[21]

At the Second Battle of Trenton on 2 January 1777 Cornwallis made three futile attempts to cross the Assunpink Creek in the face of determined American resistance. A stone bridge 'looked red as blood with their killed and wounded, and their red coats'. Nightfall rather than good judgement ended the assault. More than a hundred Americans were killed or wounded while the British suffered nearly 500 casualties, almost 8 per cent of the force that had marched from Princeton.

There is no good account of the British medical arrangements at the battle. It is very likely that buildings in Trenton were pressed into use as field hospitals and that the more severely wounded were evacuated along Cornwallis's line of communications through New Brunswick and Perth Amboy to New York. There were several noted American doctors on the field. Benjamin Rush was with John Cadwalader's brigade of Pennsylvania Associators and Jonathan Potts was serving in Thomas Mifflin's brigade of Pennsylvania militia.[22] John Cochran and John Warren were also on hand. Rush later recalled his introduction to battle in his autobiography.

> 'The first wounded man that came off the field was a New England soldier. His right hand hung a little above his wrist by nothing but a piece of skin. It had been broken by a cannon ball. I took charge of him, and directed him to a house on the river which had been appropriated for a hospital. In the evening all the wounded, about 20 in number, were brought to this hospital and dressed by Dr. Cochran, myself, and several young surgeons who acted under our direction. We all lay down upon some straw in the same room with our wounded patients. It was now for the first time war appeared to me in its awful plenitude of horrors. I want words to describe the anguish of my soul, excited by the cries and groans and convulsions of the men who lay by my side. I slept two or three hours. About 4 o'clock Dr. Cochran went up to Trenton to inquire for our army. He returned in haste, and said they were not to be found. We now procured wagons, and after putting our patients in them directed that they should follow us to Bordentown, to which place we supposed our Army had retreated.'[23]

Washington had confounded both his own doctors and the enemy. Leaving 400 men behind to keep campfires alight, he marched the remainder of his army through the night to the village of Princeton. Here, on 3 January 1777, he clashed with Cornwallis's rearguard under the command of Lieutenant Colonel Charles Mawhood. At first, the better-armed British forced their opponents back at the point of the bayonet, but the appearance of Washington and the rebels' superior numbers soon led to the breaking of Mawhood's line. This improbable victory had cost the patriots sixty to seventy casualties, perhaps half of them killed. The British forces in the village capitulated and Cornwallis's total losses were as great as 450 killed, wounded, or captured. This was nearly 50 per cent of the men who saw action, a heavy toll from a battle that lasted only fifteen minutes.[24]

Pools of blood congealed on the frozen ground. Small groups of men combed the field, seeking out the wounded by their cries. Some of the injured were taken on wagons to Princeton village but most were carried to nearby houses which acted as makeshift field hospitals for both sides.[25] A local inhabitant and his family hid in their cellar during the battle:

> 'Almost as soon as the fighting was over our house was filled and surrounded with General Washington's Men and himself on horseback at the door. They brought in with them on their Shoulders two Wounded [British] Regulars, one of them was shot in at his hip and the bullet lodged in his groin, and the other was shot through his body Just below his short ribs he was in very much pain and bled much out of both sides, and often desired to be moved from one place to another, which was done.[26]

The farmhouses of William and Thomas Clarke were also used as field hospitals. In the former, twenty wounded soldiers, mostly British, lay on straw in a single room. In the latter, the casualties included the American general, Hugh Mercer.[27]

Benjamin Rush arrived the next day and tended to the wounded in the Thomas Clarke House. Here he amputated the legs of four British soldiers, all of whom survived. Captain John McPherson of the 17th Foot had a chest injury. His condition improved despite (or, according to Rush, because of) a considerable loss of blood.[28]

Mercer was a physician soldier, in command of a brigade at Princeton. He was born and medically trained in Aberdeen and emigrated to America in 1746 after fighting for Prince Charlie at Culloden.[29] Rush inherited his management from a British surgeon's mate. The wounds were extensive, including seven bayonet stabs to the body and a head injury from a musket butt. The American doctor was cautiously optimistic but the patient anticipated his own fate, worried particularly about a penetrating wound under his right arm; '[it] is the fellow who will soon do my business'. Mercer died on 10 January. His body was removed to Philadelphia where he received a hero's public funeral.[30]

After the engagement, a hospital was opened in Princeton College's Nassau Hall. Rush and Potts helped care for the patients until the end of the month.[31] They worked with a British surgeon and five surgeon's mates who had been left behind to tend for their own and the enemy's wounded. Rush was impressed by this initiative, and he took the opportunity to converse with the British doctors. It is likely that these discussions strengthened his resolve to reorganise the American service along British lines.[32]

Cornwallis was, at least according to one of his enemies, 'in a most infernal Sweat, running, puffing & blowing & swearing at being so outwitted'. He feared for his New Brunswick cantonment, and he hurried north leaving behind the sick and wounded. The patriot army was exhausted, and Washington wisely decided to take up winter quarters in Morristown.[33] The King's soldiers spent the winter in camps along the Raritan River between New Brunswick and Perth Amboy. In New York, Howe was agitated; 'I do not see a prospect of terminating the war but by a general action and I am aware of the difficulties in our way to obtain it'.[34]

John Morgan was now under attack from all sides for the perceived failings of the American medical services. He was held responsible for the poor treatment of patients, departmental corruption, and even the low morale of regiments. In Congress it was said that 'the very air teems with complaints about him'.[35] The director general had lost power and usefulness and was a convenient scapegoat for Congressional ineptitude and poor planning. In his biographer's words, he had been blamed 'because he had not performed miracles'.[36] On 9 January, Congress announced the dismissal of Morgan and of Samuel Stringer. This decision left William Shippen in effective control of the medical department.

The movement of American sick and wounded across the Delaware necessitated hospitals outside Philadelphia. About 300 patients were divided between Easton, Allentown, Northampton, and Wilmington, and 700 were sent to Bethlehem. The Moravians of the village of Bethlehem had insisted upon a quiet neutrality but they were dragged into the War first by the arrival of 200 British prisoners and then by an avalanche of American sick. Congress overruled the community's objections, and a general hospital was opened in the Brethren's House. This was the first instance of a religious settlement being commandeered as an American army hospital.[37] The Brethren's House was a substantial structure. Shippen filled the cellars with supplies and medicines and assigned officer patients to the upper rooms. The hospital guard, surgeons and convalescents occupied shops and other buildings on the west side of the village. The hospital was closed at the end of March 1777, the patients transferred to Philadelphia. This was also the case for Easton and Allentown.[38]

Shippen continued to issue conciliatory medical reports but the conditions in the hospitals and the army's sick and mortality rates were all of concern. Bishop John Ettwein, the leader of the Moravians, described Bethlehem as a 'sewer of impurities'. By the time of its closure, the mortality rate in the hospital had risen to a frightening 25 per cent.[39] In mid-February, a total of 4,745 of the 17,449-man rebel Army was reported to be ill or unfit. High levels of sickness persisted into the spring, a quarter of the men at Morristown listed sick in May.[40] It was claimed by John Adams that 2,000 soldiers had been buried in Potter's Field.[41]

The cramped accommodation of exhausted and emaciated troops made a serious outbreak of typhus almost inevitable. Benjamin Rush was in Philadelphia:

'A fatal hospital fever was generated in the month of May in 1777 in the house of employment [a general hospital] by our sick being too much crowded. Several of the attending surgeons and mates died of it, and most of them were infected with it. I called upon the Director [Shippen] and asked for more rooms for the sick. This was denied. Here was the beginning of sufferings and mortality in the American army which had nearly destroyed it.'[42]

Henry Hallowell, a sick soldier from Massachusetts, lay on a hard floor with no change of clothing; 'I got very lousy and flesh much gone'. He was given food by local women and survived but three of his friends died.[43]

Congress responded to these shortcomings by approving Shippen's plan for the reorganisation of the medical department (see Chapter 3). Four days later, on 11 April, Shippen was elected director general. Among other appointments, John Cochran became physician and surgeon general in the Middle Department, Jonathan Potts was deputy director of the Hospital in the Northern Department, and Benjamin Rush surgeon general in the Middle Department.[44] A platitudinous notice in *The Pennsylvania Post* of 5 June signed by Shippen and Cochran declared that the hospitals were in excellent order and the army unusually healthy.[45]

In early 1777, a resident of Princeton noted that 'the Small Pox hath got into the Neighbourhood the natural way and proved very mortal both to the inhabitants and soldiers'.[46] The disease had also made its appearance among the patriot troops in Morristown and Congress ordered the Medical Committee to write to Washington to explore the propriety of large-scale inoculation.[47] The commander, whose own pock-marked face was a constant reminder of the threat, had anticipated the question. The following letter to Shippen is dated 6 January 1777.

> 'Finding the smallpox to be spreading much, and fearing that no precaution can prevent it from running through the whole of our Army, I have determined that the troops shall be inoculated.

> The expedient may be attended with some inconvenience and some disadvantages, but yet I trust in its consequences, will have the most happy effects. Necessity not only authorizes but seems to require this measure, for should the disorder infect the Army in this natural way and rage with its usual virulence, we should have more to dread from it than from the sword of the enemy... If the business is immediately begun and favored with the common success, I would fain hope they will soon be fit for duty, and that in a short space of time we shall have an Army not subject to this, the greatest of all calamities that can befall it, when taken in the natural way.'[48]

In the first months of the year, Washington demanded that all means be taken to limit the disease including the quarantining of victims in special hospitals. He had second thoughts regarding inoculation, concerned that if not properly controlled it could worsen the situation. In early February, he had regained his resolve and thousands of troops were eventually to be inoculated with few serious problems.[49] The mortality for supervised inoculation was well under 1 per cent. Most soldiers were only briefly incapacitated, the most common side-effect being a persistent sore at the site of the lancet puncture in the arm.[50]

Shippen arranged for the inoculation of recruits in Philadelphia and doctors were sent to Morristown and surrounding outposts where divisions submitted to the procedure en masse every five to six days. Guarded private houses and churches were employed as treatment and isolation facilities. By late May, new recruits were being sent to the supply base at Peekskill in New York to allow better monitoring of the process.[51]

Washington's hesitancy is understandable. Mass inoculation was a great military risk, potentially removing large numbers of rebel soldiers from active service at a crucial stage of the War. As far as possible, the debilitated condition of the Continental Army as it recovered from induced smallpox was kept a secret from the British.[52] The commander's brave initiative did not entirely remove natural smallpox from the ranks, but the enforced regimen of quarantine, isolation and inoculation almost certainly prevented a catastrophic epidemic.

Washington was also keen to minimise the impact of other diseases. His orders in the late spring and summer of 1777 refer to the location of latrines and slaughter pens, the importance of frequent bathing, and the need to supplement the soldiers' diet with vegetables and salads.[53] In May, Benjamin Rush wrote to his chief, suggesting that the health of the men would benefit if active campaigning could be delayed for a few more weeks. Washington replied politely, agreeing to wait for better weather if possible but also pointing out that the decision 'must depend upon many other considerations and circumstances'.[54] It was at this time that Rush published his manifesto designed to improve the health of the Army; 'Fatal experience has taught the people of America that a greater proportion of men perish with sickness in our armies than have fallen by the sword'.[55]

The available sick returns for the Brigade of Guards in New York show some deterioration in the health of the British Army from September 1776 onwards. There is little information as to the specific disorders, but scabies was probably prevalent, records from the 17th Regiment of Foot telling us that a 'great Many of the Men are Itched'. By December, the sick rate for the Guards in New Jersey had increased to thirteen per cent and in January 1777 it was almost seventeen per cent. On 24 February, the Brigade reported 122 sick and 17 dead for the previous month.[56] This confirms a significant outbreak of disease in their crowded winter quarters on the Raritan. The contemporary references to fever and flux suggest that the epidemic was a malignant combination of typhus and dysentery.[57]

The best witness is John Peebles, a lieutenant in the Black Watch who had previously served as a surgeon's mate. The following is excerpted from his diary which he kept while posted around Perth Amboy and New Brunswick. He spent much of his time on a transport on the river.

> 'Monday 17th. Febry. Clear weather & gentle frost wind NW… some of our men turning sick & no doctor to attend them our surgeon having left us at New York, sent for the Surgn. of the Light Infantry who comes & visits them.

Friday 7th. March... our men turning sickly our Compy. have ½ a dozen down with flux; the Regtal. Surgeons ashore take it by turns to Visit the Grrs. [grenadiers]

Tuesday 11th. March... Had the Battn. Ashore for two or 3 hours on the beach & got the ship a little clean'd, our Compy. very sickly, two men that were orderly in the Hospital on different days were taken suddenly ill, owing they think to the putrid stench of some of the rooms.

Wednesday 19th. March... There is an ugly fever seized on a good many both in Town & Transports of which several have died, & it seems to spread, a ship appointed for an Hospital Ship, pretty full already.

Saturday 29th. March... a good many of the men sick & some dying.'[58]

Peebles makes further reference to 'fluxes and fevers' in early June.[59] The seriously sick were sent to New York. In February and March, close to 70 per cent of patients presenting to the Poor House Hospital in the city had either flux, fever, or both.[60] Sick rates for the Guards Brigade in New Jersey indicate some improvement by early summer (6 per cent in May and 8 per cent in June).[61] It may be that conditions in the New York garrison were more conducive to good health than the transports and buildings on the Raritan. In late May, Captain John Bowater describes the troops swimming in the sea and competing in foot races. He claims that the soldiers were 'remarkably healthy'.[62]

Chapter 8

The Saratoga Campaign

June 1777–October 1777

Yankee Doodle came to town,
How do you think they serv'd him?
One took his bag, another his scrip,
The quicker for to starve him.

> 'Yankee Doodle' was played at the British surrender at
> Saratoga. First written by British army surgeon Richard
> Shuckburgh, it was later a song of American defiance.

In early 1777, the British General John Burgoyne, a gaming addict, embarked on his greatest gamble. He had persuaded King George to give him an army of more than 8,000 men that would invade the upper Hudson Valley by way of Lake Champlain, going all the way to Albany. There, it was hoped that he would be joined by Howe's Army from New York, although the optimistic Burgoyne believed this to be unnecessary. The capture of Ticonderoga on 5 July was uneventful but Burgoyne was soon in a losing streak. Nothing went to plan. He was beset by supply problems, the terrain was challenging, loyalist support did not materialise, and his Indian allies were unreliable. Howe remained distant. While the Anglo-German army was eroded by fighting at Hubbardton and Bennington, rebel general Horatio Gates was being constantly reinforced and soon had more than 10,000 troops. After two actions around Freeman's Farm and Bemis Heights (the battles of Saratoga) in September and October, Burgoyne found himself unable to retreat to Canada and surrounded by Continentals and militiamen. The surrender of almost 6,000 British and Germans meant that he had lost 86 per cent of the original expeditionary force. It was a turning point in the War.[1]

Inspector of hospitals and physician Robert Knox oversaw the British medical arrangements for the Saratoga Campaign. His hospital personnel included two surgeons: John Weir, who was attached to Burgoyne's staff, and John Macnamara Hayes. Additionally, there were two apothecaries, Vincent Wood and Richard Monington, and fourteen mates. In July, Knox fell ill with a fever and, after struggling with it for a few weeks, he was forced to return to Montreal. Hayes was now in effective control.[2]

There was a general hospital at Montreal into which the regimental sick were admitted at the outset of the campaign. A medical store depot was located between the city and Lake Champlain. Cantlie describes the establishment of a flying hospital equipped with 300 sets of bedding and with a further 300 sets in reserve. All its personnel and stores were carried forward along lakes and rivers in covered boats and it was to receive wounded and sick from the regimental hospitals as the army advanced. The more serious cases were to be evacuated back to Montreal.[3] On 3 July, the flying hospital was at Three Mile Point near Ticonderoga.[4] A week later, a 230-bed general hospital was opened a few miles away at Mount Independence and in August and early September there were hospital facilities at Fort Miller.[5] General orders stipulated that two women from each battalion were to help take care of the sick and wounded.[6]

In contrast to Cantlie, Kopperman makes no reference to a flying hospital (see also Chapter 2), but he acknowledges that once Burgoyne had crossed the Hudson it was not possible to maintain a fixed hospital facility. In the words of a German soldier, 'Our hospital had to follow or else it would have been captured by the enemy'. Hospitals were opened opportunistically in barracks and houses (e.g. at Schuylerville) or in large tents (ten were available).[7]

By contemporary standards, the British force was well supplied with medical personnel. There was approximately one hospital or regimental medical officer per 100 infantrymen. At the capitulation at Saratoga, seven British regimental surgeons, six regimental mates and four German surgeons were among the prisoners.[8] An eighth British regimental surgeon, Henry Seeley of the 9th Foot, had been captured earlier in fighting near Fort Anne.[9]

The Americans were again faced with the considerable challenge of maintaining a medical service while in retreat. Jonathan Potts, in immediate charge of arrangements, was little liked or helped by General Philip Schuyler (who was not superseded by Gates until mid-August).[10] When Ticonderoga was abandoned, the remaining patients and the hospital supplies were evacuated in 200 boats first to Skenesborough and then to Fort Anne. They remained in tents here until their eventual transfer by water to the principal general hospital at Albany. This was a journey of fifty-five miles in three days.[11]

Despite Potts' best efforts there were shortcomings in his department. The constant movement of sick and wounded required suitable transport. Surgeon Jonathan Bartlett, in command of the flying hospital to the Continental Army in the Northern Department, was forced to plead for more wagons, his patients' bones 'grinding on hard oaken planks'. He also complained of the lack of staff and a shortage of lint, bandages, and surgical instruments. There was 'not a crooked needle in the camp'. Regimental surgeons claimed that Bartlett was denying them vital supplies, something he vehemently denied. This exchange reflected the persistent ill-feeling between hospital and regimental medical officers. Among Bartlett's grisly tasks was the examination of the body of a frontierswoman, Jane McCrea, who had been killed and scalped by Burgoyne's Indian allies.[12]

The seriously wounded from the Campaign – Americans, British and, later, German troops – were mostly taken to the Albany facility. This is well described by Surgeon's Mate James Thacher who had accompanied his patients south.

'The hospital was erected during the late French [Indian] war; it is situated on an eminence overlooking the city. It is two stories high, having a wing at each end and a piazza in front and below. It contains forty wards, capable of accommodating five hundred patients bedsides the rooms appropriated to the use of surgeons and other officers, stores, & c.'[13]

The building was probably constructed of wood, and it disappeared shortly after the Revolutionary War.[14]

As more casualties poured in, extra hospital space was created in loyalist homes and a church.[15] Conditions in Albany were better than the average for the War. A visiting French general, Matthias Roche de Fermoy, was pleased to see the 'care, and attention and humanity' received by the soldiers in the wards. His gift of French money to the wounded was symbolic of a growing alliance.[16]

On the eve of the Campaign, Burgoyne pronounced that his troops were in a state of health 'almost unprecedented'.[17] Lieutenant Thomas Anburey agreed that he and his comrades were 'remarkably healthy'.[18] Colonel Johann Friedrich Specht attributed his well-being to the cold Canadian winter which had 'taken the place of the best physician'.[19] Returns for early May show sick rates of 7 to 8 per cent. There were a few cases of dysentery and scurvy. The latter disorder was most common in the Brunswick Regiment, but it also occurred in the British 20th and 21st Foot where it was soon cured by spruce beer and fresh provisions. On 1 July, only 4 per cent of 3,379 listed men were sick. Some afflictions were not contained in such data. Specht noted that his men were suffering from severe homesickness.[20]

In early August, the health of Burgoyne's army began to deteriorate. This is reflected in the sick rates which were soon in the range of 13–17 per cent. Interpretation of these morbidity rates is complicated by the lack of a separate column for the wounded on the returns. Thus, an indeterminate number of soldiers in hospital were there because of battle rather than illness.[21] Nevertheless, the available qualitative evidence does support a significant increase in sickness.

Knox reported that fever was very prevalent, not one in fifty men escaping it. The disorder was only rarely fatal and was successfully treated with Peruvian bark, suggesting that it was malaria.[22] It affected the garrisons at Ticonderoga and Mount Independence and subsequently followed Burgoyne's army.[23] Dysentery was ever-present, one German soldier stating that 'it raged amongst us'. There were also some hospitalisations for other diarrheal disorders.[24]

While bark might be an effective treatment for malaria there was no equivalent therapy for dysentery. As always, the management of camp disease depended on good military hygiene. Burgoyne's care for his men is reflected in his general orders. On 8 June, it was instructed that the army was to encamp in double rows about a dozen yards apart with thirty yards between the brigades' regiments. It was to front a wood and to be as near to a lake as was possible. This was all to maximise the 'benefit of Air'.[25] At the end of July, the following order was issued at Fort Edward.

> 'Each Regiment of the Line will turn out 20 men, burn and bury all old meat, rubbish, and every other nuisance *in* or *near* the Camp, under the Direction of the Provost. This is not confined merely to the ground where the Troops are encamped on, but extended to every nuisance and unwholesome thing about the Camp.'[26]

Gates' American army became healthier as the campaign unfolded. This was despite the unpropitious season, the poor provisioning of the militia, and the number of new recruits. Potts attributed the low level of sickness to the control of smallpox and the efficiency of his own department. Rush believed the hardiness of the New Englanders and the absence of typhus from the hospitals to be factors. The favourable weather, constant change of camp sites and the care of senior officers for their men – the commander was affectionately known as 'Granny Gates' – probably all played a role.[27] Sick rates after the battles of Saratoga were reported as between 6 and 9 per cent, much lower than the 17 per cent endured by Schuyler's and Gates' troops in June.[28]

A return from Jonathan Potts' papers dated August 1777 provides a useful breakdown of diseases in the Continental Army. There were 396 cases (excluding fifty-three surgical patients) of which the following were the most common disorders: dysentery eighty-one cases (20.5% of total); intermittent fever (malaria) seventy-nine (20%); diarrhoea sixty-one (15.5%); cough twenty-five (6%); rheumatism twenty-two (5.5%).

The next largest categories were the uninformative 'convalescent' and 'debility'. The remaining cases were made up of smaller numbers of the predictable afflictions of an army including venereal disease, itch, fever, dropsy, jaundice, scurvy, pleurisy, and rupture. The six cases of 'putrid fever' suggest that if typhus was present then it was not a major problem. The one case of 'hypochondria' is the only reference to disorders of the mind.[29] The two opposing armies were most affected by the same diseases.

The fall of Ticonderoga on 6 July was bloodless and the first fighting of the campaign was at Hubbardton on the following day. Here, British forces led by Brigadier Simon Fraser attacked Seth Warner's Green Mountain Boys. It was a small engagement but ferocious; historian John Ferling points out that the total losses were proportionately equal to the Battle of Waterloo. The Americans lost 350 men, nearly two-thirds taken prisoner, and the British had almost 200 killed and wounded.[30]

Soldiers carried the British wounded to the rear. Many of the casualties had multiple wounds as it was the habit of the rebels to load their muskets with three small and three larger balls. The troops fashioned small huts covered with the bark of trees to accommodate the wounded until surgeons arrived from Ticonderoga.[31]

Evacuation away from the field proved to be difficult. At first, there were limited stretchers for the return journey. The most seriously wounded were removed on the available stretchers each carried by four soldiers.[32] The road was a quagmire. On 16 July, Major General William Phillips wrote to Fraser from Ticonderoga.

'The road to Hubberton [sic] being 26 miles long is not to be repaired for carts or carriages. The wounded are being brought away as far as they are capable of being removed on horseback, but it is impossible with every wish, joined to every duty to do so, to give more assistance.'

Phillips insisted that the best policy was to 'drive the Rebels southwards' so that the wounded would be safe at Hubbardton.[33] A 200-man detachment later transported the remaining convalescents to the general hospital at Mount Independence, the wounded carried on biers.[34]

The British were driving the Americans south. The rebel forces retreated through Skenesborough and Fort Anne to the relative safety of Fort Edward. In two weeks, Burgoyne had captured Crown Point, Ticonderoga, and Fort Anne. He was only seventy-five miles from Albany. The tide was about to turn. As part of the British strategy, Colonel Barry St Leger had invaded the Mohawk Valley and invested Fort Stanwix with a force of British regulars, loyalists, and Indian allies. An ambush of this force by Colonel Nicolas Herkimer of the Tryon County Militia resulted in the bloody Battle of Oriskany on 6 August. Both sides claimed victory. The rebel militia lost half their men, but St. Leger was forced to retreat to Canada abandoned by the disillusioned Indians.[35]

The American force at Oriskany was accompanied by Surgeon Moses Younglove who was soon captured. Potts sent Surgeon Robert Johnson of the 6th Pennsylvania to treat the casualties and he is the only good witness of the medical arrangements. Ten days after the action, Johnson informed Potts that he had thirty patients. Among them was Herkimer, who had injuries of the leg and thigh which had been dressed only once since the battle. Johnson was forced to amputate but without success, 'the cause of his death God only knows'.[36]

Burgoyne now sent 750 German troops under Lieutenant Colonel Friedrich Baum to seize the large rebel supply depot at Bennington ten miles east of the Hudson. The Battle of Bennington soon developed into a hand-to-hand contest between professional soldiers and hardened frontiersmen. They fought with bayonets, the butts of muskets, sabres, and pikes. It was a signal American victory, Baum mortally wounded, and the loss of another hundred men from Burgoyne's army.[37]

Duncan states, dismissively, that Bennington was an 'impromptu affair' and therefore there was no regular American medical service.[38] Potts had sent a medical chest before the action and Surgeon Francis Hagan was despatched after the fighting. Hagan was allowed by the local authorities to use the church and the town meeting house as hospitals. He wrote to Potts, a week after the battle, telling him that the wounded were widely dispersed and difficult to find. Surgeon Samuel McKenzie was sent to help. Apart from some shortages of medicines and surgical instruments, there was apparently a good level of provision. At the end of August, McKenzie expressed hope that the hospital would soon be 'well regulated'. General Benjamin Lincoln concurred, stating that the hospital was 'very good'.[39]

There were German surgeons on the Bennington battlefield, among them Julius Wasmus. At first, he found shelter behind an oak tree and did his best to treat the wounded. He was soon discovered by rebel soldiers who pilfered his pockets before asking for his surgical assistance. After tending to some American casualties, he returned to his own men who were crying for help but was soon dragged back to deal with the enemy's wounded. His surgical instruments, still under the tree, were confiscated by a rebel soldier who told him to drink some rum.[40]

Despite Wasmus's rough handling by American troops on the field, the captured German wounded received good management. On 2 September, two weeks after the battle, Gates reassured Fraser that 'surgeons, medicines and attendants with every comfort imaginable has been amply supplied to the sick and wounded officers and soldiers, prisoners at Bennington'.[41] A temporary hospital in the town was dedicated to the hundred German casualties. Burgoyne sent back surgical instruments and one of his own medical officers, probably Vincent Wood.[42] The more seriously wounded were eventually sent to Albany while the less debilitated followed the rest of the German prisoners to Brimfield, Westminster, and Rutland.[43]

Among Wasmus's patients was Lieutenant August Wilhelm von Breva who had received a severe wound in the shoulder. His clinical course is a reminder of the chronicity of some wounds. He had a probable fractured humerus and local infection – osteomyelitis – soon developed. On 2 July 1778, almost a year later, the wound burst open and was very painful. It was still discharging pus in the autumn. In August 1779, a small piece of bone had been removed but it was expected that further operations would be necessary. Like Jeremy Lister at Boston, von Breva survived his ordeal and died in Germany in 1790.[44]

The first Battle of Saratoga (Freeman's Farm) was fought on 19 September around the land of Freeman's Farm on Bemis Heights. It was a brutal affair, one of Burgoyne's veteran officers asserting that 'the fire was heavier than

ever I saw it anywhere'.[45] The British held the field but, in the wider context of
the War, it was an American victory. British casualties were nearly 600 killed
and wounded, roughly twice that of Gates' army. Burgoyne was still thirty
miles from Albany, and he had lost all forward momentum. He conceded to a
minister in England that 'no fruits, honour excepted, were attained'.[46]

Thomas Anburey witnessed the human cost of British honour on the day
after the battle. Shock, dehydration, and pain were the immediate enemies of
the wounded.

> 'They had remained out all night, and from the loss of blood
> and want of nourishment, were upon the point of expiring with
> faintness: some of them begged they might lie and die, others were
> again insensible, some upon the least movement were put in the
> most horrible tortures, and all had near a mile to be conveyed to
> the hospitals; others at their last gasp, who for want of our timely
> assistance must have inevitably expired.'[47]

When the wounded did reach medical help, they were subjected to a crude
triage. Some were clearly for palliative management. Twenty-two-year-old
Lieutenant Stephen Harvey of the 62nd Foot received multiple wounds. His
surgeon suggested a powerful dose of opium to avoid unnecessary suffering,
a plan to which the patient quickly consented.[48] Others were remarkably
fortunate. Captain Bloomfield of the Artillery received a shot which passed
through both cheeks without injuring his mouth.[49]

The British 'hospitals' alluded to by Anburey were accommodated in a
mixture of houses and large tents. When Lieutenant James Hadden of the
Royal Artillery carried a fellow wounded officer behind the lines he found
the 'huts' to be full of wounded and he struggled to find a suitable place.[50]
Baroness von Riedesel, the wife of a German general, waited anxiously in
a deserted dwelling near the field. The house was soon commandeered by
British surgeons and orderlies fetching the wounded. The Baroness helped
care for a young British officer who refused surgery for his leg wound; 'finally
they attempted the amputation of the limb, but it was too late, and he died a
few days afterwards'.[51]

According to George Fox of the 47th, the general hospital established after
the battle was in large marquees and was crowded with wounded.[52] This
was probably at Wilbur's Basin, a small depression on the banks of the River

Hudson.[53] Returns after Freeman's Farm show more than 500 men in hospital. A quarter of Burgoyne's army was sick or wounded.[54]

The American wounded were fewer in number, but they suffered equally. Massachusetts militiaman John Glover saw 'scores of amputees'.[55] Like the British, the casualties were first carried to shelter around the field. Contemporary maps show a field hospital in the rear of the rebel entrenchments. The more seriously wounded were sent down the river to the general hospital at Albany.[56] A few days later, James Thacher wrote in his journal that there were soldiers with life-threatening injuries in the wards and that many would need major surgery.[57] A return for 29 September indicates that there were 547 wounded at Albany.[58]

The high level of cooperation between the two army's commanders was a positive feature of the medical provision for the Saratoga Campaign. Both were caring military officers, and this is reflected in their writings and actions. At the beginning of September, Gates had written to Fraser that 'it is the wish of every generous mind that the calamities of war should lay as light as possible upon the unhappy individuals who are wounded or taken'.[59] When Burgoyne later asked for the protection of his wounded, he noted that this was nothing less than he 'would show to an enemy in the same case'. Permission was obtained for both Vincent Wood and John Macnamara Hayes to visit wounded British officers behind American lines.[60]

The Battle of Bemis Heights on 7 October – sometimes called the second Battle of Saratoga – sealed the fate of Burgoyne's army. The British again sustained very heavy losses, close to 900 men killed or wounded. Gates' force had 130 casualties.[61] All hope of a British escape to Ticonderoga or even Fort Edward had evaporated.[62] The state of the of the trapped army was pitiable, the soldiers exposed to the cold, begging for food, and drinking muddy water.[63] On 17 October, Burgoyne accepted the inevitable and surrendered.

The American medical arrangements at Bemis Heights were under the supervision of Jonathan Potts, who occupied a hospital tent.[64] Connecticut militiaman Samuel Woodruff witnessed the arrival of casualties.

> 'About two hundred of our wounded men, during the afternoon, and by that time in the evening, were brought from the field of battle in wagons, and for want of tents, were placed in a circular row on the naked ground. It was a clear, but cold and frosty, night. The sufferings of the wounded were extreme, having neither beds

under them nor any kind of bed clothing to cover them. Several surgeons were busily employed during the night extracting bullets and performing other surgical operations.'[65]

Potts had been issued a dozen musket balls, presumably for the wounded to bite on during surgery.[66] Woodruff says that seventy men died before morning.[67]

Burgoyne had had a narrow escape, his hat and waistcoat having several bullet holes.[68] Fraser was less fortunate. He was carried back to Baroness von Riedesel's house. A musket ball had penetrated his bowel and, as was invariably the case in such wounds, he soon died. All the rooms of the house were full of soldiers, many sick with dysentery. The Baroness later sought shelter in another house on the opposite side of the Hudson, only to find that this was also a field hospital. The building was under American artillery fire; 'One poor soldier, whose leg they were about to amputate, having been laid upon a table for this purpose, had the other leg taken off by another cannon ball, in the very middle of the operation'.[69]

Burgoyne withdrew to Saratoga on the day after the battle, entrusting his sick and wounded to the enemy. Captain Henry Dearborn of New Hampshire noted in his journal that the British had left 'around 500 sick and wounded on the ground'.[70] Hayes entered the American lines with a white flag. A rebel officer who met him saw 300 men 'comfortably accommodated' in British hospital tents.[71] Hayes informed Potts that he had 254 casualties who required evacuation to a general hospital. The American surgeon managed to find six wagons and Hayes then requested stretchers and bearers for his wounded who would not otherwise tolerate the journey.[72]

The more seriously wounded from both sides were taken to the general hospital at Albany where Thacher and his colleagues toiled.

'Not less than one thousand wounded and sick are now in this city [24 October]... We have about thirty surgeons and mates; and all are constantly employed. I am obliged to devote the whole of my time, from eight o'clock in the morning to a late hour in the evening, to the care of our patients. Here is a fine field for professional improvement.'[73]

Some of the wounds had not been dressed on the field and were filled with maggots.[74] Among Thacher's charges was Benedict Arnold whose leg had been badly fractured by a musket ball. The doctor notes that the general was 'peevish and impatient'.[75] He refused amputation of the limb, the same as that injured at Quebec, and eventually recovered after three months in the hospital. While at Albany, Thacher also treated Captain William Greg of a New York Regiment, who had been scalped by Indians near Fort Stanwix. He too survived his injury after a long convalescence.[76]

There was a good understanding regarding the need for care of captured wounded and sick but there were limits to Gates' generosity (or perhaps his authority). He insisted that medical assistance be paid for and that, in the absence of any other agreement, the British and German surgeons and hospitalised soldiers were to be treated as prisoners of war.[77] Congress reneged on the treaty stipulation that all the defeated soldiers be returned to Britain. They were instead first marched to Boston and then to Charlottesville. Thomas Jefferson admitted that it was 'an infraction of our [American] public honour.'[78]

It was normal for the under-resourced American authorities to rely on the British Army to provide for British prisoners of war.[79] This equally applied to medical cover and so the hospitalised prisoners at Albany were tended by British and German medical officers. John Macnamara Hayes remained in charge of these patients from October 1777 until June 1778 when he was exchanged. The last available return for the hospital under his superintendence shows that during this period of nine months there had been 477 admissions, 341 discharges, and 76 deaths with 417 remaining.[80]

While British and German doctors were incarcerated, rebel medical officers had a rare cause for celebration. On 20 October, Gates informed Congress of 'the great care and attention with which Doctor Potts and ye gentlemen of the general hospital conducted the business of their department'. Congress acquiesced to the general's request for a formal recognition of the doctors' contribution; 'their Zeal, so deeply interested in the Preservation of the Health and Lives of the gallant assertors of their Country's Cause; ...Congress cannot but entertain a high Sense of the Services which they have rendered during this Campaign'.[81]

Chapter 9

The Philadelphia Campaign

July 1777–December 1777

These are dreadful times; consequences of unnatural wars.
William Shippen, September 1777

Howe had never intended to link up with Burgoyne. In July 1777, the British fleet carried his 16,000 troops to the Chesapeake with the aim of capturing Philadelphia. Washington, in a 'state of constant perplexity' as to the enemy's destination, now moved the Continental Army south. Under the pressure of public opinion, the American commander had decided to give Howe his battle. At Brandywine Creek in September, Washington was comprehensively outmanoeuvred and defeated. The British entered Philadelphia two weeks later. Another American defeat at Germantown in early October was dispiriting for the rebel cause but Howe's victories were hollow. There was an impasse. Washington was in no position to launch an attack to retake Philadelphia while Howe was distracted by the need to clear American forts on the Delaware to safeguard his supplies. At the end of the year, the British remained in the city and Washington took his men into winter quarters at nearby Valley Forge.[1]

John Mervin Nooth was in command of the British medical department for the Campaign. He accompanied Howe from New York and took up headquarters in Philadelphia after its fall. Here, he was supported by Michael Morris, the inspector of regimental infirmaries. At this time, there were seventy-three hospital staff officers in the British service and a proportion of them had sailed with the force. Transport was provided, twelve wagons being allocated to each general hospital.

Nooth was not an inspiring leader (see also Chapter 2). He was soon wrangling over the cost of staples such as vegetables and wine. Hospital stoppages were problematic; soldiers were charged 5 pence per day, but the purveyors were allowing sailors, women, children and refugees to be treated free instead of paying the regulation 4 pence. Nooth was answerable to Adair in London and money was the constant preoccupation of both men. Adair insisted that there was overstaffing in the Philadelphia hospitals. When Nooth reluctantly inspected the Hessian hospital in the city he found the accounts to be 'irregular' before complaining that his own commission for the extra work was 'paltry'.[2]

In the summer of 1777, conditions in at least some of the American hospitals had improved. Benjamin Rush, never slow to criticise, wrote from Morristown to John Adams informing him that 'great order, cleanliness and the most perfect contentment prevail in our hospitals'. He commended Thomas Bond, the assistant director of the general hospital in Philadelphia, for his humanity and zeal.[3] Washington was determined that there should be no complacency in the service. He supported the authority of the hospital physicians, ordering that military officers only visit to check on treatment and to ensure good discipline. In September, he directed that officers should not remove patients from the hospitals without the written permission of the physician in charge.[4]

Howe's army had a torrid voyage to the Chesapeake. Delayed by unfavourable winds, it took thirty-two days, four times longer than expected. The men were crammed into hot airless compartments, fed on a diet of worm-infested bread, and given stinking water to drink. The soldiers finally came ashore on 5 August 1777.[5] A return reveals the sick rate for the Guards at the end of August to be seven to eight per cent. By September, this had increased to eleven per cent, perhaps reflecting the hardships of the voyage.[6]

There was more disease in the Continental Army. On 5 August, there were 3,745 sick in hospital in a total rank and file force of 17,949. This gives a sick rate of 21 per cent. The Medical Committee asserted that sick numbers had been 'greatly increased by the use of bad bread, and the want of Vinegar, Vegetables and soap'.[7]

By the time of Howe's landing at Head of Elk in Maryland, Washington was at Wilmington. After three weeks delay, Howe finally moved on Philadelphia. The two armies clashed at the Brandywine Creek on 11 September in the longest and largest single-day engagement of the War. Washington had not properly reconnoitred the ground and Howe was able to employ the outflanking manoeuvre which had proved so effective at Long Island. It was a British triumph; the Americans had lost 1,100 men and the British about half this number. Howe had again outthought and outfought his adversary but, crucially, the Continental Army was still intact.[8]

Most of the British casualties were taken to the general hospital at the nearby crossroads village of Dilworth. Howe ordered some of the regimental surgeons and four women from each brigade to attend the hospital. Parties were sent out into the woods to search for the wounded. Two days after the battle, the following more detailed general order was issued.

> 'Thirty Waggons will be sent this evening to receive the Wounded of Lieut. Gen. Knyphausen's Division; they are to be put into the Waggons by six to-morrow morning, and proceed immediately to Wilmington great Road, escorted by Col. Loss's Battalion, where they will be joined by the rest of the Wounded from Dilworth Hospital, who are to move from thence by five in the Morning, Escorted by a Detachment of the 71st. Regiment; Waggons being also ordered to receive them.'

Guides were to be attached to each British division.[9] Cantlie describes the Wilmington facility as being a 'flying hospital'. The Hessian wounded were also treated here until their own general hospital was established.[10]

As the battle reached its conclusion, Quaker Joseph Townsend and a few other locals were curious enough to wander on to the field. Unsurprisingly, they were horrified at the scale of the bloodshed and suffering. Townsend soon approached a British field hospital in the Birmingham Meeting House. His account contains rare detail.

> 'Some of the doors of the meeting house were torn off and the wounded carried thereon into the house to be occupied for an hospital, instead of the American sick for which it had been repairing some days previously. The wounded officers were first attended to – several of distinction had fallen, and as every thing appeared to be in a state of confusion, and we being spectators and assistance required, some of our number, at the request of the surgeons, became active in removing them therein – of whom I was one. I should have been willing to have been informed who they were, but it was not a time for inquiry, and I do not recollect to have heard the name of one of them mentioned at this time. After

assisting in carrying two of them into the house I was disposed to see an operation performed by one of the surgeons, who was preparing to amputate a limb, by having a brass clamp or screw fitted thereon, a little above the knee joint, he had his knife in his hand, the blade of which was of a circular form, and was about to make the incision, when he recollected that it might be necessary for the wounded man to take something to support him during the operation. He mentioned to some of his attendants to give him a little wine or brandy to keep up his spirits, to which he replied, "No, doctor, it is not necessary, my spirits are up enough without it." He then observed, "that he had heard some of them say there was some water in the house, and if there was he would like a little to wet his mouth'".

At this point, Townsend and his fellows left and made their way home, frightened that they would soon be detained by British troops.[11]

The American medical preparations for Brandywine were undermined by uncertainties regarding Washington's strategy. Shippen had been unable to provide an adequate number of medical personnel, wagons, or stretcher-bearers. Drugs and surgical instruments were in short supply.[12] The Meeting House described by Townsend was actually an American field hospital at the start of the battle. As the casualties mounted, they were unceremoniously left in front of the hospital, the wagons returning to the front for another load. Captain Samuel Dewes of Maryland heard the 'wild and frantic' cries of the wounded as they waited for attention.[13]

Inside the house, Benjamin Rush and his colleague Dr Lewis Howell used wooden benches and an unhinged door as improvised operating tables. They had already dug a pit outside for the corpses and amputated limbs. As the battle progressed, it became obvious that the Meeting House was no longer behind American lines but was almost exactly in the middle of the field. Rush and Howell kept operating despite what Howell referred to as 'the heaviest fighting I ever heard'. A white hospital flag gave them some protection but when it became inevitable that British troops would capture the building the two made a last gasp escape.[14]

The main location for American wounded evacuated from the field was the hospital at Ephrata.[15] However, in the first days after the battle, they were very widely dispersed. Some of the walking wounded made their way to

Philadelphia while others ended up in Reading, Bethlehem, Northampton, Trenton, Burlington, and Wilmington.[16] The experience of Major Joseph Bloomfield of the Third New Jersey Regiment was probably typical:

> 'Thursday 11 [September 1777]
>
> about sunset we made a stand, when I was wounded, having a Ball with the Wad shot through my left forearm & the fuse set my coat and shirt on fire. Soon after this, I left the field & rode about two miles. By the assistance of a stranger dressed my wound with some tow from my Catorich [cartridge] box & wrapped my Arm in my handkerchief. Rode 7 miles further & lodged with in 5 miles of Chester with Mr. Periam, my Arm swelling and being Very painful all this time.'

Unable to walk due to blood loss, Bloomfield was carried across the Delaware to Trenton where his wound was properly dressed for the first time by Dr Bodo Otto. This was fifty-three hours after the injury. Two sinuses formed between the elbow and the wrist, and he became feverish. He was 'much alarmed' but made a good recovery over the following three weeks.[17]

Townsend saw the British surgeons preferentially treating senior officers and the same prioritisation prevailed in the Continental Army. The nineteen-year-old Marquis de Lafayette was a volunteer general with Washington's forces at Brandywine. Having dismounted to rally the troops, he received a rifle bullet through the calf (or possibly thigh) of his left leg. With blood pouring from the top of his boot, he was forced to the rear where he was met by John Cochran, the future director general. Cochran applied a temporary bandage and then further managed the wound at Chester Creek during the retreat. He may then have accompanied the young Frenchman to the general hospital at Bethlehem. Lafayette recovered although he was still limping a month later.[18]

The most seriously wounded rebel soldiers were left on the field and became the responsibility of the victorious British. On the 14th, Howe ordered a surgeon's mate from the 42nd Regiment to attend to wounded Americans at the Birmingham Meeting House.[19] Others were collected and taken to Wilmington. Howe and Washington had reached an agreement that American doctors should be sent across to tend their wounded. Benjamin Rush and six of his medical colleagues made the humanitarian visit to Wilmington, arriving three days after the battle.[20] The British were taken aback by the talkative Rush, who was very ready to espouse the rebel cause even when behind enemy lines. Rush was moved when British officers thanked him for the care he had given to their comrades who had been left in American hands after the Battle of Princeton.[21]

On 20 September, Colonel Charles Grey made a surprise night attack on Anthony Waynes' rebel division which was camped near Paoli Tavern. Grey ordered the use of the bayonet and American losses were staggering, close to 400 men. The affair was later to be portrayed as either a one-sided battle or a massacre.[22] There were accounts of British atrocities. London-born William Hutchinson of the Second Delaware Regiment described a rebel being repeatedly bayoneted on the ground by a group of soldiers. He survived as none of the forty-six stab wounds had affected vital organs.[23] From a British perspective, Paoli was an unqualified success, Howe congratulating his men for 'their steddiness in Bayonitting the Rebels without firing a shot'. The victors sent a flag of truce to Washington to allow the Americans to bury their dead and to provide surgeons.[24] The wounded were first cared for at Ship's Tavern in Chester County and then taken to Lancaster.[25]

The final major battle of the Philadelphia Campaign was at Germantown on 4 October. Washington took the initiative but his four-pronged assault proved to be overambitious. The British were surprised and shaken but soon recovered and pushed back the less experienced Continentals before driving them from the field. The Americans lost around 1,200 men while Howe's losses were approximately 500.[26]

Anecdotal evidence suggests that the evacuation of British casualties from the front was typically opportunistic. Able-bodied combatants carried their injured comrades to the rear as best they could. Lieutenant Richard St George Mansergh was wounded in the head and was taken to safety by Corporal George Peacock of the 52nd. The officer subsequently gave Peacock the enormous sum of fifty guineas and recommended him to a fellow officer in the corporal's new regiment.[27]

Local Jacob Miller witnessed British surgeons at work after the battle:

> 'observed a gathering at his next door neighbor's, the Mechlin's house on the Germantown Road, and entering, there found a British hospital had been improvised in the large stable in the yard. The

surgeons were beginning to arrange long tables, made of doors, on
which to lay the wounded, friends and foes alike, for amputation.'

Like Joseph Townsend at Brandywine, Miller was asked to help but he
managed to escape as he 'did not like the employment'.[28] There was also a
British field hospital in the house of the Wyck family. The good relationship
between the two medical departments was maintained at Germantown, the
British surgeons being assisted by surgeons from the nearby Medical College
of Philadelphia.[29]

British wounded were taken to both Germantown and Philadelphia in
wagons. On the day after the battle, four brigades were ordered to send a
surgeon to Philadelphia to attend the sick and wounded in the general
hospital.[30]

As was the case at Brandywine, the American wounded were widely
scattered after Germantown. A large number were evacuated on foot, on
horseback, and in wagons to the churches at Evansburg and Trappe while
others were accommodated on the retreat at Pennypacker's Mill and Skippack.
Seventy wounded were first taken to Falkner's Swamp and were eventually
moved to Reading, their wounds in a bad condition.[31]

When the Hessian soldier Johann Ewald entered Philadelphia on 5 October,
he saw British and German wounded lying on straw 'almost without any
care'. There was a shortage of medicines and bandages both of which had
first been requisitioned locally and were now awaited from the fleet.[32] A week
earlier, Howe had directed that all the sick be sent to the hospitals in the
city, accompanied by hospital surgeons and mates. A woman from each corps
was also to attend the sick. On 21 October, a general order stipulated that
regimental surgeons and mates working in the general hospital could return
to their own units, suggesting that there was no senior perception of a shortage
of army doctors in the city at this time.[33] At the end of the year, there were
1,000 sick in the wards.[34] The sick rates in the British forces in Philadelphia
had fallen from almost 15 per cent in October to 10 per cent in December.[35]

The period after the battles of Brandywine and Germantown was a perfect
storm for the American general hospitals in Pennsylvania, New Jersey, and
Maryland. In Richard Blanco's words:

'Due to the fluid nature of the campaign, the large number of
casualties, and the lack of sanctuaries for the sick and wounded,

preparations for their reception were disastrous. Never before had Pennsylvania been confronted by such masses of helpless men, nor did the state possess the quarters to house them. The British held Philadelphia and its large buildings, the Continentals were severed from many routes to the Delaware, which complicated not the housing but supply problems, and the province had few areas where casualties could be properly quartered.'[36]

Shippen was forced to reopen the hospital at Bethlehem; 'It gives me great pain to be obliged by order of Congress to send my sick and wounded soldiers to your peaceful village'.[37] The Brethren's House was soon crammed, and the wounded spilt over into tents and barns. By October, there were 500 patients in the village, a number that was to increase to 700 by December. The exhausted medical staff struggled to keep proper records of admissions.[38]

Elsewhere in Pennsylvania, hospitals were established at Reading, Lititz, Ephrata, Easton, Mannheim, Lancaster, Allentown, Rheimstown, Sheaferstown and Buckingham. Churches, barns, taverns, schoolhouses, and private homes were pressed into use.[39] In New Jersey, the hospital at Princeton was large enough for 150 men but now held 400.[40]

Numerous eyewitnesses confirm the appalling conditions in these hospitals and their environs. Sick and wounded often travelled in freezing conditions only to be denied any proper treatment. When Private Elijah Fisher of the 4th Massachusetts Regiment arrived at Reading there was no space, so he was sent on to Ephrata. Here, on Christmas Eve, a local resident saw troops arriving 'in open wagons at nighttime, almost naked, many of them without shoes, stockings or blankets to cover them'. They were dumped there by the wagon drivers, left with no nurses or other attendants. In Pennsylvania alone, there were perhaps 3,000 invalids in the hospitals and 2,000 more spread around the state.[41] Shippen appealed to Congress in late October for supplies of clothes. The hospitals, he admitted, 'were begin[ning] to feel the effects of cold and dirt'.[42]

There was no doubt that the American general hospitals were as much the problem as the solution. Rush estimated that nine out of ten soldiers who died of disease contracted the fever in a hospital.[43] With men packed together and their filthy clothes swarming with vermin, an epidemic of 'camp diseases' was inevitable. Dysentery was prevalent but the greatest threat was typhus. James Tilton noted that relatively healthy soldiers were admitted with minor disorders and soon succumbed to a 'hospital fever'.[44] Doctors and other hospital staff were not spared. Tilton was a prescribing surgeon at Princeton:

> 'The sick and wounded, flowing promiscuously without restraint into the hospital, it soon became infectious and was attended with great mortality. I caught the jail fever [typhus] myself and narrowly escaped with my life. After a tedious illness, I got leave to return home for the recovery of my health. The enemy occupying Philadelphia, at that time, it became necessary for me to take a circuitous route to the state of Delaware, through Bethlehem in Pennsylvania. At Bethlehem was another hospital and I found it convenient to rest there a day or two. During my stay, it was natural to enquire into the state of their hospital. The method I took was to propose a competition, not whose hospital had done the most good, but whose hospital had done the most mischief. I was required to give an account of Princeton hospital; I stated with all the exaggeration I could with truth, not only an affecting mortality among the sick and wounded soldiers, but that the orderly men, nurses and other attendants on the hospital were liable to the infection; that I had myself narrowly escaped death, and that five other surgeons and mates had afterwards been seized. I was answered that the malignancy and mortality of Princeton hospital bore no comparison with theirs; that at Bethlehem not an orderly man or nurse escaped, and but few of the surgeons.'

Tilton was informed that out of forty men of a Virginia volunteer regiment admitted to Bethlehem, it was expected that only three would recover sufficiently to rejoin their unit.[45] Soldiers fled the hospital at Lititz to escape disease but were driven back by snowstorms.[46] Typhus had also broken out in the American prisoners in Philadelphia. Death was so frequent 'it ceased to alarm survivors'. In three months, 400 men were interred without coffins in a mass grave.[47]

Sick rates and mortality levels in the rebel army in late 1777 are difficult to compute. Formal record-keeping was difficult or non-existent. It is likely that the extant figures underestimate the ravages of disease and wounding. Rush notes that 'many hundreds' of fatalities were buried every week in the villages of Pennsylvania and New Jersey.[48] Some of these will have been civilians. A detailed return dated late November for thirteen American general hospitals, mostly in Pennsylvania, shows totals of 1,272 sick, 284 wounded and 601 convalescents. This excludes patients in regimental and brigade hospitals.[49] Seventeen percent of the Continental Army was listed sick in October and 25 per cent in November.[50]

Washington took his men into winter quarters at Valley Forge in mid-December. The site was twenty miles from Philadelphia in populous Chester County. It was not as barren as it is often portrayed but it proved to be near impossible to feed, shelter, and clothe an army in winter.[51] The hardships experienced by the rebel soldiers are well described in the diary of Surgeon Albigence Waldo of the Continental Line:

> 'December 14 1777: The army which has been surprisingly healthy hereto, now begins to grow sickly from the continued fatigues they have suffered this Campaign. Yet they still show a spirit of Alacrity & Contentment not to be expected from so young troops. I am Sick – discontented – and out of humour. Poor food – hard lodging – Cold weather – fatigue – Nasty Cloaths – nasty cookery – Vomit half my time – smoak'd out of my senses – the Devils in't – I can't Endure it – Why are we sent here to starve and Freeze – what sweet Felicities have I left at home! A charming Wife – pretty Children – Good Beds – good food – good Cookery – all agreeable – all harmonious. Here all Confusion – smoke & Cold – hunger and filthiness – A pox on my bad luck.'[52]

Conditions in the hospitals remained so poor that General Wayne admitted that he would rather fight the British at long odds than inspect them. In addition to the normal regimental hospitals in the encampment, Washington, and Cochran, at this time the chief surgeon of the flying camp, arranged two flying hospitals for each brigade. Special diets were given to the sick whenever this was possible.[53]

A return of 23 December shows 2,898 men sick or unfit for duty on account of a lack of clothing.[54] Sick rates at the end of the year exceeded 30 per cent. It is claimed that 2,200 soldiers died at Valley Forge, but archaeological excavations have revealed no mass graves.[55] Waldo noted on 25 December that 'very few of the sick men die'.[56] A typhus-typhoid type of fever and dysentery were still sapping the army's strength. Other afflictions at Valley Forge included cold exposure, malnutrition, scurvy, scabies, venereal disease, and smallpox.

The troops were ordered to build huts but on Christmas Day most of them were still in tents.[57] Many were without blankets, shoes, and stockings; 'it was not uncommon to trace the march of the men over ice and frozen ground, by the blood from their naked feet'.[58] Amputations of feet and legs were performed for frostbite.[59] Food shortages were acute. The normal ration was a 'fire-cake' fashioned from flour and water and cooked over the fire. An order for two barrels of lime-juice suggests an outbreak of scurvy due to the lack of fresh provisions.[60]

Scabies ('Itch') was a predictable blight wherever debilitated men were forced together in the cold. It was soon 'rampant'. Those affected were sent to special huts and treated with sulphur in 'hog's lard'.[61] Venereal disease was, as usual, present but under-reported. Regulations contributed to its concealment, a fine of ten dollars payable by every officer and four dollars by every soldier sent to hospital to be cured of the disorder. Sufferers often preferred covert mercurial treatment obtained from compliant doctors.[62]

The oldest enemy of the Continental Army had made a reappearance. Washington was dismayed to discover that many of the recruits at Valley Forge had not been inoculated against smallpox. Three to four thousand men remained vulnerable to the infection and cases started to surge. In the early days of 1778, the commander ordered a fresh round of inoculations while making every effort to hide this from the enemy.[63]

During the winter and early spring, Washington also encouraged more general improvements in military hygiene in the face of persisting unsanitary practices. The freezing conditions made it difficult to enforce regulations relating to the digging and use of latrines. Dead horses littered the camp. Washington issued stern warnings.

> 'much filth and nastiness, is spread among ye Hutts, which will soon be reduced to a state of putrefaction and cause a sickly camp.'

He gave these orders, he explained, 'out of tender regard' for the lives and health of his brave soldiery and he expressed surprise that previous similar directives had not been implemented. He was eventually forced to order that all men found not using the latrines be arrested and immediately given five lashes.[64]

The poor morale in the wider army – there were numerous resignations of line officers – was shared by the regimental surgeons. Many doctors simply disappeared from Valley Forge.[65] When Albigence Waldo requested leave on the last day of 1777, he received a conciliatory letter from John Cochran.

'We shall soon have regimental Hospitals erected, and general Ones to receive the Superabundant Sick from them; if you will tarry till such regulations are made, you will have an honourable furlow; and even now, I will, if you desire it — recommend you to his Excellency [Washington] for one, but desire you would stay a little while longer, and in the meantime recommend to me some young Surgeon for a Regiment and I will immediately appoint him to a chief Surgeoncy from your recommendation. I shall still remember the rascals who have us'd me ill.'[66]

Chapter 10

Monmouth

January 1778–December 1779

We buried 245 of their dead on the field of Action – they buried several themselves... the amount of their wounded we have not learnt with any certainty; according to the common proposition of four or five to one, their [sic] should be at least a thousand or 1200.
Washington on the British losses at the Battle of Monmouth

Washington remodelled his army in the winter of 1777–78. Conscription was introduced and there were changes to promotion, pay and pensions. It was hoped that these steps would remove 'uneasiness, discord, and perplexity'.[1] Washington was much helped by the Prussian mercenary soldier Baron von Steuben. Although he was very likely not the aristocrat he claimed to be, Steuben proved effective in training and disciplining the raw rebel troops. The German also took a keen interest in their wellbeing; 'There is nothing which gains an officer the love of his soldiers more than his care of them, under the distress of sickness'.[2]

There were only limited changes in the administration of the Continental Army's medical department during this period. In February 1778, Shippen was divested of responsibility for commissary functions and Jonathan Potts was appointed to the role of purveyor general and deputy director of the Middle Department.[3] Potts was highly rated by Washington and there was an immediate improvement in the supply of hospital drugs and other essentials. By mid-April, it was possible to fill the regimental medical chests. There was also improved documentation of stores and more accurate registration of the sick.[4]

These records showed the stubborn persistence of diseases in the Valley Forge encampment in the spring of 1778. There were 3,800 men in the regimental and flying hospitals in April and May. When Washington left his winter quarters in mid-June, 2,800 sick were still at Valley Forge and another 1,200 in the general hospitals.[5]

The British garrisons of New York and Philadelphia also suffered from disease. Military returns between January and May 1778 show sick rates of 12 to 14 per cent in the two cities. Some regiments had more than 20 per cent of their men incapacitated. Other units, notably the Guards, were relatively spared. Tabitha Marshall, in her forensic analysis of the health of the British soldier during the War, suggests that sickness may have resulted from falling standards of hygiene. In April, the commander in New York noted that rubbish and waste had not been cleared from the streets. The combination of dirt and overcrowding led to outbreaks of dysentery and fever, the latter probably typhus. Records from the general hospital at Philadelphia confirm the presence of 'flux', 'fever' and 'fever and flux'. These afflictions accounted for close to 80 per cent of the deaths between January and April.[6]

More surprisingly, there were also relatively high rates of sickness in the British troops in Canada. Between January and May 1778, these varied between 8 and 11 per cent. The troops affected at Sorrel, Chambly and St Genevieve were all detachments that last served with Burgoyne in the summer of 1777. They may have contained groups of men left behind and evacuated there due to infirmity.[7]

Washington feared a British attack on Valley Forge, but this was never likely. Howe still had the carnage of Bunker Hill in his mind, and he was reluctant to attack a well-entrenched position. American morale was boosted at the start of May with the arrival of news of a treaty with France. A few days later, the cautious Howe was replaced by Sir Henry Clinton. The new British commander had orders to campaign in the South in the autumn and the dispersal of his forces made the abandonment of Philadelphia inevitable. Ships were needed to carry off the loyalists of the city and Clinton and his army set out on a march of a hundred miles to New York. After a period of irresolution, Washington opted to attack Clinton's rear-guard, and the two sides clashed on the ground around Monmouth Court House on 28 June 1778.[8]

The bloody and inconclusive Battle of Monmouth (now Freehold Township in New Jersey) is remembered for the greatest artillery barrage of the War and the acrimony between Washington and his eccentric second-in-command, Charles Lee. Clinton could claim that he had beaten off the attack and was able to resume his march to New York which he reached on 5 July. Washington emphasised and possibly exaggerated the scale of enemy losses; the British had around 500 casualties compared to the Americans' 360.[9]

Monmouth was fought in a furnace. It was an exceptionally hot summer's day, around 96 degrees Fahrenheit (35 degrees Celsius). Lafayette saw soldiers fall dead without being touched.[10] John Peebles of the Black Watch also witnessed the effects of exertion and extreme heat; 'a great number of the several Corps died upon the Spot'.[11] Perhaps sixty of the British casualties were caused by sunstroke.[12] Washington acknowledges some heat-related deaths among his men but the rebels were probably partially protected by their flimsier dress and their habit of discarding their packs.[13] Surgeon Johann David Schoepff of the Ansbach-Bayreuth troops believed the Germans to be the most vulnerable.

> 'enveloped as our men are in heavy woollen garments and tight leggings, and carrying the entire weight of a gun, sixty cartridges, knapsack, and rations, they cannot but suffer doubly from all the discomforts of such [hot] days. The English, who are more used to fighting in warm countries, provide their troops with a lighter clothing, adapted to the climate.'[14]

At Monmouth, the effects of the heat were exacerbated by a shortage of water after the battle. According to Private Greenman, it was almost as scarce as liquor '& what is got is very bad indeed'.[15]

The best narrative of the management of the British wounded at Monmouth is by an American doctor. Philadelphia educated William Read arrived while the battle was raging, his intention being to join the Continental Army as a soldier. As the fighting petered out, he entered the field with his servant. The following account is taken from his papers.

> 'At the summit of the hill, dismal indeed was the scene; there lay fifty or sixty British grenadiers – some dead, some alive, calling for "help", "water", uttering the most dreadful and severe imprecations on the "the rebels". Dr Read and his servant ran down the hill and found plenty of water; with his servant's hat, he administered many draughts of water to these poor, famished soldiers; it was busy occupation for an hour. Dr Read now found himself embarked in the business in a most remarkable manner; he proceeded to dress

wounds and apply bandages. Tearing off shirts from the dead, he made bandages, and applied them, to the best of his skill, for remedying haemorrhage.'

Read enlisted some locals to get the wounded on to wagons and to take them to Monmouth Court House. Twenty-one British soldiers with broken bones and lacerated muscles were transferred. Still receiving no other medical assistance, Read performed several amputations. He was eventually relieved by two British surgeons four days after the battle. When he explained his medical interventions, they coolly informed him that he 'had only given so many subjects to the Chelsea Hospital'. Read at least had the satisfaction of an appointment in Washington's medical department.[16]

Some British wounded were carried along with Clinton's army, but others were necessarily left behind in houses around the field.[17] This was in part due to a shortage of wagons.[18] Peebles says that most of these men were in Monmouth and that those too ill to be moved were left 'with a Surgeon & flag'.[19]

On the American side, Private Joseph Plumb Martin went off in search of water. His account well illustrates the lottery that was casualty evacuation in the battles of the Revolution.

'I found the wounded [American] captain... lying on the ground and begging his sergeant, who pretended to have the care of him, to help him off the field or he should bleed to death. The sergeant and a man or two he had with him were taken up in hunting after plunder. It grieved me to see the poor man in such distress and I asked the sergeant why he did not carry his officer to the surgeons. He said he would directly. "Directly!" said I, "why he will die directly". I then offered to assist them in carrying him to a meetinghouse [the Old Tennent Church] a short distance off, where the rest of the wounded men and the surgeons were. At length he condescended to be persuaded to carry him off. I helped him to the place, and tarried a few minutes to see the wounded and two or three limbs amputated.'[20]

John Cochran made the American medical arrangements for the battle. He was instructed to seek assistance from the quarter master and the adjutant general.[21] The American casualties were treated in the Court House and two local churches, including that of St Peters. Every room in the Court House was filled, the wounded lying on straw on the floor. Two hundred soldiers were detached to bury the dead.[22]

Monmouth was the last large-scale battle of the War in the North. Washington remained cautious, awaiting substantial French help. There were, however, some smaller campaigns fought between the summer of 1778 and autumn 1779 which will now be reviewed with reference to the medical arrangements.

In August 1778, the Americans and French agreed to attack the British garrison of Newport on Rhode Island. There was little coordination between Admiral d'Estaing's French fleet and the rebel land forces and the short siege had to be abandoned. The Americans had sustained fewer casualties than their enemy – 200 to around 300 – but the British remained in control of Newport and there was sniping between the new allies.[23]

The care of the Continental Army's wounded was entrusted to Dr Thomas Tillotson of the staff of the Northern Department. He was supplied with medicines and instruments 'necessary in the formation of a military and flying hospital'.[24] The Newport Campaign gives a first view of the French medical services. Soon after the arrival of d'Estaing's fleet, a hospital was established which is referred to as the *Hôpital de Rhode Island*. Subsequently, two more hospitals were opened near to Providence. The main role of these facilities was to care for cases of scurvy put ashore from the fleet. The sick were tended to by the ships' surgeons and assistant surgeons. When d'Estaing withdrew, the hospitals' patients were removed to Boston.[25]

Towards the end of the year, the British launched their 'Southern Strategy' with an expedition sent to seize Georgia. The American resistance at Savannah was tactically naive and there was a rout. The attackers suffered only a handful of casualties while three-quarters of the defenders fell into the hands of the enemy.[26] The British medical provision for the expedition included the American-born surgeons and assistant surgeons of the four loyalist regiments.[27]

In autumn 1779, the Americans captured the vulnerable British fort at Stony Point. It was a bloody encounter with brutal hand-to-hand fighting. The Continentals lost around a hundred men – including seventeen of the twenty in the forlorn hope – and the British sustained close to 700 losses, the total of killed, wounded, and captured. This was followed by another sharp raid on the British post at Paulus Hook.[28] These American successes contrasted with the abject failure of the rebels' largest amphibious expedition of the War at Penobscot Bay.[29]

We have limited details of the medical support for these operations. There is more information available for the Sullivan Expedition of August and September 1779. This was a short punitive campaign fought by General John Sullivan against loyalist and Iroquois forces in New York and Pennsylvania. Sullivan's troops met little real opposition. The general had been charged with the destruction of the Indian lands and he reported that his men had 'left not a single settlement or field of corn'.[30]

Despite its one-sided nature, the Sullivan Expedition is a good illustration of the functioning of the Continental Army's medical department on campaign. At the outset, general hospitals were opened at Easton and Sunbury. Sick men, mostly suffering from malaria and dysentery, were left on the wards. Sullivan, also ill, marched north. At Wyoming, the regimental surgeons were instructed to report to the 'senior surgeon to the flying hospital' and another general hospital was established. The senior surgeon with the force was ordered to remain by Sullivan's side, while the surgeons and mates of the flying hospital were to march at the rear of the force, and the regimental surgeons were to remain at the rear of their respective brigades or regiments. After fighting near the village of Newtown, casualties were sent back by water to the newly constructed Fort Sullivan at Tioga. On the return of the expeditionary force, the sick and wounded were evacuated by water to Wyoming, before being taken to Easton.[31]

We have a further insight into the organisation of the French medical services at Savannah in October 1779. The combined American-French assault was courageous but it was their own 'Bunker Hill', the doughty British garrison losing only seventy-five men while the allies suffered very heavy casualties.[32] According to Maurice Bouvet, in his *Le Service de Santé Français pendant la Guerre d'Indépendance des États-Unis*, the French losses alone were probably 150 killed and 400 wounded. D'Estaing received gunshot wounds in the arm and the leg. The French casualties were immediately taken to a hospital at the landing site of Thunderbolt Bluff around five miles from Savannah. Here, they were managed by the surgeons who had disembarked from the French fleet. As for the British and Americans, some French soldiers had prolonged complications from their wounds. Two years later, *Chef d'Escadre* Barras asked for help from the minister for one of his brave lieutenants injured in the action.

'[He] has the most pressing need to recover his health; he has a badly paralysed right arm, which he sustained at the landing at Savannah, where he was five days and nights in a boat, his body soaked with rain; he is obliged to go to Montpellier to seek treatment; from there he will go to take the waters.'[33]

The Continental Army was in winter quarters at Middlebrook in 1778–79 and at Morristown in 1779–80. There was a delay in building huts at Middlebrook camp so that the soldiers lived much of the winter in tents. Surgeon Thacher complains of exposure to cold and storms, but conditions were better than at Valley Forge and there was even time for medical education.[34] All regimental medical officers were desired to attend a course of lectures on 'physick', anatomy and surgery given by the physician general William Brown.[35]

The Morristown winter was the most severe for at least twenty years. Veterans agreed that nothing could compare with its 'cruelties'.[36] Snow fell early, the rivers froze over, and an icy wind blew from the north. The four to six feet of snow made transportation difficult and there were food and clothing shortages.[37] Thacher lay on the frozen ground, wrapped in a greatcoat with his feet to the fire. The soldiers, he explains, were so enfeebled by hunger and cold that they struggled to construct their huts or perform military duties.[38]

Director General Shippen had an increasingly antagonistic relationship with Congress and his influence was waning. When he submitted his budget for 1779, Congress halved the amount.[39] There was continued confusion in the wider American medical administration. For instance, the boundary between the Middle and Eastern Departments was poorly defined, leading to arguments between physicians regarding authority over hospitals.[40] Much of the American medical service in the South, to which our gaze must increasingly turn, was autonomous. Before March 1781, only Virginia was part of the Hospital Department and even this was contested.[41] The separation impeded the movement of medical officers from one department to another. In the summer of 1779, Cochran sent a few surgeons south following a direct order from Washington.[42]

The Continental Army's hospitals were in the usual state of flux. During the summer of 1778, as Washington moved north, general facilities were open at Trenton, Princeton, and Springfield. As several older units in Pennsylvania and New Jersey were closed, new hospitals were established to meet the demands of the army's operations, including the Sullivan Expedition. During the Morristown winter encampment, there were general hospitals at Basking Ridge and Pluckemin. A third hospital was later created in the Morristown huts.[43] A return for December 1779, very likely incomplete, shows a total of 911 sick in eleven general hospitals.[44]

It was at Basking Ridge that Dr James Tilton ordered the construction of his famed experimental hospitals. These log buildings were based on Indian huts. They had a central ward for twelve 'febrile' patients and two side wards each for eight patients who were wounded or who had 'topical affections'. Great emphasis was given to warmth and ventilation. Any residual smoke from the fire was thought to combat infection. Tilton was satisfied with his efforts, there being little spread of infection in the huts.[45] He may have been too pleased with his success, making him 'even more conceited and quite contemptuous of authority'.[46] Perhaps because of this, there is little evidence that his hospital design was replicated.

Average conditions in the American general hospitals probably improved in 1778 and 1779. A visiting chaplain, the Reverend Dr James Sproat, made inspections of the hospitals and kept notes in his journal. His observations suggest much good practice; the 'medical gentlemen' taking care of the sick in well ventilated and provisioned hospitals.[47] No doubt this proficiency was not universal. In 1779, a physician complained that in the Northern and Eastern Departments 'everything is carried on, as in the beginning, with wild anarchy and uproar'.[48] Local help remained vital. Sympathetic farmers carried the sick between hospitals in their wagons and supplied food, straw, and clothing.[49]

Despite Potts' best efforts, the deficiency of medical supplies remained a cause of concern. At Morristown, the shortages were the worst since early 1778, exacerbated by inadequate funds, uncoordinated procurement, and Congressional apathy. Cochran exonerated Potts from blame, but his frustration is obvious; 'it grieves me to see the poor worthy fellows passing away from the lack of a few comforts'. Washington raised the matter with Congress which passed the responsibility on to a vacillating Medical Committee.[50]

Disease rates in the Continental Army in the second half of 1778 and 1779 were lower than earlier in the War. After Monmouth, the incidence of sickness in Washington's forces fell from 21 per cent in July to 16 per cent in November and December. Average rates at Middlebrook were around 15 per cent and this dropped to 9 per cent in May 1779. Even the harsh conditions at Morristown were surprisingly well tolerated. In February 1780, only 3 per cent of the 11,500 men were sick enough to require hospitalisation and overall sick rates were 10–11 per cent.[51] There is no single explanation for this improvement in health. Factors probably included a higher proportion of seasoned troops, prioritisation of discipline and sanitation, and large-scale inoculation.[52]

Smallpox was significantly reduced in incidence at this time.[53] The diseases which most afflicted the troops were predictable. Records for the general hospital at Sunbury show that in September 1779 the commonest diagnosis was 'bilious fever' followed by dysentery and diarrhoea. Disorders less often leading to hospital admission included venereal disease, rheumatism and ophthalmia.[54]

A document dated 6 December 1778 gives the strength of the British Army's hospital staff at Rhode Island and New York: five physicians (including inspector and purveyor); thirteen surgeons (including chief, field inspectors and deputy purveyors); eight apothecaries (including field inspectors and deputy purveyors); thirty-nine established mates; thirty-two supernumerary mates; eleven clerks; two chaplains; one cutler.

In addition to these 111 posts, there was a physician, eight surgeons, three apothecaries, a chaplain, and an unknown number of mates in Canada.[55] In the summer of 1779, Nooth had fifty-eight staff officers at his disposal in New York. Extensive hospital supplies had arrived in the city in March. These included tents for hospital use where there were no suitable buildings.[56]

In August 1778, 13 per cent of the British troops in New York were ill.[57] Surgeon Robert Jackson had recently arrived with the 71st Regiment and he describes intermittent fevers and an epidemic form of dysentery. The latter disorder was stubborn and unpleasant, often lasting for two weeks, but Jackson could not recollect any deaths. Peruvian bark proved useful in the treatment of fevers, suggesting that these were mainly malarial in origin.[58] Malaria was also prevalent in Canada, the senior medical officer at Montreal, Hugh Kennedy, remarking that officers and soldiers admitted to the hospital 'have been visited by the universal complaint, the Ague'. The sick rate in Halifax was twice that of the remainder of Canada (16 vs 8 per cent) for reasons that are unclear. It may be that the men were poorly accommodated.[59]

The Hessian soldiers experienced the same diseases as the British while being more vulnerable to scurvy. Half of the Anspach-Bayreuth troops at Newport in 1778 were sick with the disorder and many died. In the following year, the Seyboth Regiment on Rhode Island was said to have suffered more from scurvy than any other unit. Some remedies were extreme, as is related by a German eyewitness on Long Island; 'During our sojourn at this place,

I often saw people buried up to their necks in the earth; for in this manner they cure the scurvy'.[60]

The most severe epidemic of disease in the British Army in the North struck at New York in August 1779. This was very likely a lethal mix of typhus, malaria, and dysentery. Armies were especially vulnerable to combinations of infectious diseases. The New York epidemic of 1779 has many similarities to the 'Walcheren fever' which was to decimate another British force thirty years later.

Captain John Peebles' detailed journal gives useful clues as to the underlying disorders, particularly supporting the presence of malaria and dysentery.

'Tuesday 31st [August 1779]: The Men growing very sickly within these few days, a general complaint over the whole army, they are mostly taken with a headache & universal pain, a chill & feverishness, which for the most part turns into a quotidien or tertian intermittent, & some few are taken with the flux.'

Elsewhere, Peebles describes the 'ague' and a bilious continued fever.[61]

A board of army doctors reported 'Intermittent, Bilious Fever, & Dysenteries'. They believed heavy rain to have played a role and they also implicated troops recently arrived in the city who had brought a contagious fever with them.[62] This convoy from England had reached New York at the end of August. Of the 3,868 rank and file on board, 795 men were sick with a 'malignant jail fever'. According to General Clinton, this affliction, almost certainly typhus, soon spread through the army, sending 6,000 of his best troops to hospital.[63]

The sick rate in the New York garrison was 21 per cent in September and 26 per cent in October. Individual regiments suffered terribly. In mid-October, 63 per cent of the men of the 54th Foot were listed as sick.[64] These were not the relatively benign disorders of the previous year. The 54th, 89th and 37th regiments had sixty-six, fifty, and thirty-five deaths. Sick rates were lower in the Guards despite them being described by a resident as being 'constantly drunk'.[65] The locals were not spared, many who lived in Manhattan and on Long Island falling ill.

The army's medical department was reasonably well staffed and supplied but it was soon under considerable strain. On the first day of September, Peebles saw 120 sick men loaded into two barns, 'only one Surg[eo]n to attend them, no nurses or utensils'. A month later, the number of patients was still increasing and there was only one hospital mate to attend to '130 or 40 sick'.[66] Medicines became scarce, forcing the appropriation of supplies intended for the West Indies.[67] A large ship was converted to serve as another convalescent hospital.[68] By November, there was a reduction in the numbers of sick but the recovery from the epidemic was slow with many relapses. In December, 18 per cent of the army was still listed as sick.[69]

Disease was also stalking British soldiers in the South. In July 1779, General Augustine Prevost wrote to Clinton from Savannah, explaining that a combination of sickness and heat had put an end to active operations.[70] Robert Jackson had sailed south with his regiment to Ebenezer in Georgia, and he has left a detailed description of malaria.

> 'the intermitting fever soon made its appearance, and spread so rapidly, that before the end of June [1779] very few remained, not only in the regiment, but also in the garrison [at Savannah] who had not suffered more or less from this raging disease... the type of fever was most usually double tertian or quotidian [daily] from its very commencement in the month of June.'

The paroxysms of fever were like a 'cold fit' and Jackson notes that they were interrupted by the administration of Peruvian bark. If not properly treated, then malaria was often complicated by the onset of dysentery.[71]

Sick rates at Savannah were probably even greater than in New York. Cantlie quotes a figure of 1,500 British sick out of the 3,700 strong garrison during the siege in October 1779.[72] This was a timely reminder of the dangers of campaigning in the South. The British would now be fighting a war in a region described by a medical officer as 'a Country full of Marshes & small Rivers, Woods and Insects, and a Sun so powerful in heat'.[73]

Chapter 11

Charleston and Camden

January 1780–December 1780

The life of a soldier in its best state is subject to innumerable hardships, but where they are aggravated by a want of provision and clothing his condition becomes intolerable, nor can men long contend with such complicated difficulties and distress — deaths, desertion, and the hospital must soon swallow up an army.

Nathanael Greene to Thomas Jefferson, 6 December 1780

Except for ongoing Indian conflicts, the Southern states were mostly spared the miseries of war in the first four years of the Revolution. This suddenly changed when Henry Clinton left New York in December 1779 to seize the South Carolina port of Charleston. In the greatest American reverse of the War, the city fell to the expeditionary force in May 1780. Clinton returned to New York to be replaced by Lieutenant General Charles Earl Cornwallis. The Carolinas now erupted in a brutal civil war in which backcountry patriots fought rejuvenated loyalists (often referred to as 'Tories'). The ruthless loyalist dragoons of Lieutenant Colonel Banastre Tarleton slaughtered Continental troops at Waxhaws in late May. In the major battle of the year, the American general Horatio Gates was decisively defeated by Cornwallis at Camden in August. The civil war raged on, much of it guerrilla in nature, and the merciless frontiersmen gained their revenge over the Tories at King's Mountain in October in a battle where the loyalist leader, Scotsman Patrick Ferguson, was the only non-American on the field. In the North, Washington, while underestimating the venom and significance of the Southern theatre, was waiting for French assistance in a potential strike against New York. At the end of 1780, he was forced to admit that the great revolution 'hung in the balance'.[1]

John Mervin Nooth, superintendent general of hospitals for the forces in North America, was responsible for the British medical arrangements in the South. He anticipated that the Anglo-German army of 8,000 men would require five hospital ships and he recommended a British hospital staff of a physician, three surgeons, eight mates and a deputy purveyor and clerks. The German contingent was to be similarly provided. This was all based on an assumption that during the Southern Campaign 4–5,000 men would need treatment for disease or wounding.

Nooth was an awkward individual, quick to make enemies. He intended to stay in New York and thus delegated some of the planning to physician Charles Blagden, his immediate subordinate. The two men did not get on and when Blagden was informed that he was to serve below a hospital surgeon, Alexander Grant, he successfully applied for leave to return to England. Because of these political machinations, the experienced John Macnamara Hayes was appointed physician and director of the hospitals in the South. Unlike Nooth, Hayes had an engaging personality and was popular with senior army officers.

The doctors sent with Clinton from New York were joined by fourteen hospital staff from Georgia. Approximately ninety medical officers served with the British Army at some point in the Southern Campaign. These were almost equally divided between the general hospitals and the regiments. British army doctors were generally preferred but there were loyalist doctors in Cornwallis's force, perhaps as many as half the hospital mates being American. The evidence available suggests that the men who provided the medical care in the South were mostly experienced and competent, albeit young. At the outset of the campaign, half of them had served for three years or more. This was largely a reflection of the duration of the conflict, now entering its sixth year. Paul Kopperman, who has made the most detailed study, concludes that most of the men who attended the troops in 1780 'had a meaningful degree of attachment to the life and duties of an army medical officer'. Some — notably Robert Jackson, Colin Chisholm, Robert Freer, Thompson Forster, and Hayes — would have highly distinguished medical careers.

There were early shortcomings in hospital provision and clumsy communications with the army's wider administration. The hospital ships were soon judged to be too few or too small or inadequately fitted out. In February, Hayes complained that the quarter master general was refusing to arrange quarters for hospital staff. The senior doctor was later forced to accommodate patients on the hospital ships because of the poor care given by some regimental surgeons. However, these were isolated incidents, problems were overcome, and complaints about the service were rare. In mid-March, Hayes declared the hospitals to be 'in the Compleatest Order'.

The pressures of campaigning and the sickliness of the South soon placed severe strain on Hayes's assiduous arrangements. By July, he was reporting a severe shortage of medicines and hospital stores. Personnel were also thin on the ground. Many doctors fell ill. Hayes himself suffered for thirty days with 'a most violent bilious fever'. Nooth was asked to send an apothecary, a surgeon and six mates. The regimental establishment was equally inadequate, this being most obvious at the Battle of Camden. Overall, these shortages were worse in 1780 than in 1781, suggesting a gradual improvement in the medical service in the South. Where local resources were overwhelmed, or the needs of individual cases dictated, then there was the option of sending sick and wounded men back to New York.[2]

When the American medical services were reorganised in the spring of 1777, the entire army was in the Middle and Northern Departments. This explains the autonomy of the provision in the South previously alluded to.[3] Dr William Rickman, director of hospitals in Virginia, was able to rebuff Shippen's attempts to supervise his inoculation programme. The military hospital near Williamsburg was the only State-constructed building of the War. In South Carolina, Dr David Olyphant, the State's director general, insisted that no outside oversight of his hospitals was required and, furthermore, that Southern medical men were best qualified to meet the unique challenges of the region. There was little medical cooperation among the Southern States and medical staff from the North were largely excluded.[4]

Olyphant was charged with improving this organisation by combining resources including the whole of Carolina and Georgia, but his efforts were thwarted by the British capture of Charleston. Nineteen American medical officers were incarcerated in vessels in the harbour.[5] This much disrupted an already fragile service and from the spring of 1780 onwards the medical care of troops south of the Virginia-North Carolina border was haphazard. This was almost entirely in the hands of the regimental and militia surgeons. When Gates arrived in Virginia in June, he had no medical staff, drugs, or equipment. Not even Virginia or North Carolina could give much assistance and it was not until July that Congress approved physicians and surgeons to his command. Both senior doctors and military officers complained of severe shortages and of 'wretched' hospital conditions.[6]

Neither side suffered large numbers of casualties at the siege of Charleston. The defenders lost only 4 per cent of their combatants and the British 2 per cent. However, the imprisonment of 6,700 soldiers and sailors remains one of the greatest capitulations in American military history.[7] The main British general hospital during the siege was located on James Island. There was a second hospital at Charleston Neck and hospital ships were also employed. By 18 May, the James Island Hospital contained 300 men and Hayes requested more staff. Some of the sick were treated in tents. Following the fall of the city, British and Hessian hospitals were promptly relocated. These facilities in Charleston also served the small numbers of loyalist troops and the soldiers' wives.[8]

The South was well known to be unhealthy by both doctors and the local population. In the years before the Revolution, the British naval surgeon James Lind noted that tropical fevers were more common than in the North, more comparable to the West Indies. Residents believed the British would be mad to attack in the sickly summer season.[9]

Following the siege, Charleston was extremely dirty, a situation exacerbated by the carelessness of the soldiers.[10] It was fertile ground for epidemics. Smallpox had returned at the end of 1779 after a hiatus of twenty years. Many of the troops in the American Southern Army were militia who had missed the mass inoculations of the Continental Army. They were reluctant to come to the aid of pestilential Charleston. The pox, they feared, 'would be worse to them than the enemy'. The epidemic worsened after the occupation, many children falling ill and the disease apparently growing in virulence.[11]

In contrast, the British were dismissive of the pox, their susceptible regulars already inoculated. An unplanned delay in Clinton's expedition had the benefit of allowing his army some recovery from the outbreak of disease in New York the previous autumn. Returns during March to May 1780 show sick rates of 15 to 16 per cent. These excluded sick soldiers left in New York.[12] The predominant disorder was very likely malaria. John Peebles, writing at the end of April, describes the men becoming ill with 'the ague or a lax aches and fever or diarrhoea'.[13] Another British officer documents fifty men of his regiment admitted to hospital 'suffering from the southern agues'.[14]

As always, the ordinary soldiers had their opinions as to the causes of disease and the best means of prevention. The British artificers at Charleston complained to the commander of the Royal Artillery that their rum ration had been reduced; 'an Article we humbly conceive to be essentially necessary to the health of Labouring Men in this sultry Climate'. They pointed out that they could not be expected to work twelve hours a day 'on simple Water, which is peculiarly bad in this town'.[15]

Sick rates in Cornwallis's army escalated between the fall of Charleston and the Battle of Camden. By August, 30 per cent of the force was unfit for duty. The commander reported from Camden that the sickness was 'great and truly alarming'.[16]

Some regiments were affected more than others. The 71st Foot was consistently among the worst; on 13 August, 72 per cent of the second battalion was listed as sick.[17] The regiment's surgeon's mate, Robert Jackson, attributed the soldiers' poor health to the location of the campsite on the Great Pee Dee River at Cheraw. Local advice to avoid the place had been ignored. Jackson's description of the men's symptoms is consistent with malaria, possibly with some cases of its more virulent (*falciparum*) form.

> 'In a fortnight or three weeks, the intermitting fever began to shew itself. It spread so rapidly, particularly in the second battalion, that before the end of July, when the post was abandoned, few were left who had not felt its influence. The prevailing symptoms were much similar to those of the fever of Ebenezer. The type was frequently double tertian, or quotidian; the remissions were indistinct; the bilious vomiting and purgings were often excessive, and marks of malignity [probably gangrene] appeared in several instances. The approach of the enemy made it necessary that the post should be withdrawn; but there was much difficulty in accomplishing it. Two thirds of both officers and men were unable to march; and it was not possible, in the situation in which we were placed, to find wagons sufficient to carry them, together with the necessary provisions and baggage; so that no other resource was left, than to convey some part of them to George Town by water.'[18]

St David's Church in Cheraw was used as a regimental hospital. Soldiers of the 71st were buried there and their graves remain identifiable today.

Jackson also refers to dysenteric complaints.[19] Eyewitnesses and historians have suggested the presence of other infectious diseases such as typhus, dengue (breakbone fever) and yellow fever.[20] The latter entity is unlikely as Jackson witnessed the disorder in the Caribbean and he describes nothing similar in the Southern states. Indeed, in his treatise on the fevers of the West Indies, he notes that '[yellow fever] has not, so far as I know, been described by the practitioners of any other country'.[21]

Whatever its precise nature, disease did not spare senior military officers and medical staff. A week after the Battle of Camden, Cornwallis wrote to Clinton:

> 'I am at present so hurried with business with everybody belonging to me sick... The officers are particularly affected; Doctor Hayes and almost all the hospital surgeons are laid up. Every person of my [official] family and every Publick officer of the Army is now incapable of doing duty.'[22]

Thousands of slaves had fled to the British lines to seek their freedom and by July large numbers were perishing of a malignant fever and smallpox.[23]

The defeat of Colonel Abraham Buford's Virginian Continentals by Lieutenant Colonel Banastre Tarleton's loyalist dragoons at Waxhaws at the end of May was one of the most controversial episodes of the War. Buford's men were quickly overwhelmed, and the dragoons fell among them, hacking away with their sabres. The high proportion of American killed to wounded (113 to 150) suggests a massacre. Tarleton later claimed to have been trapped under his horse and it may be that he lost control of his troops rather than having a personal bloodlust.[24] In his account of the action, Tarleton insists that the survivors were well cared for:

> 'The wounded of both parties were collected with all possible dispatch and treated with equal humanity. The American officers and soldiers who were unable to travel, were paroled the next morning, and placed at the neighbouring plantations and in a meeting house, not far from the field of battle: Surgeons were sent for from Camden and Charlotte town to assist them, and every possible convenience was provided by the British.'[25]

Tarleton's memoir of the Southern Campaigns makes unusually frequent references to the care of the wounded, perhaps a deliberate attempt to cast off his reputation as a heartless British commander. In America, he was widely known as 'Bloody Tarleton' and the phrase 'Tarleton's quarter' was used in anger.

Gates and Cornwallis fought the largest battle of 1780 at Camden on 16 August. The American general made the fatal error of arranging his line such that his untested militia were opposed by British and German regulars. The militiamen soon melted away, allowing a flank attack on the remaining Continental Army. Gates had lost more than 20 per cent of his force and his reputation. British losses were 324 of all ranks killed and wounded.[26]

Hayes oversaw the staff of the British flying hospital at Camden.[27] A count of British and loyalist regimental surgeons on the field well illustrates the mismatch between the number of combatants and the number of medical officers on an eighteenth-century battlefield, even for a victorious army. There were three regimental surgeons and three regimental mates to attend to 2,233 officers and men of the British and loyalist units.[28]

After the fighting, Cornwallis's army fell back towards to its original position at Camden. Loyalist militia were ordered to search the woods for wounded and wagons were assembled for their evacuation.[29] Four weeks later, the wounded were sent back to Charleston as is detailed in a letter written by Staff Surgeon West Hill to Cornwallis.

> 'I have the pleasure to inform your Lordship that seventy eight wounded men were embarked yesterday and fell [?] down the River at Eleven o' Clock; the Boats were well covered with tents, and plenty of good straw for them to lay on...the men are very comfortably placed, not crowded, they have two hospital mates to attend them.'

Hill reassured his commander that there was an adequate supply of dressings, medicines, wine, and food.[30]

With the American medical department of the South in disarray and the British preoccupied with the care of their own wounded, it was inevitable that the American wounded at Camden would be inadequately managed. Dr Hugh Williamson of North Carolina and his small team crossed behind enemy lines under a flag. They did their best to treat the 700 wounds of the 250 casualties.

> 'The Enemy was disposed to neglect us, and a [British] victory... did not increase their humanity. For eight or ten days after the Battle our people suffered great neglect... Our militia surgeons disappeared... and Cornwallis ignored us.'[31]

Williamson wrote to Hayes, complaining that the American wounded were crowded into six small wards without straw or coverings and were lacking the most basic supplies; 'nothing is left for us but the painful Circumstance of viewing wretches who must soon perish if not soon relieved'.[32]

The American prisoners of war after Camden joined the soldiers captured at Charleston. Large numbers, especially those in the stinking prison ships, died of diseases such as malaria, dysentery, typhus, and smallpox. The senior American physician Peter Fayssoux was among the doctors captured at Charleston and he was given access to the prison ships there. A few excerpts from his lengthy report give an insight into the miseries endured by the prisoners of war.

> 'After the defeat of General Gates [at Camden] our sufferings commenced. The unhappy men who belonged to the militia and were taken prisoner on Gates' defeat, experienced the first effects of the cruelty of the new system. These men were confined on board of prison ships, in no means proportionate to the size of the vessels; immediately after a march of 120 miles, in the sickly season of this unhappy climate.
>
> The vessels were generally infected with the small-pox, very few of the prisoners had gone through that disorder. A representation was made to the British commandant, and permission was obtained for one of our surgeons to inoculate them. This was the utmost extent of humanity — the wretched objects were still confined on board of the prison ships and fed on salt provisions, without the least medical aid, or any proper kind of nourishment. The effect that naturally followed was a small-pox with a fever of the putrid type [probably typhus]; and to such as survived the small-pox, a putrid dysentery – and from these causes, the deaths of 150 of the unhappy victims.'[33]

Most of the sick brought ashore to the general hospital at Charleston died within two or three days. Conditions on the wards, which were staffed by American doctors, were also very poor, the patients without clothing, coverings, or a proper diet. Fayssoux alleges that his concerns were rejected by Hayes; 'To my astonishment, he replied that the ships were not crowded, perfectly wholesome and no appearance of infections or disorders among the prisoners!' Such a blanket denial of all American claims by such a senior British doctor is jarring and it must be remembered, in fairness to Hayes, that the subject of prisoners of war was a source of propaganda for both sides. It cannot be denied, however, that conditions in the hulks and other British prisons were a significant cause of disease and death. The best estimate is that close to half of the 18,000 American prisoners taken during the War died in captivity. The unfortunate captives at Charleston did receive some help from the women of the city – Whig and Tory alike – who procured clothing and food for them.[34]

Cornwallis's army was now engaged in a guerrilla war, continually harassed by the American backwoodsmen and overly reliant on loyalist militia. Patrick Ferguson's 1,000-strong Loyalist Legion was annihilated by patriot frontiersmen at King's Mountain near the North and South Carolina border on 7 October. The Tories lost more than 300 killed and wounded and around 700 more were taken prisoner. Little compassion was shown to the wounded, the rebels exulting in cries of 'Tarleton's quarter!' Some of the victors urinated on Ferguson's bullet-riddled body.[35]

We have little information pertaining to the medical arrangements for either army at King's Mountain. What we do have suggests that they were primitive, verging on non-existent. It was reported that two loyalist surgeons were killed and one captured.[36] The latter must have been Uzal Johnson, surgeon of the 5th New Jersey Volunteers. His diary includes a brief account of his actions after the battle.

'Saturday, 7 October 1780.

How many of the Enemy got killed is uncertain. Not far inferior to ours if we judge from the number of their wounded, which was equal to ours [most sources state much less, possibly ninety], I being employed to dress them in preference to their own Surgeon enable[d] me to get the Number.'

Johnson, now a prisoner of war, spent the next few days dressing the wounded of both sides. His baggage was lost, and he used torn-up shirts as bandages. Thirty loyalist militiamen were hung for 'treason'. Johnson's status as a surgeon and his treatment of the rebel wounded did not guarantee his own safety. Two weeks into his captivity, he received sword wounds to the head and hand from a patriot officer who 'had found out my Villainies and had a great mind to cut me up'.[37]

According to one authority, there was not an American medical officer of any kind at King's Mountain.[38] Johnson's comment that he was 'preferred' to a rebel surgeon suggests that there was some presence. We are left to guess why the victors favoured the attention of an enemy doctor over their own. It was most likely his greater competence.

In the North, the British Army was still struggling with high rates of disease, although less than in 1779. Sick rates in New York between August and November 1780 ranged from 13 to 15 per cent. Malaria and typhus were the probable culprits.[39] On 12 September, John Peebles made the following diary entry:

> 'The Country people very sickly especially about Jamaica [now the New York borough of Queens], a good many dying. The Army keep their health better than last year, the Grenadrs. Battns. have about 60 or 70 sick each, mostly an indistinct remitting or intermitting fever, sometimes with a ague. bilious, bile at bottom at present I have but six or 7 & last year at this time had above 50.'[40]

Seven hundred miles to the south, Cornwallis was fretting at the stubbornly high level of disease in his army. His frustration is obvious from the tone of his correspondence. In September, he writes, 'We must positively get healthier, or there is no doing any thing – I find the Ague and Fever all over this country, full as much as at Camden'.[41] The 63rd, he informed Clinton, was 'so totally demolished by illness, that it [would] not be fit for actual service for some months'.[42] A monthly return for the troops in South Carolina dated 1 November showed a sick rate of 29 per cent.[43] Robert Jackson tells us that the fever still had the character of 'intermittents', but that there were more severe cases, some complicated by gangrene and more often fatal.[44] This supports the presence of potentially lethal *falciparum* malaria.

The British commander had accepted that he could not outrun the fever.

> 'They say go 40 or 50 miles farther and you will be healthy. It was the same language before we left Camden. There is no trusting such experiments.'[45]

When disease rates did start to fall in November, it was likely the effect of 'Good Doctor Frost' rather than any human intervention. On the last day of the year, Hayes reported that the troops were 'in high Spirits and health'.[46]

Cornwallis deserves credit for his constant personal support of Hayes and his medical services in the South. He allowed his senior doctor considerable autonomy in his management of the patients and was quick to address specific complaints, for instance highlighting and attempting to correct deficiencies of medicines, hospital supplies and medical personnel. He demanded that his officers cooperate with the Hospital Department. On 20 September, his deputy adjutant general was ordered to discuss the arrangements for hospital mates and medicines 'very fully' with Staff Surgeon West Hill.[47] He is maligned in contemporary American correspondence for his apparent lack of concern for the rebel wounded and sick after Camden, but his actions must be judged in the context of the period and the War. As has been described, the British had hardly enough surgeons to attend to their own casualties and the causes of the poor American provision were closer to home, including the large-scale desertion of militia surgeons. An instruction issued after the battle that the American prisoners should be divided into smaller groups to prevent the spread of disease does not suggest a British general wholly indifferent to the fate of enemy soldiers.[48]

The patriot troops were less fearful of fevers than were the British and Germans. Presumably some of them had greater levels of immunity against the diseases common in a hot climate.[49] However, Gates's army did not campaign in the South with impunity. On 25 November, the rebel general held a council of war at Hillsborough in part to address the 'increasing levels of sickness and the unwholesome situation of the camp'. There was a lack of proper accommodation for the ill men and a shortage of hospital stores. It was decided that the army should relocate to Charlotte. Out of a force of 2,045 men, 21 per cent were listed as sick. The diseases were mainly 'intermittents' (malaria) and dysentery.[50]

At the time of General Nathanael Greene's arrival in December, the general hospital had moved to Salisbury, but the situation had not much improved. Greene described the troops of the Virginia line to be 'literally naked' and totally unfit for any kind of duty.[51] He wrote to Washington, emphasising the lack of progress in the Hospital and other departments and raising the spectre of the entire destruction of his army.[52]

Shippen's acquittal at his court martial gave him official vindication but in reality his position was now untenable. The medical department reorganisation of September 1780 was very much the work of John Cochran. The numerous resolutions included the abolition of the district departments and their hierarchies, all authority to be concentrated in one medical director and three assistants. The staff was slightly reduced but the director was now allowed to appoint a chief physician to a field army to supervise the regimental medical officers. The new egalitarian rank of 'hospital physician and surgeon' caused rancour and led to some unwelcome resignations. It was directed that returns were to be sent to Congress each month. A flying hospital was to accompany the army and, as Shippen had rarely left his comfortable city quarters, it was made explicit that the director was to stay at the front. Washington made his personal recommendations for some of the reappointed posts.[53]

It must be reiterated that although this detailed legislation recognised the hospitals in the South, it did not define the relationship of these institutions to the wider medical department. The medical director of hospitals was given authority over all hospitals 'to the northward of North Carolina'. Virginia was included in the general scheme, but the Carolinas were still independent. American medical officers south of Virginia – men such as James Brown, chief physician and surgeon of the Southern Department – were little impacted by the changes. Brown was left to use volunteer doctors and to beg for supplies from Shippen.[54] The American historian Louis Duncan admits that the 'medical affairs in these [Southern] colonies do not assume great prominence'.[55]

The British medical department was not subject to equivalent change but, at the end of 1780, there were still operational issues to resolve. Hayes informed Cornwallis that many of his staff remained ill, especially the hospital mates, some of whom had been necessarily returned to Europe due to their debility.[56] He stated that the hospitals were in good order.[57] The main general hospital was established at Camden. Even when the army relocated from Charlotte to Winnsborough in late November, the sick were still transported thirty miles to the Camden facility.[58]

Chapter 12

Cowpens to Eutaw Springs

January 1781–September 1781

For God's sake, endeavour to send us some stores, and Dressings, Lint, and Lancets.
John Cochran to Purveyor Thomas Bond, 4 July 1781

William Shippen finally resigned on 3 January 1781, claiming that this was only because Congress had deemed the roles of professor of anatomy and director general to be incompatible. He returned to private practice. Two weeks later, John Cochran was formally elected as his replacement. The highly capable James Craik was promoted to Cochran's previous post of chief physician and surgeon.[1]

Cochran was the only director general of the War to emerge unscathed from the role (see also Chapter 3). This is much to his credit as the early days of his directorship were characterised by severe shortages of supplies, staff, and money.[2] Extracts from Cochran's correspondence well demonstrate the fundamental problems afflicting the medical department. On 25 March 1781, he writes to Thomas Bond, the army purveyor at Philadelphia.

'I am sorry to inform you that I found that Hospital [Albany] entirely destitute of all kinds of stores, except a little vinegar, which was good for nothing – and frequently without bread or beef for many days – so that the doctor, under the circumstances, was obliged to permit such of the patients as could walk into town to beg provisions among the inhabitants.'[3]

In his letters to Congress, he strained to convey the wider implications of the failures within his department.

'unless some speedy and effective measures are taken to relieve the sick, a number of the valuable soldiers of the American Army will perish through want of the necessaries, who would soon be serving their country in the field, could they be well supplied.'[4]

The poor staffing situation was compounded by resignations. Cochran warned that a major new campaign could overwhelm the available medical resources. In July, he informed the authorities that out of the fifteen hospital physicians and surgeons established by Congress in October 1780, there were only eight in post. As three of these were at Boston, Philadelphia and Yellow Springs, there remained only five with Washington's Continental Army in New York, a hopelessly inadequate number.[5]

The resignations were largely due to poor morale, which in turn was exacerbated by pay arrears. Many medical officers were unpaid for two years. Cochran was left to write placatory letters to his disgruntled colleagues. To Mr Nitchie, former hospital commissary at Peekskill:

'I am sorry you have not been able to keep your family from starving but on credit. Your situation is like many others in our service, for I have not received one shilling as pay in twenty-eight months, and there are few among us who have been in better circumstances.'[6]

The director general reminded Robert Morris, the superintendent of finance, that British and French army doctors were better rewarded than their colonial peers.[7] When Congress did issue warrants for pay, they proved to be almost worthless. Some relief was eventually obtained when real money in the form of gold arrived from France in September.[8] Cochran also fought against proposals for the automatic promotion of medical officers by seniority. He instead recommended the British practice of promoting men from the hospitals and regiments who had shown themselves to be 'more capable and attentive'.[9]

Legislation approved by Congress in March at long last brought the South under the jurisdiction of the Continental medical department. The regulations were to be the same as those already in operation in other areas. Cochran sent Greene some experienced northern doctors and, by the summer, prominent Southern medical officers had been released from captivity by exchange. David Olyphant was appointed deputy director of the Southern

Department and Peter Fayssoux became chief physician of the Hospital. Greene was hopeful that his doctors, still relatively few, would now be able to provide documentation of medical supplies, reports of conditions in the hospitals, and sick returns.[10] Thus, in the final year of fighting, the authority of the director general was extended to include all armies and all colonies. In further legislation in May, the long-standing supervisory Medical Committee was replaced by the Board of War.[11]

At the start of 1781, Washington was still in New York, fretting at the inactivity of his Continental Army and unable to agree a definite plan with his French allies. Morale was low. When men of the Pennsylvania line at Morristown mutinied on New Year's Day, the commander stayed at West Point, concerned that his departure might worsen the insurrection. In the South, Greene took the brave decision to divide his army, a step partly dictated by the lack of supplies. He complained to Washington that his troops were in a 'wretched condition'. Cornwallis's army was also dispirited and weary, worn down by months of hard campaigning. Nevertheless, he was determined to hunt down both of Greene's forces, ordering the army's wagons to be burnt so that he could move faster. Sick men would have to fight for space on the regimental carts.[12]

Hayes and Jackson both insist that Cornwallis's army was in good health in the winter of 1780–81 but the available sick rates are less reassuring.[13] In January, 18 per cent of the force in South Carolina was listed as sick.[14] There was a marked decline in the number of fit regulars in the country outside Charleston.[15] The prevalent disorders included those of the 'General & of the Bilious kind mostly tending to a Putrescency'. Hayes noted that the residents of the region were as much affected as the troops. Malaria was ever-present, dysentery remained a scourge, and there were a few cases of smallpox, possibly spread to the soldiery by slaves seeking refuge.[16]

Morbidity rates in the British Army in the North were lower, as was usually the case. In Canada, only 6–7 per cent of the men were sick.[17] The Hessian army doctor Johann David Schoepff confirms the good health of the troops in New York; 'scarcely one in twenty-four is sick; these affections are trifles, or attack those with feeble and decrepit bodies, as might occur anywhere'.[18]

Smallpox remained a threat to the Continental Army, albeit a diminishing one. In early 1781, Surgeon Thacher was ordered to inoculate the troops in the Highlands near West Point. His account reveals some changes in the procedure.

'All the soldiers, with the women and children, who have not had the small-pox, are now under inoculation. Of our regiment, one hundred and eighty-seven were subjects of this disease. The old practice of previous preparation by a course of mercury and low diet, has not been adopted on this occasion; a single dose of jalap [a purgative drug derived from a plant root] and calomel [mercury chloride], or of the extract of butternut, *juglans cineria*, is in general administered previous to the appearance of the symptoms. As to diet, we are so unfortunate as to be destitute of the necessary comfortable articles of food, and they subsist principally on their common rations of beef, bread and salt pork. A small quantity of rice, sugar or molasses, and tea are procured for those who are dangerously sick. Some instances have occurred of putrid fever [possible typhus] supervening, either at the first onset or at the approach of the secondary stage, and a few cases have terminated fatally. Many of our patients were improper subjects for the disease, but we were under the necessity of inoculating all, without exception, whatever might be their condition as to health. Of five hundred who have been inoculated, four only have died, but in other instances the proportion of deaths is much more considerable.'[19]

Inoculation was a risky undertaking in a force in the field. Greene's army contained many militiamen and so was particularly susceptible to smallpox. In January 1781, the disease made its appearance at Salisbury in North Carolina. Senior American officers believed systematic inoculation to be obligatory, but Greene disagreed. He was anxious that it would paralyse the militia and possibly infect other non-immune troops. It would be better, he insisted, to dismiss the militia rather than inoculate them.[20]

We have scant information regarding other diseases in Greene's Southern Army at this time. The profound shortage of basic articles very likely contributed to poor record keeping. Cochran wrote to the president of Congress in early spring alerting him that several of the hospital physicians and surgeons had omitted hospital returns as they had no paper. The director general was forced to tear leaves out of a book.[21]

Cornwallis sent Tarleton and 1,100 troopers after the detachment of Greene's army commanded by Brigadier Daniel Morgan. After a fatiguing pursuit, Tarleton caught Morgan on 17 January in an area known as the

Cowpens. The battle lasted for forty minutes and was one of the fiercest of the War. It was a catastrophe for the British. Tarleton left a hundred dead on the field – many killed after they had surrendered their arms – and 800 prisoners. Around 200 of those captured were wounded. The rebels lost seventy-three men of whom twelve were killed.[22] The surgeon's mate of the British 71st Foot, Robert Jackson, showed great bravery, riding on to the field to give his horse to Tarleton who made a last-ditch escape.[23]

Cowpens is an example of the frequent contrast between the merciless fighting, often punctuated by atrocities, and the gentlemanly nature of the arrangements for the wounded once hostilities had ceased. Realising that he was bound to be captured, Jackson tied a white handkerchief to a stick and walked into enemy lines. He was at first treated suspiciously but let through to the American rear where he spent the night attending to the British wounded, improvising bandages from his only shirt. The next day, he was allowed to also treat the American wounded.[24] The lowly surgeon's mate appears to have taken all of this in his stride, writing a note to Morgan seeking permission to contact Cornwallis to request 'some Surgeons of the General Hospital and Hospital appointments'.[25] Tarleton contacted Morgan, informing him that he was sending across with a flag his personal surgeon, John Stewart, and another regimental medical officer.[26]

At least one American doctor gave help to the British wounded. Six days after the battle, Stewart wrote to Tarleton that Morgan had left a surgeon and a commissary 'to provide for [our wounded] in the best manner possible'. Even with this laudable cooperation, resources were wholly inadequate, Stewart noting that the country was poor and wretched and the American surgeon 'so ill furnished with medicines and other necessaries' that there was much suffering.[27] John Pindell was very likely the American surgeon referred to by Stewart. Pindell informed his commander that he was 'entirely out of Brandy and Lint' and that the supply of medicines would soon be exhausted. The plan was to move the American wounded to Salisbury but there was as yet no suitable transport.[28]

Both sides were keen to arrange a quick return and subsequent exchange of the British wounded. Pindell wrote to Morgan on the 18th:

'Enclosed I send a Flagg which arrived yesterday from Colo. Tarleton. You will see his own requisitions, in addition to which Doct'r Jackson, in conjunction with the Gentlemen who came with the flagg, (finding it impossible to have the wounded properly provided for in this country) are desirous of having the men paroled and to have permission to take them within the British lines. They will give a receipt for the number of wounded men they receive and make a return of those that may recover to our Commissary of Prisoners, when they will exchange. I am of opinion also that they cannot be provided for here, and think their proposals of equal advantage to us.'[29]

When the return of the British wounded was finalised, Jackson was sent back by the grateful Americans without the requirement for any exchange for him and without asking for his parole.[30]

Washington's hope was that Greene could preserve his Southern Army through 1781 so that he and General Rochambeau could eventually make a decisive intervention. Greene was becoming bullish. He had the advantage of local help, his sick and wounded left in the care of the inhabitants.[31] By March, his army had grown significantly, and it now contained a sizeable number of hardened Continental soldiers. He was ready for a battle and the two sides clashed at Guilford Courthouse on 15 March 1781. The 'long, bloody and severe action' was technically a British victory as Cornwallis's troops held the field. However, it was, in the words of one British officer, 'that sort of Victory which ruins an Army'. Cornwallis had lost 550 men, twice the number of his enemy.[32]

Sergeant Roger Lamb saw the British wounded being collected from the field. The operation was difficult as they were scattered over a large area, the night was dark and wet, and there were insufficient tents or nearby buildings to give cover. Their cries 'exceeded all description'. He believed fifty men to have died before morning.[33]

The Quaker New Garden Meeting House was converted to a makeshift hospital. American, British and Hessian wounded were all treated there under a flag of truce.[34] Greene sent surgeons across the lines to help. Hospital Physician and Surgeon William Read assisted in the arrangements before leaving the American wounded in the care of Surgeon's Mate Robert Brownfield and 'the excellent Quaker inhabitants'.[35] An extant receipt for American wounded two days after the battle is in the hand of Surgeon James Wallace of the 2nd Virginia Regiment.[36]

The senior British doctor on the scene was Staff Surgeon West Hill. His report of the triage and management of the wounded at Guilford Courthouse, conserved in the National Archives in London, is probably the best medical account from a Revolutionary War battlefield. Hill's documentation of the nature of the wounds has an immediacy and reality which is often missing from contemporary surgical texts written in retrospect far from the action.

Hill's priority was to decide which of the British wounded could be moved with the army. Sixty-four of the more severe cases were to be left hospitalised in the Meeting House. Hill's report gives details of the sites of their wounds, the incidence of multiple wounding, the number of deaths, and the nature of the surgical interventions. The most common sites of wounds were predictable, including the limbs, chest, and abdomen. More specific but less frequent wounds were to the head, eyes, clavicle, shoulder blade, and testicle. Sixteen of the sixty-four men had sustained multiple wounds. Between 17 March and 8 April, there were seventeen deaths, a mortality rate of 27 per cent. Fourteen of these deaths were within the first two weeks.

It must be remembered that Hill had pre-selected these men according to the severity of their injuries and thus the more slightly wounded were excluded. The number of deaths is insufficient to draw definite conclusions but many of the deceased had wounds thought to be associated with a poor prognosis. These included trauma to the thigh, chest and abdomen, arterial injuries, and compound fractures. The vague description of wounding 'through the body' occurs in six of the seventeen fatalities. Hill's report underlines the infrequency of major surgical operations close to the field. Only four amputations were performed in the sixty-four cases, three of these still surviving three weeks after the battle.[37]

Cornwallis announced that fatigue and the care of the wounded precluded any immediate further military action, and he took his army to the port city of Wilmington for 'rest and refreshment'.[38] A British general order, issued the day after the battle, directed that seventeen wagons were to be made available to transport those wounded who could not ride or walk.[39] The men left in the Meeting House would become prisoners. On 8 April, Hill reported that of the forty-seven cases remaining under his care, twenty would need wagons for their evacuation.[40]

While Cornwallis recuperated at Wilmington, supplying his army by sea, the thinly spread 8,000-strong British forces in South Carolina and Georgia were left under the command of 27-year-old Lieutenant Colonel Francis Rawdon. On 25 April, Rawdon launched a surprise attack on Greene's larger army at Hobkirk's Hill, a mile north of Camden. In a confused fight, the rebels gained the initiative and were within 'three minutes' of victory but they ultimately broke and fled. It was another pyrrhic triumph for the British, their losses exceeding those of their foe. In Greene's prescient words, 'We fight, get beat, rise and fight again'. Unable to exploit his victory, Rawdon quickly withdrew from the exposed hill back to Camden.[41]

There is limited information pertaining to the medical arrangements at Hobkirk's Hill. Towards the end of the action, around 200 of Rawdon's men were captured by American dragoons trying to get into the rear of the British line. According to Lieutenant Colonel Guilford Dudley of the North Carolina Militia, these included some medical officers.

> '[at three or four o'clock in the afternoon] Rawdon was burying the dead on both sides on Hobkick's Hill and affording what relief he could to the wounded in the absence of four of his surgeons brought off by Colonel [William] Washington from the enemy's rear during the engagement.'[42]

Despite his victory, Rawdon's medical and commissary departments had ended up in enemy hands.

On the same day as Hobkirk's Hill, Cornwallis left Wilmington and headed for Virginia. This movement was against Clinton's orders. The commander-in-chief in New York remained convinced that the British priority should be to secure the South and recover North Carolina. Clinton might have relieved Cornwallis of his command, sent his subordinate back to South Carolina, or even gone to Virginia himself. In the event, he vacillated, expressing contradictory opinions before leaving Cornwallis to his own devices. Washington was finally convinced that any attack on New York would be futile, and he prepared to move to Virginia. The main American and French armies commenced their march south in mid-August. The naval battle of the Virginia Capes fought on 5 September was tactically indecisive but strategically vital, leaving the French fleet in control of the Chesapeake and preventing any British help from New York. As Washington's and Rochambeau's armies approached, Cornwallis had chances to break out from his base at Yorktown, but he remained strangely inactive. A siege was now inevitable.[43]

Clinton later defended his indolence at New York, claiming that this was partly due to a lack of manpower; 'I had not 12,000 effectives, and of these not above 9,300 fit for duty, regulars and provincials'.[44] The sick rates for the

British forces in the North at this time do not suggest that disease was a major problem. In New York in May and June, the rate was around 9 per cent and for Canada only 6 per cent.[45]

In contrast, the health of Cornwallis's army rapidly deteriorated on the march to Virginia. A general return of the army made in mid-August, shortly after the arrival at Yorktown, shows a sick rate of 29 per cent.[46] Jackson's 71st were stationed in Portsmouth, south of Yorktown. Just outside the town was a morass known as 'the Great Dismal Swamp'. The diseases affecting the troops were familiar enemies; 'an intermitting fever, complicated, or alternating with a dysenteric complaint, made its appearance soon after our arrival and continued to increase during the short time we remained in the place'.[47]

Hayes reported from Charleston in July that disease rates were on the rise, particularly in the newly arrived unseasoned regiments. Rawdon complained to Cornwallis that his troops were almost incapacitated by fatigue.[48] He was soon replaced by Lieutenant Colonel Alexander Stewart. By early September, the new commander's force had 26 per cent of its men listed sick. In the 62nd Regiment of Foot at Eutawville it was 57 per cent.[49] The impact of disease was exacerbated by the heat. Cornwallis had dispensed with most of the tents and the men's hastily constructed brush huts were intolerably hot.[50] Captain Johann Ewald believed the climate to be causing disease 'as it decomposed our blood too much'.[51] Several German soldiers died of 'extreme heat' while marching.[52]

The American armies were also troubled by disease but the extent of this is disguised by inconsistencies in the Continental Army returns, issued by Washington, and the hospital returns, made by Cochran. In May 1781, the director general reported a total of 400 men and forty women and children being treated in all types of hospital whereas the army return showed more than 700 men under the care of army doctors. The figures for June are also discrepant. In July, the overall sick rate in Washington's army was probably close to 11 per cent.[53]

A more detailed return for the general hospital at Albany for August well illustrates the nature of the more common afflictions: bilious or putrid fever (109 cases); dysentery and diarrhoea (80); intermitting fever (77); ulcers (57); rheumatism (53); venereal diseases (44); wounded (42). 'Bilious or putrid fever' was almost certainly a mix of infectious diseases including malaria. There were close to a hundred patients with 'various chronic' disorders and a similar number of convalescents. Notably, there were only two cases of smallpox. Of the total hospital population, 8 per cent were women and children. Deaths were infrequent, only five documented for the whole month.[54]

In the South, Greene's army was also having to operate in a country 'as hot as the Antechamber of Hell'. Increasing levels of disease led to desertions. The American general took his men into camp in the High Hills of Santee in South Carolina. This move very likely benefited their health, but hundreds remained sick and supplies of bark were exhausted by the autumn.[55]

There were no significant organisational changes in the British Army's medical department in the spring and summer of 1781. Hospital equipment and stores were regularly transported across the Atlantic, a further shipment arriving in August. Medicines were procured in blocks or 'divisions', each containing an amount sufficient for 5,000 men for a prescribed period. Routine hospital items such as palliasses, bolsters, sheets, blankets, coverlets, ward furniture, surgical instruments, and dressings, were accompanied by eight machines designed to impregnate water with fresh air.[56]

The American medical situation was more fluid, the rapid evolution of the War exposing persisting deficiencies. When, in the late spring of 1781, the forces of Lafayette and General Anthony Wayne were sent to Virginia, the principal hospital was moved to Williamsburg. There was also a facility in a private house at Hanover where untrained soldiers were pressed into service as nurses. When the physician died, one of the patients was left to care for his fellows. There was a dire shortage of equipment, army surgeons being expected to provide their own instruments. Local women were asked to donate old linen for dressings.[57] Washington wrote to Congress in mid-July:

> 'But should we unfortunately enter upon the Campaign without an ample supply of those necessaries and comforts which ought to be introduced in aid to medicine, and without which medicine is often of little avail, I plainly perceive that we shall again experience the same Calamities and miseries which prevailed in 1776, and which destroyed many hundred men.'[58]

Director General Cochran was frustrated by instructions from the Board of War to start closing general hospitals, including those at Yellow Springs, Pennsylvania, Albany, and Boston. He described the order as 'ridiculous', believing it to be both expensive and unsafe. He reluctantly acquiesced with respect to the Boston unit but managed to defer closing the Albany hospital. The changes were false economies and may have been initiated due to persisting concerns as to the high death rates. Cochran was dismissive, pointing out that one might equally say that it was unsafe to go to bed as so many people died there. He suspected ulterior motives in the administration; 'I fear we have some evil Counsellors who are endeavouring to lead us astray, for astray we are going as fast as the Devil can drive us'.[59]

There was one more battle in the South. Eutaw Springs, fought on 8 September, was to be overshadowed by events at Yorktown but it was a vicious and bloody encounter. After four hours, the British again held the field at a terrible cost. Greene's casualty rate was at least 25 per cent while Stewart had lost around 35 per cent of his men. As with their previous Southern 'victories', the British subsequently retreated from the field, on this occasion to Charleston.[60]

Immediately after the battle, Stewart ordered as many of his wounded as possible to be loaded into waggons and sent towards Moncks Corner ahead of the main army. Greene wrote to the British commander suggesting a 'cessation of arms' to allow burial of the dead and collection of the wounded. A distrustful Stewart turned down the proposal, preferring to leave his seriously wounded under a flag of truce. He informed Greene that Lieutenant Colonel William Washington had assured him that the Americans would allow a captured British surgeon's mate to attend the British wounded.

These exchanges could not disguise the desperate state of the badly wounded on both sides. Many were left out in the heat with no water, food, or medical assistance. Eight days after the battle, they were still awaiting help. Otho Williams, Colonel of the Sixth Maryland Regiment, witnessed their plight.

> 'The condition of the wounded was deplorable. We found them without necessarys, some of them scarcely attended, and others wholly neglected. Many had their wounds animated by fly bows [? blowflies], and all together they exhibited one of the most humiliating and distressing Scenes I ever beheld. Their moans indicating pain, want and despair, impressed the Spirits of every humane Spectator'.

The British wounded were mostly transferred to Charleston and the American wounded were taken to Laurence's and Richardson's Plantations near St Marks Church. Some casualties from both sides were still in the hospital at Camden nearly a year after the battle.[61]

Chapter 13

Yorktown and Aftermath

August 1781–1783

Let the same Prayer be Continued that the troubles of our enemies may accumulate every Hour, so may their Head never cease to Ache, as much as yours has done after a Drunken Frolick.
John Cochran to James Craik, 1 October 1781

The combined American and French forces of Washington and Rochambeau at Yorktown were more than twice the size of Cornwallis's besieged army. An immediate assault was nevertheless judged to be impractical, and the attackers instead employed the traditional arts of siege warfare, digging parallels out of the Virginia soil. The fate of the British and German garrison was sealed. Sorties against the rebel lines on 16 and 17 October saved only a little honour. The surrender began on the 19th, the besieged army marching out of the ruins of Yorktown. Brigadier Charles O'Hara performed the grim necessities, Cornwallis pleading illness. Washington refused O'Hara's sword, directing him instead to General Benjamin Lincoln, the American second-in-command.

Yorktown was the effective conclusion of the War although there was some sporadic skirmishing in the South in the following year, mostly involving rebels and Tories. Prolonged peace negotiations were concluded in Paris in September 1783 with the recognition of American independence. Washington had ordered the cessation of hostilities in April, ending eight years of fighting.

The British and Hessian defenders suffered around 500 casualties at Yorktown. The attackers lost about 700 men, just less than half American.[1] Director General Cochran remained on the banks of the Hudson and James Craik took control of the Continental Army medical department. The Scottish-born Craik had served with the Redcoats in the French and Indian War. He was ordered to keep close to the Marquis de Lafayette 'to pay the first attention to him, in case he should be wounded'. The extent to which this instruction impeded his wider duties is uncertain.[2]

The American medical provision included a flying hospital. Contemporary maps show a field hospital established at the camp before Yorktown.[3] General hospitals had been opened at the Governor's Palace in Williamsburg, and in two nearby churches. The Vineyard Hospital was outside the town and there was also a facility at Hanover. During the siege, the American hospitals at Williamsburg were the responsibility of Dr Thomas Tucker but after the surrender Dr James Tilton was left in charge of the sick and wounded. There were approximately 400 inpatients at Williamsburg and more than 200 at Hanover.[4]

A 200-man detachment from the besieging army had been left at Williamsburg to guard the main hospitals.[5] A letter from Tucker to Cornwallis in mid-August highlights the potential vulnerability of more isolated medical services:

'I have just now received information that Mr Evan Lewis, apothecary's mate in the Continental hospital [at Williamsburg] and three other men employed in the service of the said hospital, being on Saturday night last on the road with a cart coming for some of the hospital stores in this town [Williamsburg] for the use of the sick at Hickery [Hickory] Neck Church about 12 miles distant, fell in with a party of British troops, who put them under guard and sent them to York. I beg leave to inform your Lordship that the sick at Hickery Neck Church are a part of those who came lately from Charlestown and that they were, on the arrival of your army at York, removed from hence before I could get sufficient assurance that our hospital was to be considered as under the sanction of a flag. But upon being certified by Major General the Marquis de la Fayette that it was to remain sacred, and seeing the same assented to in a letter from Captain [Robert] Cooke written by your Lordship's authority, I thought it unnecessary either to remove the remainder of our sick from Williamsburg or to have those at the church conveyed farther into the country. In this situation it was impossible for our officers to do their duty to the sick at both places without being at liberty to go and return at pleasure, which I conceive to be fully authorised by your Lordship's consent.'

Cooke was a British commissary of prisoners. Tucker goes on to request that the captured men and cart be immediately returned so that they could resume their medical duties.[6]

Jean-François Coste was the chief of the French medical department (see also Chapter 3).[7] There are a number of references to French field hospitals (*ambulances*) among the front-line trenches where Rochambeau's army saw some of the fiercest fighting. *Commissaire des Guerres* Claude Blanchard notes that he visited an *ambulance* installed to the left of the American flying hospital and that there was another resource for the wounded 'close to the trench'. It is probably the latter field hospital which the army chaplain, Jean-Baptiste-Claude Robin, refers to as '*le premier dépôt pour les blessés*'. He says that this was near to a passage to the trench where the enemy was directing most of his fire. He was relieved that there was not even greater bloodshed as there was no straw for the wounded to lie on and no linen to dress their wounds. Blanchard also mentions a separate *ambulance* for the division of the Marquis de Choisy towards Gloucester.[8]

French casualties were evacuated to Williamsburg where general hospitals were opened in the College of William and Mary and at the Capitol.[9] The College had been handed over to the French in mid-September. A letter of 15 October to Washington from its president, John Blair, suggests local resistance.

> 'The French Line are now in possession of the whole, except the Library, the Apparatus Room, and the Rooms of Mr. Bellini, Professor of Modern Languages, and the only Professor who remains in the College: all this is as great a supply of conveniences as could be reasonably required from one place – but Mr. Bellini has just been with me to inform that the Commissary has demanded of him the keys of an out-building called the Granary and other houses near it, in which is a variety of useful Articles which can be removed nowhere else and which must be lost to the College if this measure be persisted in.'

Washington replied courteously that, under the circumstances, he was sure that the professor would be ready to give up the buildings.[10]

On the British side, O'Hara had arranged the transfer of all hospital patients at Portsmouth to Yorktown. The convoy was sent around the middle of August under the supervision of Staff Surgeon Alexander Grant.[11] The

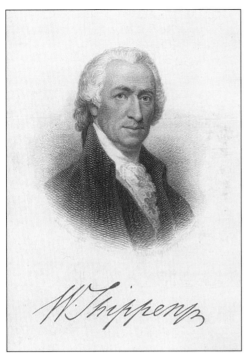

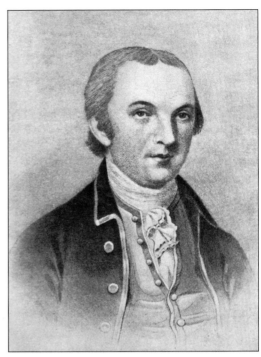

Above left: *William Shippen.*

Above right: *John Cochran.*

Right: *James Tilton.*

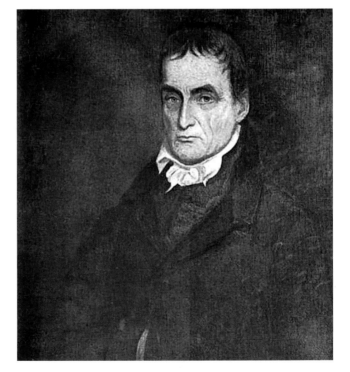

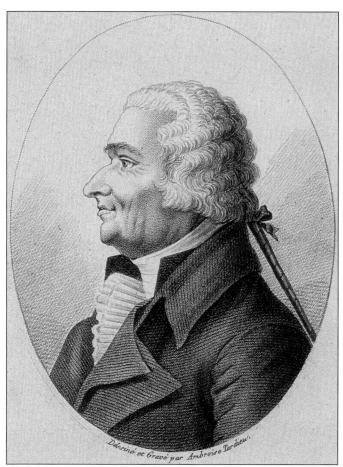

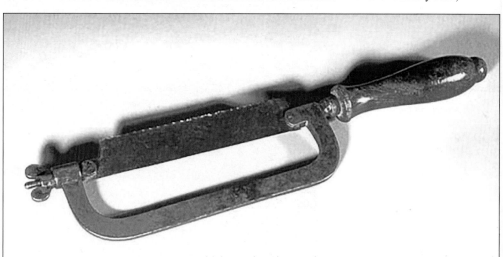

Left: *Jean-François Coste.*

Below: *Amputation saw.*
(Guilford Courthouse
National Military Park)

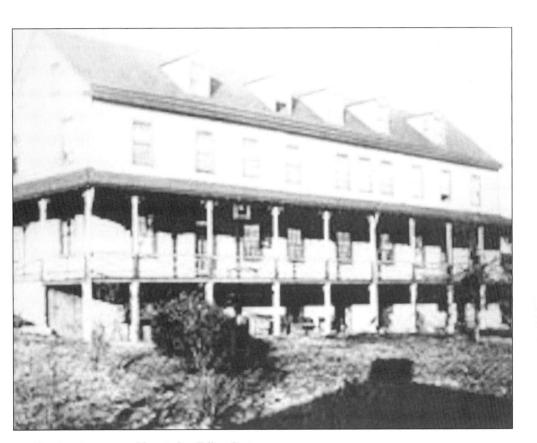

The American general hospital at Yellow Springs.

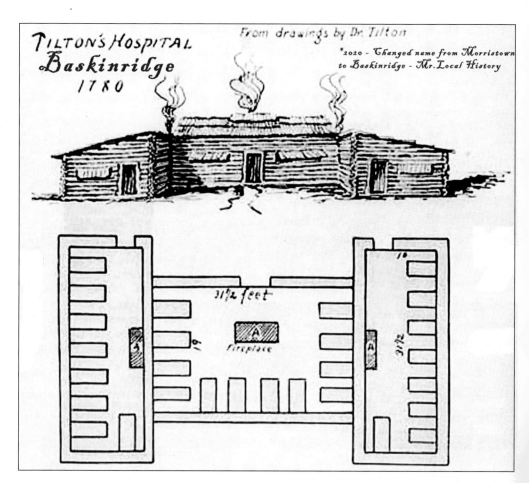

James Tilton's experimental hospital hut.

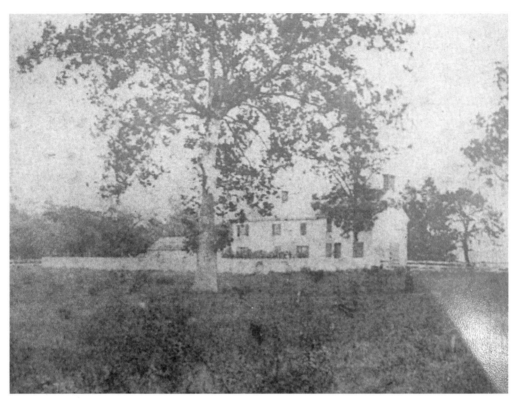

The Thomas Clarke House in 1860. Used as a field hospital by both sides at the Battle of Princeton.

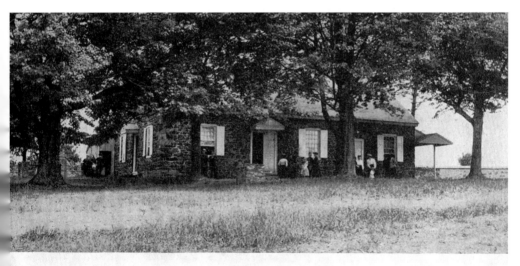

Birmingham Meeting House. The building was used as a field hospital in the Battle of Brandywine by both the Americans and British.

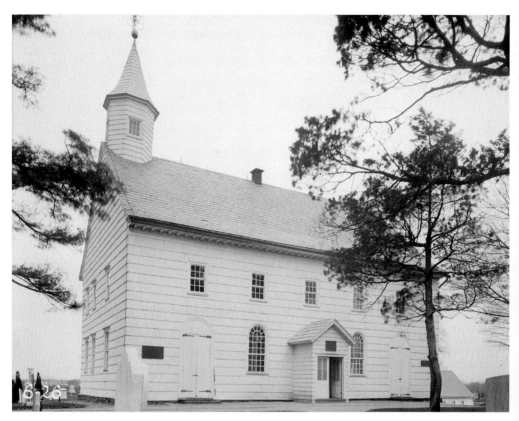

The Old Tennent Church at Manalapan served as an American field hospital during the Battle of Monmouth. A saw mark and stains on the existing pews are possible relics of Revolutionary War surgery.

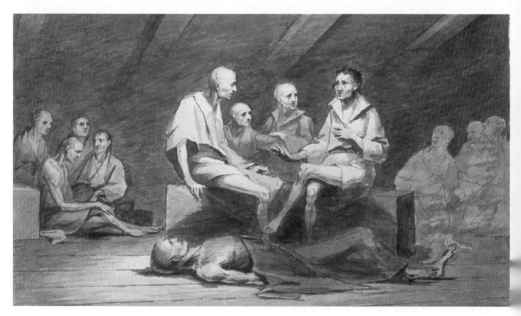

American prisoners on the British prison ship HMS Jersey *anchored off New York.*

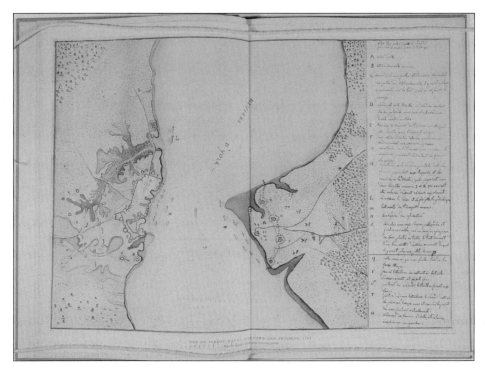

Pass issued to British Staff Surgeon West Hill to allow him to treat the wounded in the New Garden Meeting House after the Battle of Guilford Courthouse. (The National Archives)

Map of Yorktown and its environs, 1781. Drawn by French infantryman Joachim du Perron.

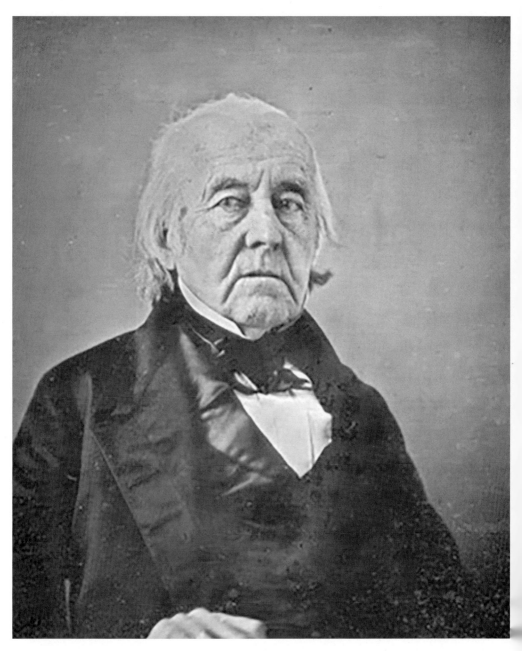

American surgeon's mate Aeneas Munson. He assisted James Thacher at the Siege of Yorktown.

senior medical officer at Yorktown was Dr Robert Smith (sometimes referred to as Smyth), his formal appointment being that of surgeon and director of British hospitals in Virginia.[12] At the time of the capitulation, his hospital staff consisted of three surgeons, two purveyors and ten hospital mates. There were, of course, also the regimental surgeons and mates, and the German medical officers. The main British hospital was located across the York River at Gloucester Point.[13]

Surgeon James Thacher provides the best eyewitness account of the American medical services during the siege. The following is his journal entry for 7 October.

'A large detachment of the allied army, under the command of Major-General Lincoln, were ordered out last evening for the purpose of opening intrenchments near the enemy's lines. This business was concluded with great silence and secrecy, and we were favoured by Providence with a night of extreme darkness and were not discovered before day-light. The working party carried on their shoulders fascines and intrenching tools, while a large part of the detachment was armed with the implements of death. Horses, drawing cannon and ordnance, and wagons loaded with bags filled with sand for constructing breastworks, followed in the rear. Thus arranged, every officer and soldier knowing his particular station, orders were given to advance in perfect silence, the distance about one mile. My station on this occasion was with Dr. [Aeneas] Munson, my mate, in the rear of the troops; and as the music was not to be employed, about twenty drummers and fifers were put under my charge to assist me in case of having wounded men to attend. I put into the hands of a drummer, a mulatto fellow, my instruments, bandages, & c., with a positive order to keep at my elbow, and not lose sight of me a moment; it was not long, however, before I found to my astonishment that he had left me, and gone in pursuit of some rum, carrying off the articles which are indispensable in time of action. In this very unpleasant predicament, unwilling to trust another, I hastened with all speed to the hospital, about one mile, to procure another supply from Dr. Craik; and he desired that if the Marquis de la Fayette should be wounded, I would devote to him my first attention. On my return I found Dr. Munson and my party waiting, but the troops had marched on and we knew not their route. We were obliged to follow at random, and in the darkness of the night, hazarding our approach to the enemy. Having advanced about half a mile, of a sudden a party of armed men in white uniform rose from the ground and ordered us to stop; they proved to be the rear-guard of the French. The officer demanded the countersign, which I was unable to give, and as we could not understand each other's language, I was detained under considerable embarrassment till an officer who could speak English was called, when producing my instruments and bandages, and assuring the French officer that I was a surgeon to the infantry, he politely conducted me to my station.'[14]

Thacher later attended the hospital, most likely the field or flying facility, where he dressed wounds and amputated a man's arm.[15]

Joseph Plumb Martin was also in the thick of the action and he makes an interesting allusion to a 'wind-of-ball' fatality. A cannon ball flew close to a soldier's face without touching it and he fell dead into the trench.

'I put my hand on his forehead and found his skull was shattered all in pieces and the blood flowing from his nose and mouth, but not a particle of skin was broken. I never saw an[other] instance like this among all the men I saw killed during the whole war.'[16]

Eyewitness accounts of other campaigns of the period describe similar wounds, serious injuries such as broken bones occurring without any apparent external damage.

We also have glimpses of the work of French surgeons at Yorktown. Some soldiers were so seriously wounded as to be beyond medical help. On the night of 5 October, Pierre Louis de la Loge, a lieutenant in the artillery, was carried by his comrades to the *ambulance*.

'he was in a coma, too enfeebled by loss of blood to be resuscitated. The surgeon covered his body with a flag in the colours of the King, red, white and blue, and the Abbot Robin, chaplain of the army, recited prayers.'[17]

On the 14th, Charles de Lameth, *aide-maréchal-général de Logis*, received gunshot wounds to both knees.

'The surgeons at first decided that he might only be saved by bilateral amputations at the thigh, but the *chirurgien en chef*, M. Robillard, rather than reduce such a hopeful young officer to a *cul-de-jatte* [person with no legs], would not permit the amputations and he trusted to nature for the cure of such serious wounds. Success crowned his confidence. Charles de Lameth quickly recovered and returned to France two months later.'[18]

We have no good eyewitness accounts of the functioning of the British medical department at the siege. The medical officers, imprisoned at the surrender, perhaps wished to forget their involvement in the debacle. Johann Conrad Döhla, a private in the Fourth Company of the Bayreuth Regiment, does give a German view of the deprivations and wounds suffered by the besieged garrison and the local population:

'10 October. We had to change our camp this morning and set up our tents in the communication trenches, because of the enemy's heavy cannonade. He threw bombs at us of 100 and 150 pounds, also of 200 pounds, and his howitzer and cannonballs were of 18-, 24-, 36-, and, a very few of 12 pounds. It was impossible to avoid the frighteningly many balls in or outside the city. Most of the inhabitants who were still to be found here fled eastward with their best possessions on the waters of the York River, and dug into the sand cliffs, but even there they were not uninjured. Many were seriously and fatally wounded by the broken pieces of the bombs that were exploding, partly in the air, partly on the ground, which broke arms and legs, or killed them. The ships in the harbour also suffered great damage because the cannonballs flew across the river and as far as the land at Gloucester. At nine o'clock in the morning our sutler [Johann Wilhelm] Seewald of Quesnoy's Company, was fatally wounded by a cannonball that struck him in the right side while he was in a small house immediately behind the front of our camp, near Yorktown, where he had his store. At noon Grenadier Dörrer, of Molitor's Company, was dangerously wounded on the left leg by a bomb, and during the evening the leg had to be amputated above the knee.'

A shell striking one of the regiment's tents immediately killed four men and fatally wounded two others. The overworked German surgeons welcomed any help. Döhla held a man down while a ball was cut out from between his shoulder blades.[19]

In early September, Cornwallis had complained to Clinton that his army was 'very sickly'.[20] At the time of the surrender of the British forces at Yorktown there were 2,037 fit and 1,260 sick or wounded men (a rate of 38 per cent). The detachment at Gloucester was a little healthier while the more recently arrived units were badly affected. The 17th, 43rd, and 80th Regiments all had more than 50 per cent of their men unfit.[21] Jackson confirms the presence of both malaria and dysentery. There was a tendency for fever to become chronic and complicated.

> 'if allowed to go on, it often degenerated into dropsy [oedema or heart failure], obstructions in the abdominal viscera, or a dysenteric complaint, which frequently proved fatal in the beginning of the following winter.'

He says that the incidence of disease increased after the capitulation with dysentery the chief cause of death.[22]

Döhla refers to dysentery, diarrhoea and 'putrid fever' in the German troops. He attributed these diseases to fatigue and to the presence of saltpetre (potassium nitrate) in the drinking water.[23] Drugs were in short supply. According to Captain Ewald, the invalids were deceived by the administration of an 'emetic' which was a mixture of earth and sugar. When he fell sick with fever, he self-medicated with a combination of China powder (probably gunpowder) and strong rum.[24]

Senior British officers were not oblivious to the gaps in their ranks resulting from disease and there were attempts at military hygiene. Soldiers were instructed to only drink from a well distant from the encampment and women were forbidden to wash at the creek. Extra stockings were provided when a regimental surgeon reported that rheumatic complaints were due to the men being too thinly clothed. These measures were particularly applied by Major Thomas Armstrong, commander of the light infantry. Despite his efforts, 40 per cent of his men were invalids.[25]

Malaria and dysentery were also the commonest diseases in the Continental Army. A return for October shows a total of 1,815 men sick or wounded in the American general hospitals. Among the 326 inpatients at Williamsburg, there were 109 cases of intermittent fever and forty-three of dysentery. The number of disease cases in the town comfortably exceeded the number of wounded (fifty-nine).[26] An October return for the flying hospital at Yorktown is similar (209 cases of intermittent fever and 103 of diarrhoea) and Thacher comments that the New England troops were suffering mostly from intermittent and remittent fevers which were prevalent in the region in the autumn months.[27]

Climate was routinely invoked as a cause of disease and soldiers often chose to blame their living conditions and diet. Water was a particular source of concern. Private Martin was on twenty-four-hour duty in the Yorktown trenches:

'The greatest inconvenience we felt was the want of good water, there being none near our camp but nasty frog ponds where all the horses in the neighbourhood were watered and we were forced to wade through the water in the skirts of the ponds, thick with mud and filth to get at water in any wise fit for use.'

Martin complained that even the fresh spring water of the country had a metallic taste.[28]

By March 1782, there were very few sick in the American hospital at Williamsburg. Washington suggested that the hospital might be broken up; 'it would be a pleasing circumstance'.[29] Farther to the south, Greene's army continued to suffer. By the summer of 1782, the number of fever cases had escalated to the point that soldiers were 'dying fast' and the hospitals were crowded. The deaths were so numerous that funeral ceremonies were dispensed with.[30] The diseases of the South were proving to be more resilient adversaries than the British.

In her detailed history of the American Army Medical Department, Mary Gillett insists that at Yorktown the French were as much affected by disease as their American allies.[31] French commentators, notable Jean-François Lemaire in his biography of Coste, make the case for relatively low mortality rates in Rochambeau's force. Basing his argument partly on the findings from a twentieth-century archaeological excavation of the cemetery at the College of William and Mary, he estimates the total loss of the French expeditionary force from disease to be around 600 men; '*pourcentage très faible pour l'époque et dans le contexte*'.[32]

Accusations of biological warfare resurfaced at Yorktown. As early as June 1781, American soldiers suspected that Cornwallis's retreating army was using the smallpox-infected black population to propagate the disease. Josiah Atkins's regiment was pursuing the British near Richmond. He saw the dead by the side of the road, their bodies 'putrefying with the smallpox'. Cornwallis, Atkins believed, had inoculated up to 500 black inhabitants to spread the disease through the country.[33] In early October, James Thacher made the same allegation; 'The British have sent from Yorktown a large number of negroes, sick with the small-pox, probably for the purpose of communicating the infection to our army'.[34] Washington advised his soldiers to avoid communicating with the locals as, he explained, 'Our ungenerous enemy, [has], as usual, propagated the smallpox'.[35]

Was this a malicious design or an inevitable consequence of the War? The British might have argued that it was impossible for them to support so many camp-followers and that the American charges were propaganda. The following short extract from a letter written by General Alexander Leslie to Cornwallis from Portsmouth in July 1781 is not conclusive but it does suggest a degree of intent; 'Above 700 Negroes are come down the River in the Small Pox. I shall distribute them about the Rebell Plantations'.[36]

Duncan's assertion that after Yorktown the Continental Army marched away and the sick and wounded were 'practically abandoned' may be exaggerated but the American medical services were still compromised by many of the deficiencies first experienced in 1776.[37] Doctors paint a sorry picture of grim hospitals and desperate shortages. In December, the situation became even worse when the palace in Williamsburg burnt to the ground. Fortunately, there was only one casualty.[38] In January 1782, Dr Monroe wrote from the town complaining of the 'improper direction of public affairs'. He had hardly enough provisions 'to keep the Hospital from Starving'. Conditions were no better elsewhere. At Richmond, Surgeon Matthew Pope was responsible for a hospital in an unfinished log house. Ten men were confined to a small room and water poured through the roof. They had no clothes or blankets. Pope described them as 'wretched'; 'when it rains the sick might as well be out of doors'.[39]

Washington was well informed. Two days before the British surrender, he had written to Governor Blair informing him that the number of sick and wounded was increasing so fast as to exhaust the room necessary for their 'Cover and Conveniences'.[40] At his moment of victory, the American commander could only hope that captured funds would allow the necessary improvements.[41]

There was still the need for specialist hospitals. In late October, Washington approved a request from Craik for a dedicated smallpox facility in Williamsburg. The quarter master general was ordered to secure any necessary houses in the town.[42]

The demand for general hospitals in Virginia persisted over the next few months. Those at Williamsburg were not disbanded until March 1782.[43] Other temporary hospitals were opened to give care to American troops returning north from Yorktown. These included units at The Head of Elk and at Wilmington. The general hospital at Philadelphia housed more than 300 patients in November.[44] It remained easier to open hospitals than to properly supply them. In January 1782, Major Dick was still complaining of a scarcity of food and supplies for the hospital at Portsmouth.[45]

The French hospital at the College in Williamsburg was also affected by a fire, one wing being destroyed.[46] James Tilton had a low opinion of the hospital and the wider French medical services:

'Being thus in a French garrison [Williamsburg], I had some opportunity of observing the French practice and management of their sick. In passing the wards of their hospital their patients appear very neat and clean, above all examples I had ever seen. Each patient was accommodated with every thing necessary, even to a night cap. Nevertheless, they were not more successful than we were. Even their wounded, with all the boasted dexterity of the French to help them, were no more fortunate than ours. I was led to attribute their failure principally to two causes. For ease and convenience, they had contrived a common necessary [toilet] for the whole hospital, the college, a large building, three stories high, by erecting a half hexagon, of common boards, reaching from the roof down to a pit in the earth. From this perpendicular conduit doors opened upon each floor of the hospital; and all manner of filth and excrementitious matters were dropped and thrown down this common sewer, into the pit below. This sink of nastiness perfumed the whole house very sensibly and, without doubt, vitiated all the air within the wards.'

The second French shortcoming, Tilton opined, was their reluctance to prescribe medication. They used little bark or opium and their hospital pharmacy consisted chiefly of herbal remedies ('decoctions') and watery drinks. Tilton's criticism of Coste was, in retrospect, unjustified. It is likely that the French physician's conservatism did more good than harm.[47]

Articles eleven and twelve of the capitulation agreement made provision for the captured British and German sick and wounded. 'Proper hospitals' were to be furnished and the patients were to be tended by their own surgeons on parole. The American victors were expected to provide medicines, stores, and wagons. It was intended that the necessary hospital supplies would be obtained in Yorktown, Williamsburg and possibly from New York.[48] Those too unfit to be moved, around 1,500 men, were housed in the main British hospital at Gloucester Point where Robert Smith remained in charge.[49] Smith corresponded with the local governor in a vain attempt to obtain the promised provisions and medical supplies.[50] Captain Ewald saw the resultant suffering and filth; 'amputated arms and legs lay around in every corner and were eaten by the dogs.'[51]

When French soldier Lieutenant Joachim du Perron walked along the beach at Gloucester Point on 21 October, he saw the large tents of the British hospital. '[We] found at our feet several dead bodies that stank horribly... so many of them died that there was no time to bury them, and they simply threw the dead out of the tents as they expired'.[52]

The British prisoners were marched to Winchester after the surrender. On 9 November, 350 of the sick and convalescents in the hospital at Gloucester Point were taken to Ladd's Bridge and 250 were then sent up the river to Fredericksburg. When another 200 were discharged on the 17th, many were abandoned in the country, nobody taking responsibility for their care. A large party of sick were marooned at Aylett near Richmond due to a lack of wagons and 200 more ended up at New Castle. Towards the end of the month there were only 300 left at Gloucester. These inpatients were nominally under a French guard but 'those able to walk did as they pleased, while the sick suffered'. The main diseases were smallpox and dysentery.[53]

Smallpox continued to disproportionately affect the black population. On the day of the capitulation, Pennsylvania soldier Ebenezer Denny noted in his journal that, 'Negroes lie about, sick and dying in every stage of the smallpox. Never was in so filthy a place'. The American camp contained a sizeable number of susceptible white regulars and militia who had missed out on the Continental Army's inoculations. Despite efforts to isolate those infected, soldiers from Yorktown spread the disease to Cumberland County where a serious outbreak resulted. By December, troops marching north had carried the virus as far as West Point. Here, in January 1782, another 2,000 men were inoculated.[54]

Although there was no fighting after 1782, British troops remained in America until after the peace of 1783. During this period, there were the British general hospitals at New York and Boston and smaller hospital staff detachments at Rhode Island, at St Augustin in Florida, and in South Carolina. When these hospitals closed, any surplus equipment was either disposed of locally or sent to Canada where there were still general facilities at Trois-Rivières, Montreal, Halifax, and Newfoundland. As there had been no military operations in the region since Burgoyne's surrender, there were only a few inpatients, mostly suffering from fevers and scurvy. The general hospital at Quebec closed in 1781. It had previously been moved out of the Augustinian convent, the medical officer in charge accusing the nuns of killing some patients by attempting to convert them from Protestantism, 'when in a state of great weakness of body and mind'. To support the remaining general hospitals, there were small detachments with a hospital mate in isolated places such as St Johns and on Lake Champlain.[55]

Washington remained near New York City until the end of the War and Greene's Southern Army finally left for home in the summer of 1783. As has been noted, Congress had ordered the closure of some major hospitals even before the end of 1781. The general hospital at Boston was disbanded in the spring of 1782 but others continued. At Philadelphia, it was as late as 1783 before remaining patients were transferred to the city's civilian institutions. The hospital at Albany, under threat for some time, was shut early in 1782 but then later reopened, still staffed by a surgeon and mate, towards the end of 1783. Women and children made up around a third to a half of the inpatients at both Philadelphia and Albany.[56] Washington inspected those hospitals still open. A general order of May 1782 stipulates that they be 'ampliy supplyed with Medicines, refreshments and accommodations'.[57]

The dismantling of the Continental Army left large numbers of invalided, homeless, and helpless men still reliant on the government for support.[58] These veterans were often disappointed. In February 1783, Director General Cochran writes to Quarter Master General Timothy Pickering regarding 50-year-old Captain Gershom Mott of the 2nd Continental Artillery:

> 'whose situation for several Years has been very distressing on Account of this Health, few have suffered more or made a

greater struggle for life than he has done, & I believe his present circumstances are equally as bad as he paints them. He appears to merit relief but that is out of my Power to afford him, as I know of no provision made for sick or wounded officers, unless they are put into the Hospitals allotted for the privates or they are billeted by the Magistrate.'[59]

In September 1783, the granting of furloughs to all medical staff whose services were no longer necessary was effectively a disbandment of the American Army Hospital Department.[60] In the following month, a proposal was made for a peacetime hospital establishment, but this was not acted upon.[61]

Medicine and
The Revolution

Chapter 14

Disease and the American Revolution

Two questions are addressed. Firstly, what was the total loss of life in the American Revolution? Secondly, did disease materially affect the outcome of the conflict?

Estimation of the mortality of the War is not straightforward. We have seen that the Continental Army made efforts to collect returns but that these were often omitted or of doubtful accuracy. Many ill American troops walked away from the ranks. Thousands of these 'absent sick' regularly departed for their homes or elsewhere and there is no way of knowing how many eventually succumbed to wounds and disease.[1] Most of the deficiencies in the returns were very likely accidental but there may also have been deliberate manipulation of the figures. Washington noted frequent discrepancies between the hospital returns and the number of sick reported absent by regimental officers. He believed Director General Shippen's reports to be overly optimistic.[2] Benjamin Rush was in no doubt as to Shippen's culpability. He wrote in sarcastic vein to Nathanael Greene that he had assumed that the coffins he counted going into the ground contained dead soldiers due to their 'weight and smell'. If Shippen's numbers were correct, then soldiers were being 'buried alive'.[3]

British army returns were also incomplete. The evangelical data collector, Thomas Dickson Reide, struggled to keep a continuous record; 'The regiment being much divided, and having made frequent movements, I could not keep records so well as could be wished, or fit to lay before the public'.[4] There was a relative wealth of returns from Canada but fewer for regiments actively campaigning in the South. Where returns are available, the calculation of mortality is compromised by the absence of a column listing the number of dead in more than 65 per cent of cases.[5] The French and German army returns are plagued by similar shortcomings and the information pertaining to disease, wounding, and death in the white civilian, black, and American Indian populations is even thinner.

There was interest in the human cost of the War as early as 1777 when Thomas Jefferson assessed British casualties and assumed the American losses to be half as many. Most early estimates of the total mortality were little more than wild guesses. Continental Army doctor James Thacher believed American deaths to amount to 70,000. Perhaps the best calculation of American mortality is that of Howard H. Peckham, published in 1974. Peckham asserts that around 25,000 American soldiers died: 6,800 in battle, 8,500 in British prisons, and 10,000 in camps and hospitals. If this figure is accurate – and it is probably an underestimate – then this represents just less than 1 per cent of the total population of America at the time of the Revolution (2,781,000 in 1780). This might be compared to 1.6 per cent of the population in the American Civil War, 0.12 per cent in the First World War and 0.28 per cent in the Second World War. Of the 200,000 American men who fought during the Revolution, 12.5 per cent died. This is very close to the 13 per cent of the Civil War.[6] French losses are even more difficult to compute. The most detailed study suggests 2,000 deaths in America between the years 1777 and 1783.[7]

In his *History of the British Army Medical Department*, Sir Neil Cantlie gives the total British deaths between 1775 and 1780 as 6,107. This was an average rate of 1,000 per year or 2.6 per cent. The total toll of the War in North America was likely close to 10,000 men, roughly a quarter of the British troops sent across the Atlantic.[8] For the German forces, Cantlie states 7,774 deaths over a six-year period.[9] The losses of the loyalist forces are obscure but extrapolation from the 20 per cent mortality recorded in the New Jersey Volunteers gives very approximate provincial unit losses of 4,000 men.[10]

More soldiers perished from disease than from wounds. Contemporary observers believed disease deaths to considerably outnumber wound deaths. James Tilton wrote that the American forces 'lost not less than from ten to twenty of camp diseases, for one by the weapons of the enemy'.[11] British surgeon Robert Hamilton commented that in the American War fevers had killed eight times more men than had succumbed to their wounds.[12] Some modern researchers support these opinions.[13] Marshall suggests that more than 80 per cent of British deaths were disease related. This figure is based on a study of the Brigade of Guards between 1776 and 1779.[14] Cantlie quotes a similar proportion of disease deaths in the German troops (77 per cent).[15] There were variations dependant on the state of the warring armies and other interpretations are possible. Kopperman proposes a lower proportion of disease deaths for a wider period in North America, close to two-thirds between 1755 and 1781.[16]

One reason for the relative infrequency of death from battle or accidents was the apparent favourable prognosis of many wounds. We have limited data, and this pertains to the British Army. Reide quotes a remarkably low (1 in 300) 'surgical mortality' for his regiment between 1777 and 1786. This presumably reflects the trivial nature of the great majority of the injuries or other surgical complaints that he was dealing with.[17] Historian Don H. Hagist presents more meaningful information derived from British regiments. Over a period of 45 months, the Brigade of Guards suffered forty deaths due to combat, including twenty-two killed in battle and eighteen who died of wounds, only 3 per cent of those serving. After the Battle of Rhode Island in 1778, the 22nd Regiment had around fifty men wounded. Only five of these men died in the subsequent four months. Three regiments storming Fort Clinton and Fort Montgomery in October 1777 suffered sixty-one wounded but by the end of the year only eleven had died of any cause. The survival chances of a wounded British soldier were surprisingly good.[18]

The figures available allow a comparison of the disease morbidity in the American and British armies. Sick returns in the Continental Army between 1775 and 1783 show an average morbidity of 16 per cent. The actual rate was probably greater as few returns exist for the Canadian Expedition and the Southern theatre, both notoriously unhealthy campaigns. This is significantly greater than the British Army average morbidity of just less than 11 per cent.[19] Duncan believed that twice as many American soldiers died of diseases compared with their British counterparts and Surgeon Johann David Schoepff noted that the German troops were also relatively spared compared with their enemy; 'disease has frequently been rife among them [the Americans] when our men have been enjoying the best of health'.[20]

This gap in disease morbidity probably had a multifactorial aetiology. Many British soldiers came from large cities, and they had the advantage of some immunity against the prevalent infectious diseases. They were particularly more protected against smallpox than the ranks of the Continental Army who were largely recruited from isolated country districts. In America, the British troops were often quartered in cities such as Philadelphia, New York, and Charleston. These were not always healthy locations, but the men were more warmly clothed and better sheltered than the rebels who were routinely accommodated in poorly supplied camps such as at Valley Forge. The greater discipline of the British regular, especially early in the War, facilitated the enforcement of regulations regarding personal and military hygiene.[21]

These are average figures and there were variations in sick rates within armies with respect to individual units and ranks. It was common knowledge that new recruits were more vulnerable to disease than 'seasoned' veterans. Medical examinations were not mandatory in the British Army until 1790 and many soldiers were unhealthy at the time of enlistment. Approximately 8 per cent of the men embarked on British transports during the American War died in transit.[22] The recruits continued to suffer an excess of morbidity and mortality after their arrival in America. More than half of the Royal Welch Fusiliers' 'poor, raw, country soldiers' who were recruited in 1779 died within two years of their arrival in the country.[23] The same was true of the German forces, as is testified by Schoepff; 'During the first twelve months we lost many men, but during the next twelve months barely thirty, and now, as a rule, hardly more than we lose in our fatherland… most of the patients in the hospitals are usually recruits'.[24]

Officers had better access to medical advice and treatment than the private soldiers. Cornwallis was in receipt of a document from his surgeon, Robert Knox. Undated, this gives meticulous instructions. The general is advised to take bark once or twice a day, to drink spruce beer, and to avoid highly seasoned meats and any excessive consumption of punch.[25] In the Continental Army, officers had first call on medical services because of their status as 'gentlemen'. Major Henry Sherburne of the Rhode Island Continentals asked Jonathan Potts to give special attention to his sick cousin, a young militia officer. The overworked Potts was even expected to accommodate the patient in his own house, 'as it is impossible for him to be taken that Care of in the General Hospital that his Tender Years Require'.[26] It is difficult to quantify the extent to which this preferential attention translated into lower morbidity and mortality in the officer class as there is only anecdotal information. In the Royal Welch Fusiliers, eighty-eight officers served during the war, most being present for only one or two campaigns. Thirteen died from disease and five from wounds.[27]

Army doctors were more vulnerable to disease than military officers. Tilton concluded that the increased mortality in his colleagues provided 'strong evidence that infection is more dangerous in military life than the weapons of war'.[28] John Cochran calculated that the 'fatigue, Hardship and

Inconveniences' experienced by his hospital surgeons led them to have a three times greater risk of contracting disease.[29]

Smallpox dominates much of the medical literature of the War. It was particularly a cause of heavy mortality in the American forces in the earlier years, the miserable statistics only capturing a proportion of the 'untold numbers' of deaths.[30] The episodic and catastrophic nature of smallpox means that the affliction tends to overshadow the more pervasive influence of other infectious diseases. American historian John Duffy claims that malaria and dysentery took first place among the colonial infections. The destructive effect of dysentery on the warring armies is difficult to overstate. Duffy thought the disorder to be so extensive 'as to prevent a statistical measurement in terms of cases and fatalities'.[31] Its harm was often indirect, men already debilitated by dysentery more likely to die of other diseases, especially malaria and typhus.[32] Reide gives numerical support to the very high incidence of 'severe fluxes' in the British troops. Dysentery made up 21 per cent of the diseases he saw during the War, and it was the leading cause of death in his regiment.[33]

The toll of the War in the non-combatants of the armies and the white civilian population must have been considerable but is impossible to quantify. In the British Army, the ordinary soldiers' wives and children who fell ill were not guaranteed admission to the general hospitals. Many would have been managed by the regimental medical officers. In New Jersey in February 1777, Captain John Peebles sent a Ms Gennes, presumably a soldier's wife, to the hospital, 'but they would not admit a sick Woman'.[34] In August 1781, there were 888 soldiers in the British base hospital at New York but only twenty women and thirty-seven children.[35]

As soldiers marched through the colonies, it was inevitable that the diseases they carried would be transmitted to the local population. Civilians were unable to escape the torrent of pathogens, including *Variola*. In just one example, rebel troops returning home from the New York lakes in the winter of 1776–77 triggered smallpox epidemics in Pennsylvania and Connecticut. The governor of the latter was in no doubt that veterans who had 'taken the infection' in the retreat from Canada were the cause of the worsening contagion. He made efforts to inspect 'suspected Soldiers and Travellers' and those with the pox were quarantined.[36] Similar steps were taken in Virginia, where rumours of smallpox and typhus were likely to induce panic (unlike dysentery and various fevers which were accepted as part of life). The shacks of smallpox sufferers were burnt after their recovery or death and 'pest houses' were opened in the towns.[37]

There was an understanding that soldiers and civilians of different ethnicities were not equally vulnerable to disease. David Ramsay, a respected American physician who served as a surgeon in the War, observed that the disorders of the black population in Carolina differed from those of the whites.

'The treatment of blacks labouring under these novel diseases puzzled the physicians; for the symptoms were so various in different attacks that the best informed could not always trust former experiences, and were sometimes obliged in the first cases to grope their way.'[38]

Duffy states that epidemics in the colonies affected blacks much the same as whites but accounts of the War suggest an excess mortality in black soldiers and slaves, particularly due to smallpox.[39] The distressing epidemics of smallpox affecting Lord Dunmore's Ethiopian Regiment in 1775–76 and in Virginia in 1781 have been described. Thomas Jefferson later estimated that out of 30,000 Virginian slaves who had joined the British, about 27,000 perished from infectious disorders.[40] Blacks under British protection in the South were not inoculated and they were often denied medical treatment, being simply expelled from the ranks.[41] Serving black soldiers in the American lines were included in the mass inoculations. Nevertheless, they were probably also more affected by the pox than their white comrades. When smallpox broke out in the Rhode Island Regiment in the winter of 1781–82, the black troops suffered a higher mortality rate, approximately 58 per cent of the total deaths in November and December.[42]

Jefferson attributed the large number of deaths in the black slaves who joined the British Army to a combination of smallpox and 'camp fever'.[43] Typhus was also a major killer. In his *Observations* of diseases occurring in the American hospitals, Benjamin Rush wrote that, 'Those black soldiers who had been previously slaves, died in a greater proportion by this fever [typhus], or had a much slower recovery from it, than the same number of white soldiers'.[44]

Sick black soldiers had access to the Continental Army's hospitals and medical treatments.[45] They also had their own medical culture. The sporadic and low-quality 'physicking' administered to slaves by lay plantation owners encouraged a self-reliance and an enduring confidence in traditional West

African medical practices. Many slaves, and presumably black soldiers, took their medical care into their own hands. So active was this movement in the eighteenth century, that colonial lawmakers approved legislation in 1748 designed to curb the number of slaves claiming to be doctors and dispensing drugs.[46]

Benjamin Rush took a keen interest in American Indian diseases and medicine.[47] His statement in his *Observations* that American Indians were 'more sickly' than the natives of Europe might be regarded as an understatement.[48] The horrific disease mortality suffered by the American Indian population during the Revolutionary War was just part of a larger and long-standing biological catastrophe. European and African people brought with them Old World diseases previously unknown in America. These included smallpox, plague, measles, tuberculosis, influenza, and yellow fever.[49] The impact of these newly arrived diseases during the years of the Revolution is well summarised by historian Colin Calloway.

> 'An epidemic swept away many Schoharie Mohawks in 1775; another appears to have been present in Shawnee villages in 1776. Smallpox raged at Onondaga in the winter of 1776–7, struck Indians wintering near Michilimackinac in 1777, was killing Creeks and Cherokees again in 1783. It visited the Oneida refugees at Schenectady in December 1780 and hit the Genesee Senecas the following winter. Smallpox reduced the Wyandots to a hundred warriors by 1781. Cold and disease killed three hundred Indians in the refugee camps at Niagara in the winter of 1779–80. While redcoats and rebels killed each other by the hundreds on the eastern seaboard, a huge smallpox pandemic slaughtered Indian people by the thousands in western America. Between 1779 and 1782 the contagion, which also ravaged central Mexico and the Guatemalan highlands, travelled north across the Rockies and the plains, then spread into the forests of eastern Canada.'[50]

Eyewitness accounts confirm very high mortality rates. Fur-trader Samuel Hearne estimated that the epidemic of 1781 caused the deaths of 'nine-tenths' of the Chipewyan Indians northwest of Hudson Bay. A worker of the North West Company believed the same pestilence to have killed 'three fourths' of the American Indians of the Canadian plains.[51] American government records show fatalities among various American Indian peoples to range from 55 to more than 90 per cent.[52]

The central reason for this frightening mortality was the American Indians' lack of resistance to the imported infectious diseases. Not only did they mostly have little acquired immunity, but their previous isolation from the plagues of Europe also meant that they had not undergone the necessary genetic adaptions necessary for significant 'innate immunity', a group of biological characteristics giving some disease protection.[53]

American Indian medicine had made several notable advances independent of the Old World. These included the use of cotton and rubber in surgery, methods of manipulation in childbirth, and the use of anaesthetics and antiseptics.[54] However, some interventions were likely to have been harmful. Scottish doctor John Ferdinand Dalziel Smith toured America in 1784. He witnessed the American Indians of Carolina attempting to ward off smallpox.

> 'Their injudicious treatment of that infectious malady generally renders it fatal, for they make use of hot stimulating medicines to promote a most profuse diaphoresis [sweating], in the height of which, while reeking with sweat and dissolving in streams of warm moisture, they rush out into the open air, quite naked, and suddenly plunge in to the deepest and coldest stream of running water that can be found, immersing their whole body in the chilling flood.'[55]

These misguided practices were not unique to American Indian medicine. The 'antiphlogistic' regimens used by the military and civilian doctors of the period commonly included cold-water therapies and the administration of drugs to induce sweating.

An analysis of the total disease-related losses of the War leads naturally to a discussion of the possible impact of disease on the outcome of the conflict. The thinning of the ranks by infectious diseases inevitably reduced the military effectiveness of individual regiments and even whole armies. Although disease deaths were greatest in the Continental Army, the British Army was most vulnerable. Whereas the American leaders might be prepared to subject their mostly short-service troops to high levels of deprivation and risk of disease, the need to preserve the Crown's forces so far from home exerted a restraining influence on the British. They could not afford to lose men to sickness in the same proportion as their enemy.[56]

In addition to its direct impact on morbidity and mortality, disease could also deter enlistment and increase desertion. This was especially so in the rebel army where there was a widespread fear of smallpox and other disorders. In July 1776, Connecticut governor Jonathan Trumbull wrote to Washington informing him that 'Fear of the infection operates strongly to prevent soldiers from engaging in the service'. As a result, the colony's battalions were only filling up slowly.[57]

Once soldiers joined the ranks, the sight of their fellows perishing from disease was a powerful inducement to desert. Horatio Gates wrote to Washington in August 1776 from Ticonderoga; 'The very great desertion rate from this Army has, I believe, been principally occasioned by the dread of the smallpox'. He was concerned that he would not be able to retain soldiers for another campaign.[58] In the South in later years, Greene's men threatened to desert rather than having to serve through another fever season. An officer warned the commander that some would prefer to face a military court than risk the 'destructive climate'.[59] A reluctance to enlist and a propensity to desert may have been further encouraged by Continental Army orders against inoculation. During the periods when these applied, troops faced disciplining for trying to protect themselves.[60]

Individual afflictions might have disproportionate effects. When senior commanders and inspirational officers fell seriously ill this potentially caused a leadership vacuum. Conversely, infection may on occasion have conveniently removed an incompetent officer from the field.

Disease had an erosive effect on both sides during the years of fighting but there are particularly two campaigns where it can be argued that that it was a major factor in the denouement. Firstly, the failed American invasion of Canada in 1775–76 and, secondly, Cornwallis's defeat in the South.

It was the contemporary American view that disease, and especially smallpox, was largely responsible for their Canadian debacle. John Adams declared that smallpox had been 'ten times more terrible than the Britons, Canadians, and Indians together'. It was, he continued, the cause of the precipitate retreat from Quebec. General Gates complained that the disease had 'entirely ruined' the army and a subsequent Congressional Committee investigation into the defeat in Canada concluded that a 'still greater, and more fatal, source of misfortune has been the prevalence of smallpox in the army; a great proportion whereof has thereby been usually kept unfit for duty'.[61]

This opinion was supported by the heavy mortality of smallpox (see Chapter 5) and its undoubted role in impeding recruitment and encouraging desertion. The troops' fear of the disorder created a vicious spiral of unsupervised self-inoculation unaccompanied by quarantine. Smallpox invaded the ranks and the rebel army's commanders lost control of the health and wellbeing of their men.[62] The shortage of experienced physicians with the expeditionary force meant that good medical advice was hard to find.[63] When Montgomery made the doomed assault on Quebec in December 1775, there were 200–300 men sick and only 800 fit for duty. His decision to bring forward the attack may have been influenced by the destructive effects of *Variola*.[64]

Smallpox might have changed some operational decisions but was it the main reason for the American reverse in Canada? Ann Becker, who has made a study of the strategic implications of smallpox in the American Army of the War, believed it to be significant; 'Contemporary evidence is overwhelming: smallpox destroyed the Northern Army and all hope of persuading the Canadians to join the Revolution'.[65] Other historians have disagreed regarding the role of smallpox, one believing it to be 'the greatest contributing factor' in the failed invasion and another thinking it 'of little consequence' at the time of the pivotal attack on Quebec.[66] Although smallpox was obviously deleterious to the American effort, the disaster was at least as much caused by purely military factors. Historian Rick Atkinson describes a botched operation 'laden with miscalculation and marred by mishap'.[67] Smallpox contributed to American failure, but it was only one factor. The disease had shown itself to be a real danger to the American forces in the remainder of the War.[68]

The very substantial losses of Cornwallis's Army in the South have been described in chapters 11 to 13. Disease, particularly malaria, was perhaps more harmful to the British than the arms of the patriots. Contemporary accounts suggest that the unremittingly high level of sickness impacted on several operational decisions. Cornwallis's resolution to fight the Battle of Camden was at least in part because a retreat would have left many sick in the hands of the rebels.[69] His intended advance into North Carolina was delayed by the struggle to secure sufficient wagons to carry soldiers too ill to march. The commissary was ill and his position filled by an aide-de-camp.[70] John Macnamara Hayes claimed that sickness was the main reason for the rebels' hold on the colony.[71] The fateful transfer to Virginia was made as only by moving north could Cornwallis 'hope to preserve the troops, from the fatal sickness, which so nearly ruined the army last autumn'.[72] Once entrenched at Yorktown, he was reluctant to evacuate the place as this would have meant abandoning 800 sick.[73] He later invoked high levels of sickness in his men as a reason for surrender.[74]

The British suffered not only from much sickness in the ranks but also from the debilitating effects of illness in the army's upper echelons. Many valued senior officers were struck down by the Southern fevers. The depressing list includes Augustine Prevost, John Maitland, Banastre Tarleton, William Phillips, Alexander Leslie, Lord Rawdon, and Cornwallis himself. The temporary loss of Tarleton's services, due to a severe fever contracted in September 1781, caused near panic, such was his reputation. His perceived irreplaceability may have contributed to Ferguson's defeat at King's Mountain, Cornwallis later stating that Tarleton's absence was a reason for his decision not to send reinforcements. Cornwallis was also ill, and it is possible that his judgement and communication were both impaired. For more than a fortnight he was too incapacitated to write and was hardly able to move.[75] He must have relied on his staff, but they were often much depleted. In late August 1780, every high-ranking officer in Cornwallis's command was unfit for duty.[76]

All this appears to make a cogent case for fever being the British Army's greatest enemy in the region. Two historians who have made the most detailed medical studies of the campaign, Peter McCandless and Paul Kopperman, both fully acknowledge the destructive effects of disease on Cornwallis's forces, but they are reluctant to cite it as the central determinant of British failure.[77] The notoriously unhealthy South was poisonous to British troops but, as for the Americans in Canada, the humiliation of Yorktown had wider causes. The uncoordinated British high command made repeated poor decisions and underestimated American and French resolve. The loyalist waves of support never materialised, and Cornwallis had too few men and resources to succeed. Disease tortured an army already destined for defeat.

Chapter 15

Medicine and the American Revolution

In this concluding chapter, the impact of the Revolution on the development of military medicine and the also on the state of civilian medicine in America is assessed. Parallels are drawn between the medical challenges of the late eighteenth century and the twenty-first century.

At the commencement of hostilities, the British Army at least had a functioning medical department, but its efficacy was limited by wider contemporary views on disease causation and treatment. In the first half of the eighteenth century, medical advancement was stalled by misguided theories, 'metaphysical speculations' which led astray the most powerful intellects.[1] As the century unfolded, there were some systematic changes which offered the possibility of improvement in war medicine. As Garrison points out in his classic *Notes on the History of Military Medicine*, the administration of medical care to soldiers became a definite function of government and army medical departments also profited from the eighteenth-century culture of formal systems and better described routine.[2] The work of James Lind and others anticipated a more logical approach to the assessment of medical therapy.[3]

In her review of British medicine in the Seven Years War (1756–1763), Erica Charters argues that although there was administrative change, and some lessons from previous wars, there was no great medical innovation arising out of the European campaigns. If there was progress, it was in the form of a gradual transformation through the frequent experience of warfare.[4] This narrative – a lack of 'decisive change' – may be extended to the British Army medical department of the American Revolutionary War. There was adaptation to colonial warfare but no obvious fundamental reform. Lack of money was probably the single most vital factor. Potentially beneficial interventions such as increased medical salaries were expensive and the authorities at home were satisfied to maintain the status quo.[5]

The British were not again involved in major conflict in North America until the War of 1812. Poor medical practice persisted in British garrisons in the country until the mid-nineteenth century. This suggests that the Revolutionary War led to little long-term health benefit for British soldiers in the region.[6] When John Hunter became surgeon general in 1790, his priority was to improve the quality of the regimental surgeons who had been criticised during the American War. This was no easy task, Hunter himself commenting that 'It is hardly necessary for a regimental surgeon to practice in the army anything of surgery'.[7] The neglect of the British Army's medical services continued through the French Revolutionary, Napoleonic and Crimean Wars.

It was inevitable that the Continental Army's medical department would mostly emulate the services of European armies and especially that of its protagonist. The embryonic department of 1775 was born out of a country which had only rudimentary medical provision. At the onset of the fighting, colonial laws relating to 'physic' had limited influence on the qualifications of practitioners or the limits of their practice. Apprenticeships were poorly regulated and the early examining boards of doubtful quality, some lacking any medical members. There were only two medical colleges, in Philadelphia and New York, and only one State medical society, that of New Jersey. The existence of these institutions reflected some improvement in the status of American medicine in the immediate pre-War years (see also Chapter 1).[8]

Under the circumstances, it was an achievement to rapidly create a credible medical service for the fledgling American Army. It is also the case that opportunities for improvement were missed. Congress was unable to decide the best form of supervision for the newly formed department and its functioning was compromised by constant disputes between army doctors and the chronic shortages of drugs, hospital supplies, and surgical instruments.[9]

The period between the end of the Revolutionary War and the War of 1812 was a nadir in the history of the medical services of the United States Army. According to Gillett, physicians were 'unable to offer their patients anything of a value to rival that of their compassion and concern'.[10] The concept of a regular standing army was suspect and during these years there was reliance on militia and volunteer units. Such a limited force did not require a formal medical department and there was no proper central organisation, any suggested structure existing mostly on paper. The legislation of 1799 was not much enacted but the inclusion of more explicit lines of medical responsibility, the better-defined relationship between medical and army officers, the more detailed directions for hospital discipline and sanitation, the creation of medical boards to examine candidates, and the inclusion of a purveyor, all suggest that the failures of the Revolutionary War had not been entirely forgotten.[11]

Writing in 1781, British surgeon John Ranby outlined a scheme for the management of wounded in battle. He proposed that all the surgeons of every three to four regiments be grouped together in the rear where they could give immediate care. By treating the wounded 'on the spot' there would be less need to convey the injured 'from place to place, under the extreme misery of large, lacerated wounds, bleeding arteries, or fractured limbs'. The more distant removal of badly wounded soldiers was, he explained, 'preposterous' and a cause of 'terrible distress'.[12]

There was other well-meaning guidance pertaining to battlefield medicine, notably John Morgan's written instructions to American regimental surgeons in 1776, but the management of casualties in both armies remained haphazard. Indeed, there was still no proper evacuation system in place during the Napoleonic period. British surgeon William Fergusson enviously compared the British arrangements with the French; 'Our means of transporting sick and wounded have ever been deficient and cruel'.[13] American surgeon James Mann was aware of Dominique Larrey's flying ambulance but, in the War of 1812, he was forced to improvise, the wounded and sick moved in litters made of blankets hung from poles, and in local wagons and sleighs.[14]

In the eighteenth century, there was a tendency for general hospitals to improve during wars. This is unsurprising as the hospitals were reduced during periods of peace and had to be rapidly re-established at the recommencement of hostilities.[15] British hospitals in the Revolutionary War no doubt benefitted from this sudden concentration of resources but, as for battlefield medicine, one searches in vain for real and sustained systematic improvement. Requisitioned buildings were often of poor quality and too small, and staffing was still mostly left to chance, the lack of a professional nursing corps leading to the employment of untrained soldiers' wives and orderlies.[16] Few lessons were learnt. In the Flanders Campaign of 1793, British soldiers dreaded admission to the general hospital; 'Ah, poor fellow, we shall see thee no more for thou art under orders for the shambles!'.[17]

There was some development of American general hospitals during the Revolutionary War although James Tilton's assertion that 'the success of the hospitals was much improved' was perhaps overly optimistic.[18] As for the

British, any gains were short-lived. Eyewitness accounts of the hospitals of the War of 1812 are reminiscent of those of the Revolution, naked men packed together on cold ground in a 'wretched condition'. Where good hospitals existed, this appeared more due to the initiatives of individual physicians than to any wider change.[19] Whatever their state, the army hospitals of the Revolution were clearly necessary. The war had underlined their importance and was followed by a rapid expansion of civilian hospitals through the colonies.[20] There was also a rapid increase in the number of hospitals in Britain in the later years of George III's rule although this was more due to local factors than events across the Atlantic.[21]

The Revolution lacked a great army surgeon, a man of the stature of Dominique Larrey. No novel surgical techniques emerged despite a growing interest in the practice of surgery.[22] During the eighteenth century, 500 anatomical works were published in Britain.[23] Although there was no dramatic step forward in battle surgery, there was, as in other areas of army medicine, a continuum of slow learning. The Revolutionary War was fought in an era when surgical controversies – for instance the optimal methodology and timing of amputation – were being debated by European surgeons such as Henri François Le Dran, Jean Faure, John Ranby and Johann Ulrich Bilguer. Many of these questions were still unresolved at the outbreak of the French Revolutionary Wars in the 1790s.[24]

The American Revolutionary War, like other conflicts, provided unparalleled opportunities to operate on wounded men. Such ample surgical practice must have led to improvements in anatomical knowledge and surgical skill.[25] Independent of remote debates regarding surgical interventions, ordinary army surgeons reached their own conclusions. Tilton's comment that amputations became less common may have been just one example of everyday practice changing on the front line.[26]

The most experienced operators attempted complex procedures. John Warren successfully performed the first amputation at the shoulder joint in America.[27] Some would eventually document their more modest efforts. Surgeon Barnabas Binney submitted a report of his conservative management of an abdominal musket ball wound in 1782 to the *New York Medical and Physical Journal* of 1828. Binney concluded, very likely correctly, that 'the case was one in which the officiousness of the surgeon might have done great injury'.[28]

Although American surgeons remained indebted to the more mature military experience of British and French medical officers, a distinct

American surgical culture was appearing. John Jones's text of 1776 was largely a compilation of European views, but it was noteworthy as being both a useful surgical manual and the first surgical textbook published in America. Jones, who had previous army experience in the French and Indian War, expressed his ambition in a dedication. He had 'endeavoured to select the sentiments of the best modern surgeons upon the treatment of those accidents, which are most likely to attend our present unnatural contest'.[29]

An itinerary for an American surgeon's medicine chest drawn up in 1776 contains the following list of drugs; twenty-six botanicals, five of animal origin, twenty-three chemicals, three tinctures, four spirits, five ointments, and eight miscellaneous products.[30] Only a handful of these agents had any efficacy (e.g. bark, opiates) and many were harmful. There was, however, progress in the standardisation and production of medicines and in the development of pharmacopoeias. Authors such as Thomas Dickson Reide and Gerhard van Swieten appended 'formulas' and 'recipes' to their monographs on the diseases of armies, thus better defining the nature of individual drugs and preparations.[31] Dr William Brown's *Lititz Pharmacopoeia* of 1778 was an emergency American military hospital formulary. It was produced in a manner 'especially adapted to our poverty and straightened circumstances, and by the ferocious inhumanity of the enemy'. The author also explained that it contained two types of formulae. One was those medicaments which had to be produced in a 'general laboratory' and the second was those which could be mixed on demand in hospital dispensaries.[32] The manufacture of drugs at army laboratories in 1778 in Philadelphia eventually led to large-scale American production in the city. Brown's work was to spawn other American pharmacopoeias in the early nineteenth century.[33]

The Revolution also provided a stimulus for the recognition of the distinct role of the American apothecary, twenty-five of whom fought in the war. They became increasingly responsible for drug standards and for the preparation and dispensing of medication. In 1784, former Tory pharmacist Thomas Atwood of New York City advertised for 'a man of abilities', one who must 'understand pharmacy thoroughly, and should be grounded in chemistry'.[34]

Apart from the specific initiatives taken to prevent the spread of smallpox (to which we shall return), there were the broader measures to enforce the principles of 'military hygiene', well understood from the works of Pringle, Monro, and Brocklesby. American army doctors and senior officers such as Rush and Steuben spread the word in their writings. They had a powerful ally in Washington, a man who was both abstemious in his own habits and forward-thinking regarding the possible sources of contagion (see also Chapter 3). His orders of the War contain frequent references to the importance of hygiene. As early as July 1775, general orders specify that '[n]ext to cleanliness, nothing is more conducive to a Soldier's health, than dressing his provisions in a decent and proper manner'.[35] No detail was too small. Three years later, he notes, again in general orders, 'that notwithstanding there is three Women who draw Rations... the men receive no benefit by Washing from them'.[36] Such interventions must have saved lives although modern historians have tended to play down the impact of preventative measures in the American Revolutionary Army, choosing to stress the impediments of a lack of engagement of the officer class and ignorance of the regulations.[37]

British doctors faced similar challenges. Most military officers were aware of the need to promote regulations pertaining to hygiene. This is reflected by the importance attached to the construction of privies as the first task in a new camp or town. Attempts were made to enforce the rules, for instance sentries patrolling barracks to prevent the soldiers relieving themselves in the living quarters and stairways. According to Marshall, these laudable efforts were often undermined by the military realities of the War, the scarcity of good accommodation, and the concentration of large numbers of troops in cramped urban areas. Above all, successful prevention was limited by ignorance, the British Army 'fighting blind-folded' against the disease-causing organisms pursuing it.[38]

Attempts were made to better understand disease and to improve treatment. In the second half of the eighteenth century, it was becoming apparent that 'arithmetic' might be applied to clinical medicine.[39] Thomas Dickson Reide declared that 'Theory is a rock on which too many practitioners split'. He demanded 'proper registers of diseases' to allow the comparison of the efficacy of different therapies.[40] The concept of 'trials' was not novel. In the Seven Years War, the British navy's Sick and Hurt Board oversaw a surprisingly sophisticated system of trial supervision. A small trial in a hospital ashore might be eventually extended to a widely administered trial at sea, dependent on surgeons' evaluations and reports. Results were disappointing but the procedures were standardised and scientific.[41]

British army doctors undertook simple trials of drug treatment during the Revolutionary War. These arose partly from necessity. Richard McCausland had been stationed at Niagara since 1774 as surgeon in the 8th Regiment of

Foot. Between 1775 and 1781, there were shortages of Peruvian bark and McCausland instead treated intermittent fevers (presumably mainly malaria) with tartar emetic in the form of pills or solutions. He later reported in *Duncan's Medical Commentaries* that tartar emetic was more effective than Peruvian bark and that the pills were the best preparation. He justified his conclusions in statistical tables; the ratio of cures to relapses was 4:1 for tartar emetic and approximately 2:1 for bark. Commendably, McCausland was cautious in his interpretation of the results, noting possible confounding factors such as the season and the loss of some patients to follow up. He emphasised the dangers of drawing conclusions from a limited number of experiments. Unlike Lind's earlier trials of treatments for scurvy, McCausland's study was retrospective. The apparent lack of efficacy of bark very likely reflected the variable anti-malarial properties of different preparations.[42]

Robert Robertson entered the Royal Navy's medical department as a surgeon's mate in 1760 and served in both the Seven Years War and the American War. When he was surgeon on HMS *Juno* in 1776, his supply of bark ran out and he was forced to treat 'ship fever' (probably mainly typhus) with other methods including antimony preparations, camphor, and blisters. In statistical tables, Robertson demonstrated that whereas there were six deaths among the 296 patients of the latter group (2 per cent), there was only one death in 216 fever patients (0.5 per cent) who had received bark. These figures referred to sailors treated on board the *Juno*, excluding the sixty-two men sent ashore to New York and Rhode Island. In these hospitals, bark was also in short supply and patients treated with antimonial preparations or camphor had a death rate of 15 per cent. Based on these combined results, Robertson became an advocate of early and ample administration of bark in a wide range of fevers. He believed his methods to have given 'proof' of the superiority of bark and he would only submit to objections based on similar large comparative trials.[43]

American medical science was in its early years, and it was variably affected by the War. Scientific activity probably fell away because of the interruption of professional and personal connections with Europe. Foreign academic books and journals were suddenly more difficult to obtain and learned societies lost momentum. More positively, the War allowed doctors of the thirteen states to come together to share new experiences.[44]

Whereas American army doctors may not have embraced 'medical arithmetic' to the same extent as their British counterparts, there was understanding of the need for therapeutic innovation. In 1765, John Morgan encouraged physicians to 'dive into the bottom of things' by experiments.[45] Continental Army doctors committed their ideas and research to paper. Beyond the widely read monographs of Benjamin Rush, John Jones and James Tilton, there were the case reports of Ebenezer Beardsley and Barnabas Binney. Less well known, but not lacking in ambition, was Pennsylvania regimental surgeon Hugh Martin's *A Narrative of a Discovery of a Sovereign Specific for the Cure of Cancers*, published in Philadelphia in 1782.

In addition to their purely medical contributions, American doctors played prominent military and political roles in the Revolution. Many were dedicated patriots. Six doctors signed the Declaration of Independence, and others became brigadiers (e.g. Hugh Mercer) and major generals (e.g. Joseph Warren).[46] This medical influence persisted in the formative years of the new Republic. Of the first seven commanders of the United States Army, three had been educated as physicians, and three medical men served as early secretaries of war. Others became governors of states and filled all positions of senior rank except that of President. Duncan's claim that the American doctors of the Revolution played a more vital role than the doctors of any other war is credible.[47] It must be remembered, however, that history is largely written by the victors. Not all American medical men were winners. Most leading doctors in New York were Tories or loyalists.[48]

Just as America's doctors helped fashion the Revolution, the seismic political and military events of the period impacted on the development of medicine in the country. Several factors promoted professionalisation. As previously alluded to in the discussion of American science, army surgeons from isolated parts of America were able to meet with other military medical officers to exchange ideas. A list of doctors practising in Philadelphia in 1783 contains the names of twenty-three who had served in the Continental Army.[49] Some French and British surgeons remained to practice after the War.[50] The immediate result was a breach in medical provincialism and the encouragement of progressive thinking. The conflict had demonstrated the value of examination boards for doctors and, because of the military experience, several states soon enacted legislation to protect the public from incompetents and quacks. The opening of new medical colleges reduced the traditional dependence on Edinburgh for advanced medical training. There was a sudden profusion of medical societies and American medical journals. The War had begun to break down the Old-World dominance of medical science.[51]

It must also be conceded that any improvement in medicine in the early years of the Republic was slow and fragile. The 'professional euphoria' of medical men such as Benjamin Rush and the optimism of the medically aware founders – George and Martha Washington, Benjamin Franklin, Thomas Jefferson, John and Abigail Adams, and James and Dolly Maddison – was quickly diluted.[52] The army doctors who returned to civilian practice still tackled diseases with 'the lancet, the purge, the expectorant, and the blister'.[53] Their heroic and ineffectual remedies were challenged by American citizens and the profession risked losing respect. Historian Ronald L. Numbers describes American medicine of the mid-nineteenth century as a 'shambles'. Despite Washington's significant preventative health initiatives of the War, government was slow to enact national public health measures. The epidemics of the early Republic led to limited reform and Congress only created the short-lived National Board of Health in 1879.[54]

The American founders would no doubt approve of the transformation in modern medicine with its deep understanding of disease mechanisms and increasingly targeted and successful therapies. These profound advances should not obscure the parallels between the medical practices of the Revolution and today, particularly with respect to the control of epidemics.

Quarantine and inoculation for smallpox were the two great preventative interventions of the War but neither was easy to regulate or enforce, especially on the American side. Obligatory quarantine was unpopular, and the authorities had to take decisive steps to maintain it; by the late 1700s, Pennsylvania was the only state not using local quarantine laws.[55] Inoculation engendered much fear and was even more resisted. When Cotton Mather supported its use in Boston in 1721, his home was fire-bombed. Sceptical American colonists rioted and closed inoculation hospitals.[56] The risks of inoculation were obvious and even its supporters were cautious. Martha Washington expressed anxiety at the possibility of her son succumbing to smallpox after inoculation in 1771 and it was another five years before she was inoculated.[57]

Strategies were employed by civilian and military leaders to refine quarantine and promote inoculation. The 'six-feet rule' was just one form of isolation; a family with an infected member had to hang a six-foot pole carrying a red cloth from a public part of the house. Communities closed schools during smallpox outbreaks.[58] At least some American soldiers received certificates attesting to official inoculation. Enforcement was variable. Washington's mass-inoculations were apparently compulsory and there is no evidence of large-scale refusal.[59] The British Army instituted a voluntary inoculation programme in Boston in 1775, those soldiers who refused being quarantined. On other occasions, for instance in Canada in 1776, it was made mandatory.[60]

These efforts at disease control have resonance, being strikingly similar to the strategies of isolation and vaccination employed against the Covid-19 pandemic of the early twenty-first century. The two viral diseases are distinct in their symptomatology and mortality, and Covid-19 vaccination is a much safer procedure than smallpox inoculation. Even so, the choices which had to be made by the politicians, soldiers and doctors of the Revolution are not much different to those faced by societies 250 years later.

Notes

Chapter 1

1. Jones, *Medicine in Virginia in Revolutionary Times*, p. 253.
2. Abrams, *Revolutionary Medicine*, p. 9.
3. Shryock, *Medicine and Society in America*, pp. 96, 111.
4. Brownlee, *The Health of London in the Eighteenth Century*, p. 76.
5. Abrams, *Revolutionary Medicine*, pp. 9, 13.
6. Chaplin, *Medicine in England during the Reign of George III*, p. 8; Shryock, *Medicine and Society in America*, pp. 2–4; Kaufman, *Surgeons at War*, p. 8.
7. Chaplin, *Medicine in England during the Reign of George III*, pp. 8–9.
8. Chaplin, *Medicine in England during the Reign of George III*, p. 20.
9. Blanco, *Physician of the American Revolution*, p. 17.
10. Shryock, *Medicine and Society in America*, p. 7.
11. Blanco, *Medicine in the Continental Army*, pp. 678–9.
12. Cash, *Medical Men at the Siege of Boston*, pp. 1–2.
13. Abrams, *Revolutionary Medicine*, p. 13.
14. Blanco, *Medicine in the Continental Army*, pp. 677–8; Duffy, *Epidemics in Colonial America*, p. 7.
15. Blanco, *Physician of the American Revolution*, p. 17.
16. Blanco, *Physician of the American Revolution*, p. 17.
17. Blanco, *Medicine in the Continental Army*, p. 679.
18. Blanco, *Medicine in the Continental Army*, pp. 700–1.
19. Duncan, *Medical Men in the American Revolution*, p. 19.
20. Corner, *The Autobiography of Benjamin Rush*, p. 112.
21. Lind, *An Essay on Diseases*, p. 15.
22. Cash, *Medical Men at the Siege of Boston*, p. 10; Tröhler, *To Improve the Evidence of Medicine*, p. 23.
23. Tröhler, *To Improve the Evidence of Medicine*, pp. 23–4.
24. Pringle, *Observations of the Diseases of the Army*, pp. 70–1.

25. Duffy, *Epidemics in Colonial America*, pp. 202, 232, 237–8, 243–4.
26. Howard, *Wellington's Doctors*, p. 182.
27. Monro, *An Account of the Diseases*, p. 58.
28. Jackson, *A Treatise on the Fevers of Jamaica*, pp. 77–8.
29. Abrams, *Revolutionary Medicine*, p. 89.
30. Dickson Reide, *A View of the Diseases of the Army*, pp. 14–15.
31. Jackson, *A Treatise on the Fevers of Jamaica*, p. 101.
32. Rush, *Medical Inquiries and Observations*, p. 209.
33. Howard, *Wellington's Doctors*, p. 162.
34. Shryock, *Medicine and Society in America*, p. 52.
35. Griffenhagen, *Drug Supplies in the American Revolution*, pp. 126–7.
36. Abrams, *Revolutionary Medicine*, p. 16.
37. Rush, *Medical Inquiries and Observations*, p. 211.
38. Dickson Reide, *A View of the Diseases of the Army*, p. xi.
39. *Advice to the Officers of the British Army*, pp. 59–60.
40. Shryock, *Medicine and Society in America*, pp. 97–8.
41. Frey, *The British Soldier in America*, p. 41.
42. Simes, *The Military Guide for Young Officers*, p. 213.
43. Fenn, *Pox Americana*, pp. 29–30.
44. Dohla, *A Hessian Diary of the American Revolution*, p. 97.
45. Fenn, *Pox Americana*, pp. 31–3.
46. Gibson, *Bodo Otto and the Medical Background of the American Revolution*, pp. 84–5.
47. Fenn, *Pox Americana*, pp. 93–4.
48. Kopperman, *The British Army in North America*, p. 69.
49. Gooch, *A Practical Treatise on Wounds*, vol. 1, p. 95.
50. Kaufman, *Surgeons at War*, p. 9; Blanco, *Physician of the American Revolution*, pp. 43–4; Gillett, *The Army Medical Department*, p. 15.
51. Ravitch, *Surgery in 1776*, p. 293; Griesemer, *John Jones MD*, pp. 605–8.
52. Garrison, *Notes on the History of Military Medicine*, p. 137.
53. Hume, *1775: Another Part of the Field*, p. 436.
54. Hunter, *A Treatise on the Blood, Inflammation and Gun-shot wounds*, pp. 525–6.
55. Howard, *Wellington's Doctors*, pp. 126–7; Blanco, *Physician of the American Revolution*, p. 72; Duncan, *Medical Men in the American Revolution*, p. 12.
56. Hughes, *Firepower*, p. 29.

57. Spring, *With Zeal and with Bayonets Only*, p. 192.
58. Ranby, *Nature and Treatment of Gunshot Wounds*, pp. 37–8.
59. Jones, *Plain Concise Practical Remarks*, pp. 15–16, 21.
60. Gooch, *A Practical Treatise on Wounds*, vol. 1, p. 96.
61. Thacher, *Military Journal during the American Revolution*, p. 192.
62. Hamilton, *The duties of a regimental surgeon considered*, vol. 1, pp. 254–5.
63. Ranby, *Nature and Treatment of Gunshot Wounds*, pp. 4–10.
64. Jones, *Plain Concise Practical Remarks*, p. 17.
65. Jones, *Plain Concise Practical Remarks*, p. 19.
66. Hunter, *A Treatise on the Blood, Inflammation and Gun-shot wounds*, pp. 563–4.
67. Jones, *Plain Concise Practical Remarks*, pp. 30–56.
68. Tröhler, *To Improve the Evidence of Medicine*, p. 97.
69. Tilton, *Economical observations on Military Hospitals*, p. 62.
70. Tröhler, *To Improve the Evidence of Medicine*, p.96.
71. Ranby, *Nature and Treatment of Gunshot Wounds*, pp. 29–30.
72. Hunter, *A Treatise on the Blood, Inflammation and Gun-shot wounds*, p. 562.
73. Jones, *Plain Concise Practical Remarks*, pp. 58–62.
74. Wooden, *The Wounds and Weapons of the Revolutionary War*, p. 64.
75. Johnson, *Uzal Johnson, Loyalist*, p. 61.
76. Hunter, *A Treatise on the Blood, Inflammation and Gun-shot wounds*, pp. 551–2; Jones, *Plain Concise Practical Remarks*, p. 28.
77. Hunter, *A Treatise on the Blood, Inflammation and Gun-shot wounds*, p. 543.
78. Sabourin, *The War of Independence: a surgical algorithm for treatment of head injury*, pp. 236–41; Robertson, *Remarks on the Management of the Scalped-Head*, p. 28.
79. Lloyd, Coulter, *Medicine and the Navy 1200–1900*, vol. 3, p. 361.
80. Ranby, *Nature and Treatment of Gunshot Wounds*, p. 80.
81. Jones, *Plain Concise Practical Remarks*, p. 46.
82. Dickson Reide, *A View of the Diseases of the Army*, p. 164.
83. Tröhler, *To Improve the Evidence of Medicine*, p. 95.
84. Gillett, *The Army Medical Department*, p. 18.
85. Tröhler, *To Improve the Evidence of Medicine*, p. 100.
86. Brocklesby, *Oeconomical and Medical Observations*, pp. 105–6.
87. Pringle, *Observations on the Diseases of the Army*, p. 70.

88. Howard, *Wellington's Doctors*, p. 167.
89. Duffy, *Epidemics in Colonial America*, p. 229; Marshall, *Hygiene and Disease*, p. 314.
90. Monro, *An Account of the Diseases*, pp. 10–18.
91. Marshall, *Hygiene and Disease*, pp. 314–15.
92. Lenihan, *Fluxes, Fevers, and Fighting Men*, pp. 25–6.
93. Howard, *Wellington's Doctors*, p. 168.
94. Duffy, *Epidemics in Colonial America*, p. 221.
95. Van Swieten, *The Diseases Incident to Armies*, p. 68.
96. Tilton, *Economical observations on Military Hospitals*, p. 61.
97. Gillett, *The Army Medical Department*, pp. 4–5.
98. Tilton, *Economical observations on Military Hospitals*, 61.
99. Fenn, *Pox Americana*, pp. 16–18.
100. Dickson Reide, *A View of the Diseases of the Army*, p. 89.
101. Fenn, *Pox Americana*, pp. 27–8, 43.
102. Fenn, *Pox Americana*, p. 21.
103. Brocklesby, *Oeconomical and Medical Observations*, p. 232.
104. Fenn, *Pox Americana*, pp. 16, 108.
105. Duffy, *Epidemics in Colonial America*, p. 244.
106. Urban, *Fusilers*, p. 189.
107. Reiss, *Medicine and the American Revolution*, pp. 205–6.
108. Howard, *Wellington's Doctors*, pp. 161, 166.
109. Jackson, *A Treatise on the Fevers of Jamaica*, pp. 285–330.
110. Kiple, *Plague, Pox & Pestilence*, p. 68.
111. Van Swieten, *The Diseases Incident to Armies*, pp. 89–92.
112. Pringle, *Observations on the Diseases of the Army*, pp. 344–6.
113. Hamilton, *The duties of a regimental surgeon considered*, vol. 1, p. 71.
114. Duffy, *Epidemics in Colonial America*, p. 235; Stacy, *Venereal Disease*, p. 239.
115. Colombier, *Preceptes sur la Santé des gens de guerre*, p. 73.
116. Kopperman, *The Cheapest Pay*, p. 116.
117. Bloomfield, *Citizen Soldier*, p. 103.
118. Duffy, *Epidemics in Colonial America*, p. 162.
119. *Advice to Officers*, p. 38.
120. Van Swieten, *The Diseases Incident to Armies*, p. 7.
121. Hamilton, *The duties of a regimental surgeon considered*, vol. 1, p. 127.
122. Duncan, *Medical Men in the American Revolution*, p. 309.

123. Pringle, *Observations on the Diseases of the Army*, p. 123.

124. Colombier, *Preceptes sur la Santé des gens de guerre*, p. xxi.

125. Rush, *Medical Inquiries and Observations*, p. 214.

126. Marshall, *Hygiene and Disease*, p. 321.

127. Tröhler, *To Improve the Evidence of Medicine*, p. 115.

128. Dickson Reide, *A View of the Diseases of the Army*, p. 95.

129. Blanco, *Henry Marshall*, p. 260.

130. Marshall, *The Health of the British Soldier in America*, p. 9.

131. Toner, *The Medical Men of the Revolution*, p. 60.

132. Saffron, *Surgeon to Washington*, pp. 68–9, 112.

Chapter 2

1. Chaplin, *Medicine in England during the Reign of George III*, pp. 76–7.

2. Kopperman, *Medical Services in the British Army*, pp. 428–9.

3. Kopperman, *Medical Services in the British Army*, pp. 447–8; Marshall, *Surgeons Reconsidered*, p. 301.

4. Chaplin, *Medicine in England during the Reign of George III*, p. 77.

5. Cantlie, *A History of the Army Medical Department*, vol. 1, p. 103.

6. Cantlie, *A History of the Army Medical Department*, vol. 1, pp. 102–4.

7. Kopperman, *Medical Services in the British Army*, p. 451.

8. Drew, *Commissioned Officers in the Medical Services of the British Army*, pp. xxxviii–xxxix.

9. Frey, *The British Soldier in America*, p. 48.

10. Kopperman, *Medical Services in the British Army*, p. 433.

11. Cantlie, *A History of the Army Medical Department*, vol. 1, p. 149.

12. Howell, *The Story of the Army Surgeon*, p. 321

13. Kopperman, *The British Army in North America and the West Indies*, pp. 53–4.

14. Drew, *Commissioned Officers in the Medical Services of the British Army*, pp. 15–61; Marshall, *The Health of the British Soldier in America*, pp. 59–62.

15. Kopperman, *Medical Services in the British Army*, p. 450.

16. Frey, *The British Soldier in America*, p. 48.

17. Drew, *Commissioned Officers in the Medical Services of the British Army*, p. xxxvii; Cash, *Medical Men at the Siege of Boston*, p. 79.

18. Kopperman, *Medical Services in the British Army*, p. 431.

19. Cantlie, *A History of the Army Medical Department*, vol. 1, pp. 142–3.

20. Blanco, *The Prestige of British Army Surgeons*, p. 334.
21. Cantlie, *A History of the Army Medical Department*, vol. 1, p. 143.
22. Drew, *Commissioned Officers in the Medical Services of the British Army*, p. xxxv.
23. Kopperman, *Medical Services in the British Army*, p. 431.
24. Forster, *Diary of Thompson Forster*, p. 109.
25. Drew, *Commissioned Officers in the Medical Services of the British Army*, p. xxxii; Kopperman, *Medical Services in the British Army*, pp. 432, 434.
26. Marshall, *Surgeons Reconsidered*, p. 311.
27. Marshall, *Surgeons Reconsidered*, p. 311–12.
28. Cantlie, *A History of the Army Medical Department*, vol. 1, pp. 161–2.
29. Marshall, *Surgeons Reconsidered*, p. 312.
30. Marshall, *Surgeons Reconsidered*, p. 312–13.
31. Cantlie, *A History of the Army Medical Department*, vol. 1, p. 160.
32. Drew, *Commissioned Officers in the Medical Services of the British Army*, p. xxxiii.
33. Drew, *Commissioned Officers in the Medical Services of the British Army*, p. xxxiv; Blanco, *The Prestige of British Army Surgeons*, p. 334; Kopperman, *Medical Services in the British Army*, pp. 432, 434–5.
34. Curtis, *The Organization of the British Army in the American Revolution*, p. 10; Kopperman, *The British Army in North America and the West Indies*, p. 52.
35. Kopperman, *Medical Services in the British Army*, p. 445; Cash, *Medical Men at the Siege of Boston*, p. 73; Frey, *The British Soldier in America*, p. 49.
36. Frey, *The British Soldier in America*, pp. 49, 162; Drew, *Commissioned Officers in the Medical Services of the British Army*, p. 41.
37. Drew, *Commissioned Officers in the Medical Services of the British Army*, p. xxv; Kopperman, *Medical Services in the British Army*, pp. 443–4; Cash, *Medical Men at the Siege of Boston*, p. 75.
38. Kopperman, *The British Army in North America and the West Indies*, p. 56.
39. Hamilton, *The duties of a regimental surgeon considered*, vol. 1, pp. 5–6.
40. Kopperman, *Medical Services in the British Army*, p. 443.
41. Hamilton, *The duties of a regimental surgeon considered*, vol. 1, pp. 94–5; Kopperman, *Medical Services in the British Army*, p. 446.
42. Peebles, *John Peebles' American War*, pp. 290, 296.

43. Cash, *Medical Men at the Siege of Boston*, pp. 73–5.
44. Kopperman, *Medical Services in the British Army*, p. 445.
45. Kopperman, *Medical Services in the British Army*, p. 445–6; Marshall, *Surgeons Reconsidered*, pp. 305–6.
46. Marshall, *Surgeons Reconsidered*, p. 305.
47. Marshall, *Surgeons Reconsidered*, p. 305.
48. Frey, *The British Soldier in America*, p. 49.
49. Hamilton, *The duties of a regimental surgeon considered*, vol. 1, p. ii.
50. Hamilton, *The duties of a regimental surgeon considered*, vol. 1, pp. 139–40.
51. Kopperman, *Medical Services in the British Army*, p. 445.
52. Kopperman, *The British Army in North America and the West Indies*, pp. 57–8.
53. Hamilton, *The duties of a regimental surgeon considered*, vol. 1, pp. ii–iii.
54. Marshall, *Surgeons Reconsidered*, p. 300.
55. Blanco, *The Prestige of British Army Surgeons*, p. 336.
56. Kopperman, *The British Army in North America and the West Indies*, pp. 67–8.
57. Kopperman, *The British Army in North America and the West Indies*, p. 68.
58. *Advice to Officers of the British Army*, p. 58.
59. Lamb, *Memoir of his Own Life*, p. 290.
60. Lamb, *An Original and Authentic Journal*, pp. 338–9.
61. Cash, *Medical Men at the Siege of Boston*, pp. 78–9; Marshall, *Surgeons Reconsidered*, p. 303.
62. Monro, *Observations on the Means of Preserving the Health of Soldiers*, vol. 1, pp. 87–8.
63. Marshall, *Surgeons Reconsidered*, p. 301.
64. Pringle, *Observations on the Diseases of the Army*, p. 100.
65. Ranby, *Nature and Treatment of Gunshot Wounds*, p. 91.
66. Marshall, *Surgeons Reconsidered*, p. 301.
67. Jackson, *A Treatise on the Fevers of Jamaica*, pp. 420–4; Jackson, *A Systematic View*, pp. 54–60.
68. Marshall, *Surgeons Reconsidered*, p. 302.
69. Marshall, *Surgeons Reconsidered*, pp. 302–3.
70. Brocklesby, *Oeconomical and Medical Observations*, pp. 54–5.
71. Frey, *The British Soldier in America*, p. 50.
72. Howard, *Wellington's Doctors*, p. 117.
73. Kopperman, *Medical Services in the British Army*, pp. 436–9.

74. Kopperman, *Medical Services in the British Army*, p. 439.
75. Howe, *General Sir William Howe's Orderly Book*, pp. 30, 33; Guerra, *American Medical Bibliography*, pp. 567, 582.
76. Kopperman, *Medical Services in the British Army*, p. 440; Monro, *Observations on the Means of Preserving the Health of Soldiers*, vol. 1, pp. 121–4.
77. Cantlie, *A History of the Army Medical Department*, vol. 1, p. 156.
78. Monro, *Observations on the Means of Preserving the Health of Soldiers*, vol. 1, pp. 87–9.
79. Cantlie, *A History of the Army Medical Department*, vol. 1, pp. 144, 147; Kopperman, *Medical Services in the British Army*, pp. 428–9.
80. Hagist, *Noble Volunteers*, p. 210; Spring, *With Zeal and with Bayonets Only*, p. 159.
81. Lamb, *An Original and Authentic Journal*, p. 143.
82. Kopperman, *The British Army in North America and the West Indies*, p. 62.
83. Blanco, *Physician of the American Revolution*, pp. 153–4.
84. Curtis, *The Organization of the British Army in the American Revolution*, p. 137.
85. Newsome, *A British Orderly Book*, p. 291.
86. Urban, *Fusiliers*, p. 227.
87. Hagist, *Noble Volunteers*, pp. 233–4.
88. Cantlie, *A History of the Army Medical Department*, vol. 1, p. 151.
89. Jackson, *A Systematic View*, p. 297.
90. Cantlie, *A History of the Army Medical Department*, vol. 1, p. 151.
91. Kopperman, *The Medical Dimension in Cornwallis's Army*, pp. 381–6.
92. Frey, *The British Soldier in America*, p. 47.
93. Hamilton, *The duties of a regimental surgeon considered*, vol. 1, pp. 179–81; Cash, *Medical Men at the Siege of Boston*, pp. 74–5.
94. Jackson, *A Systematic View*, p. 84.
95. Fried, *Rush*, p. 224.
96. Schmitz, *The Medical and Pharmaceutical Care of the Hessian Troops*, pp. 38–9.
97. Schmitz, *The Medical and Pharmaceutical Care of the Hessian Troops*, pp. 40–1.
98. Schmitz, *The Medical and Pharmaceutical Care of the Hessian Troops*, p. 44.

99. Schmitz, *The Medical and Pharmaceutical Care of the Hessian Troops*, pp. 44–5.

100. Gibson, *Bodo Otto and the Medical Background of the American Revolution*, pp. 127–8.

101. Brocklesby, *Oeconomical and Medical Observations*, pp. 86–7.

102. Nadeau, *A German Military Surgeon in Rutland*, p. 278.

103. Schmitz, *The Medical and Pharmaceutical Care of the Hessian Troops*, p. 44.

104. Thacher, *Military Journal during the American Revolution*, p. 104.

105. Döhla, *A Hessian Diary of the American Revolution*, p. 231.

106. Johnson, *Uzal Johnson, Loyalist*, pp. xxiii, 75–6.

107. Kopperman, *The Medical Dimension in Cornwallis's Army*, p. 381.

108. Chaplin, *Medicine in England during the Reign of George III*, pp 101–5; Lloyd, *Medicine and the Navy*, vol. 3, p. 3.

109. Lloyd, *Medicine and the Navy*, vol. 3, p. 122.

110. Lloyd, *Medicine and the Navy*, vol. 3, p. 20.

111. Lloyd, *Medicine and the Navy*, vol. 3, p. 10.

112. Blanco, *Wellington's Surgeon General*, pp. 22–4; Lloyd, *Medicine and the Navy*, vol. 3, p. 10.

113. Lloyd, *Medicine and the Navy*, vol. 3, pp. 21–3.

114. Van Swieten, *The Diseases Incident to Armies*, pp. 131–3.

115. Lloyd, *Medicine and the Navy*, vol. 3, p. 68.

116. Lloyd, *Medicine and the Navy*, vol. 3, p. 213.

Chapter 3

1. Applegate, *The American Revolutionary War Hospital Department*, p. 296.

2. Owen, *Medical Department of the United States Army*, p. 2.

3. Gillett, *The Army Medical Department*, p. 22.

4. Gillett, *The Army Medical Department*, p. 22.

5. Applegate, *The American Revolutionary War Hospital Department*, p. 297; Gillett, *The Army Medical Department*, p. 23.

6. Applegate, *The American Revolutionary War Hospital Department*, pp. 297–8; Blanco, *Medicine in the Continental Army*, p. 686; Gillett, *The Army Medical Department*, p. 37.

7. Applegate, *The American Revolutionary War Hospital Department*, p. 298; Blanco, *Medicine in the Continental Army*, p. 689.

8. Applegate, *The American Revolutionary War Hospital Department*, p. 298.
9. Blanco, *Medicine in the Continental Army*, p. 693.
10. Applegate, *The American Revolutionary War Hospital Department*, p. 298.
11. Blanco, *Medicine in the Continental Army*, pp. 691, 695.
12. Gillett, *The Army Medical Department*, p. 26; Duncan, *Medical Men in the American Revolution*, pp. 61–4; Brown, *The Medical Department of the United States Army*, pp. 8–11.
13. Bell, *John Morgan Continental Doctor*, p. 179; Gillett, *The Army Medical Department*, p. 29; Duncan, *Medical Men in the American Revolution*, pp. 64, 69; Brown, *The Medical Department of the United States Army*, p. 11.
14. Gillett, *The Army Medical Department*, p. 38; Duncan, *Medical Men in the American Revolution*, pp. 299–300; Saffron, *Surgeon to Washington*, p. 30.
15. Gillett, *The Army Medical Department*, p. 44; Duncan, *Medical Men in the American Revolution*, pp. 345–6; Brown, *The Medical Department of the United States Army*, pp. 41–2.
16. Brown, *The Medical Department of the United States Army*, p. 41.
17. Gillett, *The Army Medical Department*, pp. 19–20.
18. Gillett, *The Army Medical Department*, pp. 33–5.
19. Morgan, *A Vindication*, p. xxv.
20. Blanco, *Physician of the American Revolution*, pp. 198–201; Duncan, *Medical Men in the American Revolution*, pp. 291–9; Bell, *John Morgan Continental Doctor*, pp. 230–9.
21. Fried, *Rush*, p. 255.
22. Saffron, *Surgeon to Washington*, pp. 66, 69.
23. Thacher, *Military Journal during the American Revolution*, pp. 7, 13–14.
24. Warren, *The Life of John Warren*, p. 191.
25. Gillett, *The Army Medical Department*, p. 20.
26. Cash, *Medical Men at the Siege of Boston*, pp. 47, 141–2.
27. Applegate, *The American Revolutionary War Hospital Department*, p. 300.
28. Thacher, *Military Journal during the American Revolution*, p. 21.
29. Saffron, *Surgeon to Washington*, p. 55.
30. Blanco, *Medicine in the Continental Army*, p. 680.
31. Gillett, *The Army Medical Department*, p. 26.

32. Martin, *Private Yankee Doodle*, p. 51.

33. Martin, *Private Yankee Doodle*, p. 70.

34. Saffron, *Surgeon to Washington*, p. 43.

35. Blanco, *Physician of the American Revolution*, pp. 211–12.

36. Gillett, *The Army Medical Department*, p. 31.

37. Duncan, *Medical Men in the American Revolution*, p. 53.

38. Duncan, *Medical Men in the American Revolution*, pp. 379–414.

39. Gillett, *The Army Medical Department*, p. 69.

40. Saffron, *Surgeon to Washington*, p. 137.

41. Cash, *Medical Men at the Siege of Boston*, p. 70.

42. Gibson, *Bodo Otto and the Medical Background of the American Revolution*, p. 106.

43. Duncan, *Medical Men in the American Revolution*, pp. 53–4.

44. Owen, *Medical Department of the United States Army*, pp. 70–1.

45. Saffron, *Surgeon to Washington*, p. 137.

46. Gillett, *The Army Medical Department*, pp. 26–7; Bell, *John Morgan Continental Doctor*, pp. 185–6.

47. Blanco, *Physician of the American Revolution*, p. 114.

48. Founders Online: Washington to John Hancock, 25 September 1776.

49. Gillett, *The Army Medical Department*, p. 32.

50. Applegate, *The American Revolutionary War Hospital Department*, p. 299.

51. Morgan, *A Vindication*, pp. 116–18.

52. Gibson, *Bodo Otto and the Medical Background of the American Revolution*, p. 140; Cash, *Medical Men at the Siege of Boston*, p. 70.

53. Applegate, *The American Revolutionary War Hospital Department*, p. 303.

54. Blanco, *American Army Hospitals in Pennsylvania*, pp. 359, 363.

55. Founders Online: Rush to Washington, 26 December 1777.

56. Dann, *Revolution Remembered*, p. 184.

57. Blanco, *American Army Hospitals in Pennsylvania*, pp. 364–5; Gillett, *The Army Medical Department*, pp. 87–8.

58. Tilton, *Economical Observations on Military Hospitals*, p. 47.

59. Tilton, *Economical Observations on Military Hospitals*, pp. 49–53; Blanco, *Medicine in the Continental Army*, p. 690.

60. Blanco, *Medicine in the Continental Army*, p. 690.

61. Applegate, *The American Revolutionary War Hospital Department*, p. 299.

62. Brown, *The Medical Department of the United States Army*, p. 25.

63. Duncan, *Medical Men in the American Revolution*, p. 141.

64. Saffron, *Surgeon to Washington*, p. 74.
65. Applegate, *The American Revolutionary War Hospital Department*, p. 299.
66. Blanco, *American Army Hospitals in Pennsylvania*, p. 363.
67. Applegate, *The American Revolutionary War Hospital Department*, pp. 300–1.
68. Tilton, *Economical Observations on Military Hospitals*, p. 26.
69. Gillett, *The Army Medical Department*, p. 85.
70. Blanco, *American Army Hospitals in Pennsylvania*, p. 363.
71. Gillett, *The Army Medical Department*, p. 56; Duncan, *Medical Men in the American Revolution*, p. 53; Becker, *Smallpox in Washington's Army*, p. 394.
72. Gillett, *The Army Medical Department*, pp. 51–2; Cash, *Medical Men at the Siege of Boston*, pp. 132–3; Cox, *A Proper Sense of Honor*, pp. 146–7.
73. Morgan, *A Vindication*, pp. 56–7.
74. Morgan, *A Vindication*, p. 58.
75. Duncan, *Medical Men in the American Revolution*, p. 143.
76. Dann, *Revolution Remembered*, pp. 150–1.
77. Duncan, *Medical Men in the American Revolution*, p. 196.
78. Applegate, *The American Revolutionary War Hospital Department*, pp. 300–1.
79. Applegate, *The American Revolutionary War Hospital Department*, pp. 301–2.
80. Griffenhagen, *Drug Supplies in the American Revolution*, pp. 110–30.
81. Toner, *The Medical Men of the Revolution*, p. 56.
82. Applegate, *The American Revolutionary War Hospital Department*, p. 303.
83. Blanco, *Medicine in the Continental Army*, pp. 689, 696.
84. Fenn, *Pox Americana*, pp. 15–16.
85. Ford, *The Writings of George Washington*, vol. 3, p. 35.
86. Saffron, *Surgeon to Washington*, pp. 56–7.
87. Gillett, *The Army Medical Department*, pp. 127–8.
88. Toner, *The Medical Men of the Revolution*, p. 64.
89. Jones, *Medicine in Virginia in Revolutionary Times*, p. 267.
90. Reiss, *Medicine and the American Revolution*, p. 145.
91. Reiss, *Medicine and the American Revolution*, p. 145.
92. Peckham, *The Toll of Independence*, p. 122.
93. Barnes, *Fanning's Narrative*, p. 58.

94. Bouvet, *Le Service de Santé Français pendant la guerre d'indépendance des Etats-Unis*, p. 3.
95. Bouvet, *Le Service de Santé Français pendant la guerre d'indépendance des Etats-Unis*, pp. 26–7.
96. Bouvet, *Le Service de Santé Français pendant la guerre d'indépendance des Etats-Unis*, p. 41.
97. Bouvet, *Le Service de Santé Français pendant la guerre d'indépendance des Etats-Unis*, p. 48.
98. Bouvet, *Le Service de Santé Français pendant la guerre d'indépendance des Etats-Unis*, p. 3.
99. Lemaire, *Coste*, p. 93.
100. Bouvet, *Le Service de Santé Français pendant la guerre d'indépendance des Etats-Unis*, p. 89.
101. Lemaire, *Coste*, pp. 73–4.
102. Lemaire, *Coste*, p. 71; Bouvet, *Le Service de Santé Français pendant la guerre d'indépendance des Etats-Unis*, pp. 38, 46–7; Trenard, *Un défenseur des hôpitaux militaires*, pp. 154–5.
103. Trenard, *Un défenseur des hôpitaux militaires*, pp. 155–6.
104. Founders Online: Washington to Coste, 7 October 1782.

Chapter 4

1. Frothingham, *History of the Siege of Boston*, p. 181.
2. Drew, *Commissioned Officers in the Medical Services of the British Army*.
3. Drew, *Commissioned Officers in the Medical Services of the British Army*, pp. 25, 41.
4. Lister, *The Concord Fight*, pp. 21–54; Cash, *Medical Men at the Siege of Boston*, pp. 21–2.
5. Atkinson, *The British are Coming*, p. 77: Cash, *Medical Men at the Siege of Boston*, pp. 22–4.
6. Chase, *The Beginnings of the American Revolution*, vol. 3, p. 186.
7. Chase, *The Beginnings of the American Revolution*, vol. 3, p. 186.
8. Chase, *The Beginnings of the American Revolution*, vol. 3, pp. 187–8.
9. Mackenzie, *A British Fusilier*, p. 61.
10. Chase, *The Beginnings of the American Revolution*, vol. 3, pp. 147–8.
11. Atkinson, *The British are Coming*, p. 77.
12. Chase, *The Beginnings of the American Revolution*, vol. 3, pp. 151–2.

13. Chase, *The Beginnings of the American Revolution*, vol. 3, p. 144; Atkinson, *The British are Coming*, p. 77.

14. Duncan, *Medical Men in the American Revolution*, p. 36.

15. Chase, *The Beginnings of the American Revolution*, vol. 3, p. 164.

16. Toner, *The Medical Men of the Revolution*, pp. 11–13; Duncan, *Medical Men in the American Revolution*, pp. 36–7; Cash, *Medical Men at the Siege of Boston*, pp. 17–19.

17. Owen, *Medical Department of the United States Army*, p. 23.

18. Chase, *The Beginnings of the American Revolution*, vol. 3, p. 147.

19. Cash, *Medical Men at the Siege of Boston*, pp. 24–5.

20. Cash, *Medical Men at the Siege of Boston*, pp. 19–20.

21. Duncan, *Medical Men in the American Revolution*, p. 36.

22. Cash, *Medical Men at the Siege of Boston*, pp. 19–20.

23. Chase, *The Beginnings of the American Revolution*, vol. 3, pp. 93–4, 96–7; Duncan, *Medical Men in the American Revolution*, pp. 36–7.

24. Mackenzie, *A British Fusilier*, p. 68.

25. Chase, *The Beginnings of the American Revolution*, vol. 3, p. 196.

26. Cash, *Medical Men at the Siege of Boston*, p. 24.

27. Chase, *The Beginnings of the American Revolution*, vol. 3, p. 164.

28. Cash, *Medical Men at the Siege of Boston*, p. 24.

29. Atkinson, *The British are Coming*, p. 78.

30. Chase, *The Beginnings of the American Revolution*, vol. 3, pp. 136–7.

31. Atkinson, *The British are Coming*, p. 83.

32. Drew, *Commissioned Officers in the Medical Services of the British Army*, pp. 25, 30, 38, 46; Barker, *The British in Boston*, p. 42; Cantlie, *A History of the Army Medical Department*, vol. 1, p. 119.

33. Duncan, *Medical Men in the American Revolution*, p. 51; Cash, *Medical Men at the Siege of Boston*, pp. 45–6.

34. Cash, *Medical Men at the Siege of Boston*, p. 157.

35. Duncan, *Medical Men in the American Revolution*, p. 40.

36. Duncan, *Medical Men in the American Revolution*, pp. 40–41.

37. Duncan, *Medical Men of the American Revolution*, pp. 40–41; Cash, *Medical Men at the Siege of Boston*, pp. 43–5.

38. Cantlie, *A History of the Army Medical Department*, vol. 1, pp. 139–40.

39. Griffenhagen, *Drug Supplies in the American Revolution*, p. 111; Owen, *Medical Department of the United States Army*, p. 12.

40. Cash, *Medical Men at the Siege of Boston*, pp. 31–2.
41. Ketchum, *The Battle for Bunker Hill*, p. 50.
42. Ketchum, *The Battle for Bunker Hill*, p. 50.
43. Cash, *Medical Men at the Siege of Boston*, pp. 34–5.
44. Howe, *General Sir William Howe's Orderly Book*, pp. 5, 18.
45. Willard, *Letters on the American Revolution*, pp. 52, 57–8.
46. Barker, *The British in Boston*, p. 25.
47. Mackenzie, *A British Fusilier*, pp. 72–3.
48. Cash, *Medical Men at the Siege of Boston*, pp. 37, 155.
49. Ketchum, *The Battle for Bunker Hill*, p. 144.
50. Lamb, *An Original and Authentic Journal*, p. 32; Ketchum, *The Battle for Bunker Hill*, p. 145.
51. Cash, *Medical Men at the Siege of Boston*, p. 60.
52. Cash, *Medical Men at the Siege of Boston*, pp. 55–6.
53. Atkinson, *The British are Coming*, p. 108.
54. Ketchum, *The Battle for Bunker Hill*, p. 129.
55. Ketchum, *The Battle for Bunker Hill*, p. 132; Lushington, *The Life and Services of General Lord Harris*, p. 55.
56. Howe, *General Sir William Howe's Orderly Book*, p. 9.
57. Willard, *Letters on the American Revolution*, p. 137.
58. Clarke, *An Impartial and Authentic Narrative*, p. 16.
59. Duncan, *Medical Men of the American Revolution*, p. 51; Cash, *Medical Men at the Siege of Boston*, p. 61.
60. Dawson, *Bunker's Hill*, pp. 374–5.
61. Clarke, *An Impartial and Authentic Narrative*, p. 16.
62. Cantlie, *A History of the Army Medical Department*, vol. 1, p. 139.
63. Howe, *General Sir William Howe's Orderly Book*, p. 7.
64. Howe, *General Sir William Howe's Orderly Book*, pp. 11, 23.
65. Atkinson, *The British are Coming*, p. 115.
66. Toner, *The Medical Men of the Revolution*, pp. 20–21; Duncan, *Medical Men of the American Revolution*, pp. 49–50; Cash, *Medical Men at the Siege of Boston*, pp. 56–7; Ketchum, *The Battle for Bunker Hill*, pp. 128–9.
67. Hope, TNA, PRO 30/39/1.
68. Dawson, *Bunker's Hill*, p. 358.
69. Spring, *With Zeal and Bayonets Only*, p. 171.
70. Ferling, *Almost a Miracle*, p. 58.

71. Ketchum, *The Battle for Bunker Hill*, p. 134; Farnsworth, *Amos Farnsworth's Diary*, pp. 83–4.

72. Estes, *A Disagreeable and Dangerous Employment*, p. 273.

73. Willard, *Letters on the American Revolution*, p. 141; Sullivan, *From Redcoat to Rebel*, p. 20.

74. Estes, *A Disagreeable and Dangerous Employment*, pp. 273–4.

75. Lushington, *The Life and Services of General Lord Harris*, pp. 55–6.

76. Duncan, *Medical Men of the American Revolution*, p. 50; Cash, *Medical Men at the Siege of Boston*, p. 62.

77. Atkinson, *The British are Coming*, p. 86.

78. Cash, *Medical Men at the Siege of Boston*, pp. 58–9; Ketchum, *The Battle for Bunker Hill*, pp. 151–2.

79. Duncan, *Medical Men of the American Revolution*, p. 59.

80. Blanco, *Medicine in the Continental Army*, p. 682; Gillett, *The Army Medical Department*, pp. 50–52.

81. Duncan, *Medical Men of the American Revolution*, p. 54.

82. Estes, *A Disagreeable and Dangerous Employment*, pp. 275–6.

83. Cash, *Medical Men at the Siege of Boston*, p. 51.

84. Duncan, *Medical Men of the American Revolution*, p. 67; Thacher, *Military Journal during the American Revolution*, pp. 25–6.

85. Bell, *John Morgan Continental Doctor*, p. 184.

86. Howe, *General Sir William Howe's Orderly Book*, pp. 26–7, 30, 96.

87. Cantlie, *A History of the Army Medical Department*, vol. 1, p. 140.

88. Willard, *Letters on the American Revolution*, p. 205.

89. Willard, *Letters on the American Revolution*, p. 191.

90. Willard, *Letters on the American Revolution*, p. 191.

91. Howe, *General Sir William Howe's Orderly Book*, p. 94.

92. Willard, *Letters on the American Revolution*, p. 191.

93. Cash, *Medical Men at the Siege of Boston*, p. 101.

94. Cash, *Medical Men at the Siege of Boston*, p. 97.

95. Bangs, *Journal of Lieutenant Isaac Bangs*, p. 17.

96. Frey, *The British Soldier in America*, p. 33.

97. Fenn, *Pox Americana*, p. 49; Becker, *Smallpox in Washington's Army*, pp. 394–6; Howe, *General Sir William Howe's Orderly Book*, pp. 148, 156.

98. Fenn, *Pox Americana*, pp. 50–51; Becker, *Smallpox in Washington's Army*, pp. 396–7; Gillett, *The Army Medical Department*, p. 56.

99. Marshall, *Hygiene and Disease*, p. 314.

100. Willard, *Letters on the American Revolution*, p. 191.

101. Marshall, *Hygiene and Disease*, p. 314.

102. Bangs, *Journal of Lieutenant Isaac Bangs*, p. 16.

103. Cash, *Medical Men at the Siege of Boston*, pp. 109–10.

104. Evelyn, *Memoirs and Letters of Captain W Glanville Evelyn*, p. 72.

105. Balderston, *Letters from British Officers*, p. 59.

106. Howe, *General Sir William Howe's Orderly Book*, pp. 85, 193.

107. Mackenzie, *A British Fusilier*, p. 32.

108. Cash, *Medical Men at the Siege of Boston*, pp. 96–7.

109. Howe, *General Sir William Howe's Orderly Book*, pp. 322–3; Estes, *A Disagreeable and Dangerous Employment*, pp. 288–9; Cash, *Medical Men at the Siege of Boston*, pp. 115–16, 156.

110. Cash, *Medical Men at the Siege of Boston*, pp. 105, 155.

111. Estes, *A Dangerous and Disagreeable Employment*, p. 290.

112. Blanco, *Medicine in the Continental Army*, pp. 682–3; Gibson, *Bodo Otto and the Medical Background of the American Revolution*, p. 93; Gillett, *The Army Medical Department*, p. 53.

113. Fenn, *Biological Warfare in Eighteenth-Century North America*, p. 1568.

114. Fenn, *Biological Warfare in Eighteenth-Century North America*, pp. 1567–9; Becker, *Smallpox in Washington's Army*, pp. 399–400; Gibson, *Bodo Otto and the Medical Background of the American Revolution*, pp. 88–90; Cash, *Medical Men at the Siege of Boston*, pp. 111–12.

115. Thacher, *Military Journal during the American Revolution*, pp. 30–31.

116. Cash, *Medical Men at the Siege of Boston*, pp. 144–5.

117. Bell, *John Morgan Continental Doctor*, p. 187.

118. Cash, *Medical Men at the Siege of Boston*, p. 145.

119. Atkinson, *The British are Coming*, p. 260.

120. Atkinson, *The British are Coming*, p. 262.

121. Howe, *General Sir William Howe's Orderly Book*, p. 230.

122. Howe, *General Sir William Howe's Orderly Book*, pp. 260, 278, 291, 324.

123. Fenn, *Pox Americana*, p. 51.

124. Warren, *The Life of John Warren*, pp. 74–6; Griffenhagen, *Drug Supplies in the American Revolution*, p. 114; Gillett, *The Army Medical Department*, p. 57.

125. Thacher, *Military Journal during the American Revolution*, p. 37; Fenn, *Pox Americana*, pp. 51–4; Blanco, *Physician of the American Revolution*, p. 79.

126. Duncan, *Medical Men of the American Revolution*, p. 114.

127. Duncan, *Medical Men of the American Revolution*, pp. 114–15; Brown, *The Medical Department of the United States Army*, pp. 16–18.

Chapter 5

1. Atkinson, *The British are Coming*, p. 143.

2. Lengel, *The 10 Key Campaigns*, p. 21.

3. Ferling, *Almost a Miracle*, p. 83.

4. Mackesy, *The War for America*, p. 79.

5. Cantlie, *A History of the Army Medical Department*, vol. 1, p. 144; Hayes, Me C 29/13/1–2.

6. Drew, *Commissioned Officers in the Medical Services of the British Army*, pp. 33, 36.

7. Atkinson, *The British are Coming*, p. 203.

8. Brown, *The Medical Department of the Unites States Army*, p. 12.

9. Gillett, *The Army Medical Department*, p. 57.

10. Blanco, *Physician of the American Revolution*, p. 86.

11. Blanco, *Physician of the American Revolution*, pp. 86–7.

12. Gibson, *Bodo Otto and the Medical Background of the American Revolution*, p. 95.

13. Blanco, *Physician of the American Revolution*, p. 87.

14. Duncan, *Medical Men in the American Revolution*, p. 86; Cash, *The Canadian Military Campaign*, pp. 52–3.

15. Senter, *The Journal of Isaac Senter*, pp. 11–12.

16. Greenman, *Diary of a Common Soldier*, p. 18.

17. Senter, *The Journal of Isaac Senter*, p. 21.

18. Senter, *The Journal of Isaac Senter*, p. 18.

19. Greenman, *Diary of a Common Soldier*, p. 18.

20. Senter, *The Journal of Isaac Senter*, p. 22.

21. Senter, *The Journal of Isaac Senter*, p. 11.

22. Cash, *The Canadian Military Campaign*, p. 53.

23. Roberts, *March to Quebec*, pp. 83, 98–9.

24. Senter, *The Journal of Isaac Senter*, p. 29; Cash, *The Canadian Military Campaign*, p. 54.

25. Roberts, *March to Quebec*, p. 692.
26. Wurtele, *Blockade of Quebec*, pp. 21–2, 25, 27.
27. Senter, *The Journal of Isaac Senter*, pp. 29, 31; Roberts, *March to Quebec*, p. 703.
28. Roberts, *March to Quebec*, p. 482.
29. Greenman, *Diary of a Common Soldier*, pp. 22–3.
30. Senter, *The Journal of Isaac Senter*, p. 31.
31. Cash, *The Canadian Military Campaign*, pp. 54–5.
32. Roberts, *March to Quebec*, pp. 374–5.
33. Senter, *The Journal of Isaac Senter*, p. 31.
34. Fenn, *Pox Americana*, p. 64.
35. Wurtele, *Blockade of Quebec*, pp. 22, 27.
36. Roberts, *March to Quebec*, pp. 374–5.
37. Roberts, *March to Quebec*, p. 482.
38. Becker, *Smallpox in Washington's Army*, pp. 408–9.
39. Fenn, *Biological Warfare in Eighteenth-Century North America*, pp. 1569–70.
40. Roberts, *March to Quebec*, p. 704.
41. Atkinson, *The British are Coming*, pp. 211–12.
42. Duncan, *Medical Men in the American Revolution*, p. 92.
43. Senter, *The Journal of Isaac Senter*, pp. 33–4.
44. Atkinson, *The British are Coming*, p. 211.
45. Roberts, *March to Quebec*, p. 108.
46. Senter, *The Journal of Isaac Senter*, p. 34.
47. Roberts, *March to Quebec*, p. 123.
48. Roberts, *March to Quebec*, pp. 389–90.
49. Roberts, *March to Quebec*, pp. 705–7.
50. Roberts, *March to Quebec*, p. 156.
51. Greenman, *Diary of a Common Soldier*, p. 25; Roberts, *March to Quebec*, p. 566.
52. Roberts, *March to Quebec*, p. 592.
53. Roberts, *March to Quebec*, p. 707.
54. Greenman, *Diary of a Common Soldier*, p. 25.
55. Roberts, *March to Quebec*, pp. 592–3.
56. Roberts, *March to Quebec*, p. 566.
57. Roberts, *March to Quebec*, pp. 411–14.
58. Duncan, *Medical Men in the American Revolution*, p. 94.

59. Blanco, *Physician of the American Revolution*, p. 89.
60. Blanco, *Physician of the American Revolution*, p. 91.
61. Cash, *The Canadian Military Campaign*, p. 55.
62. Dann, *Revolution Remembered*, p. 19.
63. Senter, *The Journal of Isaac Senter*, p. 37.
64. Fenn, *Pox Americana*, p. 67.
65. Reide, *A View of the Diseases of the Army*, p. 4.
66. Wurtele, *Blockade of Quebec*, p. 52.
67. Atkinson, *The British are Coming*, pp. 280–3.
68. Senter, *The Journal of Isaac Senter*, p. 38.
69. Wurtele, *Blockade of Quebec*, p. 84.
70. Fenn, *Pox Americana*, p. 68.
71. Senter, *The Journal of Isaac Senter*, pp. 38–9.
72. Cash, *The Canadian Military Campaign*, p. 55.
73. Duncan, *Medical Men in the American Revolution*, p. 97; Blanco, *Physician of the American Revolution*, p. 92.
74. Gillett, *The Army Medical Department*, p. 59.
75. Cantlie, *A History of the Army Medical Department*, vol. 1, p. 144.
76. Duncan, *Medical Men in the American Revolution*, p. 98.
77. Fenn, *Pox Americana*, p. 75.
78. Cash, *The Canadian Military Campaign*, p. 56.
79. Kirkland, *Journal of a Physician Lewis Beebe*, pp. 335–6.
80. Atkinson, *The British are Coming*, p. 292.
81. Blanco, *Physician of the American Revolution*, p. 93.
82. Cash, *The Canadian Military Campaign*, p. 56.
83. Cantlie, *A History of the Army Medical Department*, vol. 1, p. 144.
84. Cantlie, *A History of the Army Medical Department*, vol. 1, p. 144.
85. Reide, *A View of the Diseases of the Army*, pp. 4–6.
86. Blanco, *Physician of the American Revolution*, p. 94.
87. Blanco, *Physician of the American Revolution*, pp. 94–6.
88. Blanco, *Physician of the American Revolution*, pp. 96–7.
89. Davis, *Medicine in the Canadian Campaign of the Revolutionary War*, p. 471.
90. Blanco, *Physician of the American Revolution*, p. 104.
91. Kirkland, *Journal of a Physician Lewis Beebe*, p. 346.
92. Kennedy, *Letters of Dr Samuel Kennedy*, p. 115.
93. Atkinson, *The British are Coming*, p. 410.

94. Blanco, *Physician of the American Revolution*, pp. 100–102.
95. Blanco, *Medicine in the Continental Army*, p. 684.
96. Blanco, *Physician of the American Revolution*, pp. 105–6.
97. Kirkland, *Journal of a Physician Lewis Beebe*, p. 350.
98. Blanco, *Physician of the American Revolution*, p. 106.
99. Marshall, *The Health of the British Soldier in America*, p. 27; Reide, *A View of the Diseases of the Army*, pp. 6–8.
100. Doblin, *An Eyewitness Account of the American Revolution*, p. 32.
101. Reide, *A View of the Diseases of the Army*, p. 8.
102. Fenn, *Pox Americana*, pp. 57–62.

Chapter 6

1. Atkinson, *The British are Coming*, pp. 297–304.
2. Blanco, *Physician of the American Revolution*, pp. 115–17; Blanco, *Medicine in the Continental Army*, p. 685.
3. Symonds, *A Battlefield Atlas of the American Revolution*, p. 27; Ferling, *Almost a Miracle*, pp. 125–6.
4. Bell, *John Morgan Continental Doctor*, p. 195.
5. Blanco, *Physician of the American Revolution*, p. 114.
6. Gillett, *The Army Medical Department*, pp. 65–7; Duncan, *Medical Men in the American Revolution*, pp. 117–18; Morgan, *A Vindication*, pp. 116–18.
7. Guerra, *American Medical Bibliography*, pp. 567, 582.
8. Gillett, *The Army Medical Department*, p. 66.
9. Griffenhagen, *Drug Supplies in the American Revolution*, p.116.
10. Morgan, *A Vindication*, p. 118
11. Blanco, *Physician of the American Revolution*, p. 114.
12. Duncan, *Medical Men in the American Revolution*, pp. 117–18.
13. Duncan, *Medical Men in the American Revolution*, pp. 128–9.
14. Cantlie, *A History of the Army Medical Department*, vol. 1, p. 142; Drew, *Commissioned Officers in the Medical Services of the British Army*, pp. 25, 38.
15. Lloyd, *Medicine and the Navy*, vol. 3, pp. 67–8.
16. Warren, *The Life of John Warren*, p. 78; Blanco, *Medicine in the Continental Army*, p. 685.
17. Blanco, *Physician of the American Revolution*, p. 117.
18. Bangs, *Journal of Lieutenant Isaac Bangs*, pp. 60, 64.
19. Beardsley, *History of a Dysentery*, pp. 249–50.

20. Bangs, *Journal of Lieutenant Isaac Bangs*, pp. 34–5.

21. Bangs, *Journal of Lieutenant Isaac Bangs*, pp. 29–30.

22. Kennedy, *Letters of Dr Samuel Kennedy*, p. 112.

23. Curtis, *The Organization of the British Army in the American Revolution*, p. 125.

24. Rowley, *Medical Advice for the use of the army and navy*; Lamb, *Memoir of His Own Life*, pp. 114–17.

25. Blanco, *The Soldier's Friend*, p. 408.

26. Reiss, *Medicine and the American Revolution*, p. 155.

27. Pfister, *The Voyage of the First Hessian Army*, pp. 25–6.

28. Bender, *American Pharmacy in the Colonial and Revolutionary Periods*, p. 41.

29. Symonds, *A Battlefield Atlas of the American Revolution*, p. 27; Peckham, *The Toll of Independence*, p. 22.

30. Morgan, *A Vindication*, pp. 55–6; Duncan, *Medical Men in the American Revolution*, p. 120.

31. Duncan, *Medical Men in the American Revolution*, pp. 130–1.

32. Warren, *The Life of John Warren*, p. 99.

33. Duncan, *Medical Men in the American Revolution*, p. 134.

34. Gibson, *Bodo Otto and the Medical Background of the American Revolution*, p. 71.

35. Gillett, *The Army Medical Department*, p. 67; Duncan, *Medical Men in the American Revolution*, p. 134.

36. Forster, *Diary of Thompson Forster*, pp. 94–6.

37. Forster, *Diary of Thompson Forster*, p. 97.

38. Atkinson, *The British are Coming*, pp. 388–9.

39. Blanco, *Physician of the American Revolution*, pp. 118–19; Morgan, *A Vindication*, pp. 12–13.

40. Gillett, *The Army Medical Department*, p. 67.

41. Duncan, *Medical Men in the American Revolution*, p. 144.

42. Gillett, *The Army Medical Department*, p. 67.

43. Ferling, *Almost a Miracle*, pp. 145–6.

44. Tilton, *Economical Observations on Military Hospitals*, pp. 32–3.

45. Atkinson, *The British are Coming*, p. 432.

46. Gibson, *Bodo Otto and the Medical Background of the American Revolution*, p. 120.

47. Balderston, *The Lost War*, p. 101.

48. Forster, *Diary of Thompson Forster*, p. 102; Drew, *Commissioned Officers in the Medical Services of the British Army*, p. 35.
49. Atkinson, *The British are Coming*, p. 396.
50. Cantlie, Foster, *A History of the Army Medical Department*, vol. 1, p. 141; *Diary of Thompson Forster*, pp. 104–6.
51. Atkinson, *The British are Coming*, p. 396.
52. Gillman, *Military Surgery in the American Revolution*, p. 492.
53. Symonds, *A Battlefield Atlas of the American Revolution*, p. 29.
54. Forster, *Diary of Thompson Forster*, p. 108.
55. Symonds, *A Battlefield Atlas of the American Revolution*, p. 29.
56. Evelyn, *Memoirs and Letters*, pp. 9–11.
57. Ferling, *Almost a Miracle*, p. 57.
58. Forster, *Diary of Thompson Forster*, pp. 109–10; Hagist, *British Soldiers American War*, pp. 255–6.
59. Duncan, *Medical Men in the American Revolution*, p. 143.
60. Duncan, *Medical Men in the American Revolution*, p. 145; Blanco, *Physician of the American Revolution*, pp. 118–19.
61. Morgan, *A Vindication*, p. 17.
62. Morgan, *A Vindication*, p. 17.
63. Duncan, *Medical Men in the American Revolution*, p. 148.
64. Forster, *Diary of Thompson Forster*, pp. 112–13, (a)–(d).
65. Dann, *Revolution Remembered*, p. 120.
66. Duncan, *Medical Men in the American Revolution*, p. 148.
67. Dann, *Revolution Remembered*, p. 118.
68. Cantlie, *A History of the Army Medical Department*, vol. 1, p. 142.
69. Blanco, *Physician of the American Revolution*, p. 119.
70. Morgan, *A Vindication*, pp. xxi–xxiii; Blanco, *Physician of the American Revolution*, pp. 120–1; Bell, *John Morgan Continental Doctor*, pp. 202–3; Gillett, *The Army Medical Department*, p. 69.
71. Blanco, *Physician of the American Revolution*, p. 119.
72. Morgan, *A Vindication*, p. 45.
73. Bell, *John Morgan Continental Doctor*, p. 201.
74. Bell, *John Morgan Continental Doctor*, p. 200.
75. Bell, *John Morgan Continental Doctor*, p. 201.
76. Bell, *John Morgan Continental Doctor*, p. 201.
77. Duncan, *Medical Men in the American Revolution*, p. 148.
78. Martin, *Private Yankee Doodle*, pp. 54–6.

79. Duncan, *Medical Men in the American Revolution*, pp. 151–3; Atkinson, *The British are Coming*, p. 508; Cantlie, *A History of the Army Medical Department*, vol. 1, p. 158.

80. Marston, *The American Revolution*, p. 40; Ferling, *Almost a Miracle*, p. 123; Atkinson, *The British are Coming*, p. 341.

81. Forster, *Diary of Thompson Forster*, p. 78.

82. Willard, *Letters on the American Revolution*, p. 332.

83. Atkinson, *The British are Coming*, p. 341.

84. Gillett, *The Army Medical Department*, p. 117.

85. Atkinson, *The British are Coming*, p. 323.

86. Hagist, *Noble Volunteers*, p. 131.

87. Forster, *Diary of Thompson Forster*, p. 66; Willard, *Letters on the American Revolution*, p. 332.

88. Hagist, *Noble Volunteers*, p. 148.

89. Symonds, *A Battlefield Atlas of the American Revolution*, p. 25.

90. Blanco, *Physician of the American Revolution*, p. 108.

91. Stewart, *A Most Unsettled Time on Lake Champlain*, p. 92.

92. Blanco, *Physician of the American Revolution*, p. 109.

93. Drew, *Commissioned Officers in the Medical Services of the British Army*, p. 33.

94. Cohn, *An Incident not Known to History*, p. 106.

95. Cohn, *An Incident not Known to History*, pp. 109–10.

Chapter 7

1. Atkinson, *The British are Coming*, pp. 485–96; Ferling, *Almost a Miracle*, pp. 162–72.

2. Atkinson, *The British are Coming*, p. 492.

3. Duncan, *Medical Men of the American Revolution*, p. 168.

4. Ferling, *Almost a Miracle*, p. 165.

5. Gillett, *The Army Medical Department*, p. 77.

6. Gibson, *Bodo Otto and the Medical Background of the American Revolution*, p. 123.

7. Blanco, *Physician of the American Revolution*, pp. 121–2; Duncan, *Medical Men of the American Revolution*, pp. 168–71.

8. Gillett, *The Army Medical Department*, p. 70.

9. Gibson, *Bodo Otto and the Medical Background of the American Revolution*, pp. 123–4, 126–7.

10. Gillett, *The Army Medical Department*, p. 69.

11. Duncan, *Medical Men of the American Revolution*, p. 171.

12. Duncan, *Medical Men of the American Revolution*, p. 171.

13. Tilton, *Economical Observations on Military Hospitals*, p. 29.

14. Atkinson, *The British are Coming*, pp. 500–1.

15. Ketchum, *The Winter Soldiers*, p. 315.

16. Atkinson, *The British are Coming*, pp. 511–21; Ferling, *Almost a Miracle*, pp. 172–9; Peckham, *The Toll of Independence*, p. 27.

17. Duncan, *Medical Men of the American Revolution*, p. 176.

18. Gibson, *Bodo Otto and the Medical Background of the American Revolution*, pp. 127–8.

19. Founders Online: General Orders, 29 December 1776.

20. Young, *Journal of Sergeant William Young*, p. 260.

21. Gibson, *Bodo Otto and the Medical Background of the American Revolution*, p. 128.

22. Blanco, *Physician of the American Revolution*, p. 125; Saffron, *Surgeon to Washington*, pp. 27–8.

23. Corner, *The Autobiography of Benjamin Rush*, p. 128.

24. Ferling, *Almost a Miracle*, p. 185; Atkinson, *The British are Coming*, p. 549.

25. Ketchum, *The Winter Soldiers*, p. 372.

26. Collins, *A Brief Narrative*, pp. 36–7.

27. Collins, *A Brief Narrative*, pp. 17, 38.

28. Corner, *The Autobiography of Benjamin Rush*, pp. 128–30.

29. Duncan, *Medical Men of the American Revolution*, p. 187.

30. Corner, *The Autobiography of Benjamin Rush*, pp. 128–9; Fried, *Rush*, p. 186; Blanco, *Physician of the American Revolution*, p. 128.

31. Gillett, *The Army Medical Department*, p. 72.

32. Fried, *Rush*, p. 191.

33. Ferling, *Almost a Miracle*, p. 186; Ewald, *Diary of the American War*, p. 50.

34. Atkinson, *The British are Coming*, pp. 551–2.

35. Blanco, *Physician of the American Revolution*, p. 129.

36. Bell, *John Morgan Continental Doctor*, pp. 204–5.

37. Blanco, *American Army Hospitals*, pp. 353–4.

38. Gillett, *The Army Medical Department*, pp. 70–1.

39. Blanco, *American Army Hospitals*, p. 354.

40. Gillett, *The Army Medical Department*, pp. 70, 75–6.

41. Blanco, *American Army Hospitals*, p. 353.

42. Corner, *The Autobiography of Benjamin Rush*, p. 131.

43. Blanco, *Physician of the American Revolution*, pp. 122–3.

44. Bell, *John Morgan Continental Doctor*, pp. 221–2; Gillett, *The Army Medical Department*, p. 38.

45. Gillett, *The Army Medical Department*, p. 38.

46. Collins, *A Brief Narrative*, p. 51.

47. Duncan, *Medical Men of the American Revolution*, p. 181.

48. Gibson, *Bodo Otto and the Medical Background of the American Revolution*, pp. 131–2.

49. Becker, *Smallpox in Washington's Army*, p. 424.

50. Fenn, *Pox Americana*, p. 95; Blanco, *Physician of the American Revolution*, p. 134.

51. Becker, *Smallpox in Washington's Army*, p. 424.

52. Becker, *Smallpox in Washington's Army*, pp. 424–5.

53. Bell, *John Morgan Continental Doctor*, pp. 222–3.

54. Founders Online: Rush to Washington, 13 May 1777; Washington to Rush, 16 May 1777.

55. Rush, *Directions for Preserving the Health of Soldiers*, p. 3; Fried, *Rush*, pp. 201–2.

56. Marshall, *The Health of the British Soldier in America*, pp. 27–9.

57. Marshall, *Hygiene and Disease*, p. 314.

58. Peebles, *John Peebles' American War*, pp. 94–106.

59. Peebles, *John Peebles' American War*, p. 115.

60. Marshall, *Hygiene and Disease*, p. 316.

61. Marshall, *The Health of the British Soldier in America*, p. 29.

62. Balderston, *The Lost War*, p. 126.

Chapter 8

1. Ferling, *Almost a Miracle*, pp. 211–41, Rhodehamel, *George Washington*, pp. 148–54; Ketchum, *Saratoga*, p. 437.

2. Kopperman, *The Numbers Game*, pp. 269–71; Cantlie, *A History of the Army Medical Department*, vol. 1, p. 145; Drew, *Commissioned Officers in the Medical Services of the British Army*, pp. 33, 40, 41, 46, 48.

3. Cantlie, *A History of the Army Medical Department*, vol. 1, p. 145.

4. Callaghan, *Orderly Book of Lieut. Gen. John Burgoyne*, p. 26.

5. Kopperman, *The Numbers Game*, pp. 271–2.
6. Callaghan, *Orderly Book of Lieut. Gen. John Burgoyne*, p. 45.
7. Kopperman, *The Numbers Game*, p. 272.
8. Callaghan, *Orderly Book of Lieut. Gen. John Burgoyne*, pp. 179–80.
9. Kopperman, *The Numbers Game*, p. 271; Drew, *Commissioned Officers in the Medical Services of the British Army*, p. 50.
10. Blanco, *Physician of the American Revolution*, p. 40.
11. Gillett, *The Army Medical Department*, p. 94.
12. Blanco, *Physician of the American Revolution*, pp. 144–5; Gillett, *The Army Medical Department*, p. 95.
13. Thacher, *Military Journal during the American Revolution*, p. 82.
14. Duncan, *Medical Men in the American Revolution*, p. 251.
15. Blanco, *Physician of the American Revolution*, p. 154.
16. Blanco, *Physician of the American Revolution*, p. 158.
17. Kopperman, *The Numbers Game*, p. 236.
18. Anburey, *With Burgoyne from Quebec*, p. 133.
19. Ferling, *Almost a Miracle*, p. 213.
20. Kopperman, *The Numbers Game*, pp. 262–4.
21. Marshall, *The Health of the British Soldier in America*, pp. 30–1; Kopperman, *The Numbers Game*, pp. 265–6.
22. Cantlie, *A History of the Army Medical Department*, vol. 1, p. 145.
23. Kopperman, *The Numbers Game*, p. 266.
24. Kopperman, *The Numbers Game*, p. 266.
25. Hagist, *Noble Volunteers*, p. 127.
26. Callaghan, *Orderly Book of Lieut. Gen. John Burgoyne*, p. 60.
27. Blanco, *Military Medicine in Northern New York*, pp. 56–7; Duncan, *Medical Men in the American Revolution*, p. 259.
28. Kopperman, *The Numbers Game*, p. 278; Blanco, *Physician of the American Revolution*, p. 139.
29. Gillett, *The Army Medical Department*, p. 96.
30. Ferling, *Almost a Miracle*, pp. 221–2.
31. Ketchum, *Saratoga*, pp. 199, 212–13.
32. Ketchum, *Saratoga*, p. 213.
33. Atkinson, *Some Evidence for Burgoyne's Expedition*, pp. 141–2.
34. Ketchum, *Saratoga*, p. 242.
35. Ferling, *Almost a Miracle*, pp. 229–31.
36. Blanco, *Physician of the American Revolution*, pp. 146–7.

37. Ferling, *Almost a Miracle*, p. 228.

38. Duncan, *Medical Men in the American Revolution*, pp. 248–9.

39. Blanco, *Physician of the American Revolution*, pp. 145–6.

40. Ketchum, *Saratoga*, pp. 309–10.

41. Atkinson, *Some Evidence for Burgoyne's Expedition*, p. 142.

42. Nadeau, *A German Military Surgeon*, p. 288.

43. Nadeau, *A German Military Surgeon*, p. 273.

44. Nadeau, *A German Military Surgeon*, p. 273.

45. Ferling, *Almost a Miracle*, p. 233.

46. Lengel, *The 10 Key Campaigns*, pp. 102–3; Ferling, *Almost a Miracle*, p. 235.

47. Anburey, *With Burgoyne from Quebec*, p. 176.

48. Anburey, *With Burgoyne from Quebec*, p. 177.

49. Lamb, *An Original and Authentic Journal*, p. 180.

50. Hadden, *A Journal Kept in Canada*, pp. 165–6.

51. Riedesel, *Letters and Journals*, pp. 113–5.

52. Hagist, *Noble Volunteers*, p. 207.

53. Duncan, *Medical Men in the American Revolution*, p. 252.

54. Kopperman, *The Numbers Game*, p. 267.

55. Ketchum, *Saratoga*, p. 371.

56. Duncan, *Medical Men in the American Revolution*, p. 252.

57. Thacher, *Military Journal during the American Revolution*, p. 89.

58. Blanco, *Military Medicine in Northern New York*, p. 57.

59. Atkinson, *Some Evidence for Burgoyne's Expedition*, p. 142.

60. Blanco, *Physician of the American Revolution*, p. 153.

61. Ketchum, *Saratoga*, p. 405.

62. Ferling, *Almost a Miracle*, p. 239.

63. Frey, *The British Soldier in America*, p. 105.

64. Blanco, *Physician of the American Revolution*, pp. 148–9.

65. Dann, *Revolution Remembered*, p. 103.

66. Blanco, *Physician of the American Revolution*, pp. 148–9.

67. Dann, *Revolution Remembered*, p. 103.

68. Ferling, *Almost a Miracle*, p. 238.

69. Riedesel, *Letters and Journals*, pp. 119–20, 127–9.

70. Blanco, *Physician of the American Revolution*, p. 148.

71. Duncan, *Medical Men in the American Revolution*, pp. 254–5.

72. Blanco, *Physician of the American Revolution*, p. 154.

73. Thacher, *Military Journal during the American Revolution*, p. 104.
74. Duncan, *Medical Men in the American Revolution*, p. 257.
75. Thacher, *Military Journal during the American Revolution*, p. 95.
76. Thacher, *Military Journal during the American Revolution*, pp. 105–6.
77. Kopperman, *The Numbers Game*, p. 276.
78. Ketchum, *Saratoga*, pp. 435–6.
79. Ferling, *Almost a Miracle*, pp. 431–2.
80. Cantlie, *A History of the Army Medical Department*, vol. 1, p. 147.
81. Owen, *Medical Department of the United States Army*, pp. 87–8; Blanco, *Physician of the American Revolution*, pp. 158–9.

Chapter 9

1. Ferling, *Almost a Miracle*, pp. 242–58.
2. Cantlie, *A History of the Army Medical Department*, vol. 1, pp. 148–9.
3. Founders Online: Rush to Adams, 8 August 1777.
4. Gillett, *The Army Medical Department*, p. 79.
5. Ferling, *Almost a Miracle*, pp. 244–5.
6. Marshall, *The Health of the British Soldier in America*, p. 30.
7. Duncan, *Medical Men in the American Revolution*, p. 212.
8. Ferling, *Almost a Miracle*, pp. 246–51; Lengel, *The 10 Key Campaigns*, pp. 115–16.
9. Howe, *General Orders*, pp. 492–5; Peebles, *John Peebles's American War*, p. 134.
10. Cantlie, *A History of the Army Medical Department*, vol. 1, p. 147.
11. Townsend, *Some Account of the British Army*, p. 26.
12. Blanco, *American Army Hospitals*, p. 355.
13. Blanco, *Physician of the American Revolution*, p. 163.
14. Fried, *Rush*, pp. 216–9; Duncan, *Medical Men in the American Revolution*, p. 214.
15. Gibson, *Bodo Otto and the Medical Background of the American Revolution*, p. 142; Duncan, *Medical Men in the American Revolution*, p. 214.
16. Blanco, *Physician of the American Revolution*, p. 163.
17. Bloomfield, *Citizen Soldier*, pp. 127–8.
18. Saffron, *Surgeon to Washington*, p. 42; Wooden, *The Wounds and Weapons of the Revolutionary War*, pp. 63–4.
19. Howe, *General Orders*, p. 495.

20. Duncan, *Medical Men in the American Revolution*, pp. 213–14.
21. Fried, *Rush*, pp. 220–1; Corner, *The Autobiography of Benjamin Rush*, p. 132.
22. Ferling, *Almost a Miracle*, pp. 251–2; Symonds, *A Battlefield Atlas of the American Revolution*, p. 55.
23. Dann, *Revolution Remembered*, pp. 149–50.
24. Peebles, *John Peebles's American War*, pp. 136–7.
25. Duncan, *Medical Men in the American Revolution*, p. 226.
26. Ferling, *Almost a Miracle*, pp. 253–6; Lengel, *The 10 Key Campaigns*, pp. 123–4.
27. Hagist, *Noble Volunteers*, p. 205.
28. Duncan, *Medical Men in the American Revolution*, pp. 216–7.
29. Cantlie, *A History of the Army Medical Department*, vol. 1, p. 148.
30. Howe, *General Orders*, pp. 509, 511.
31. Duncan, *Medical Men in the American Revolution*, pp. 217–18, 226; Gibson, *Bodo Otto and the Medical Background of the American Revolution*, p. 142.
32. Ewald, *Diary of the American War*, p. 96.
33. Howe, *General Orders*, pp. 505–6, 507, 524.
34. Cantlie, *A History of the Army Medical Department*, vol. 1, p. 149.
35. Marshall, *The Health of the British Soldier in America*, pp. 30–1.
36. Blanco, *American Army Hospitals*, pp. 356–7.
37. Duncan, *Medical Men in the American Revolution*, p. 219.
38. Blanco, *American Army Hospitals*, p. 357.
39. Blanco, *American Army Hospitals*, p. 358.
40. Gillett, *The Army Medical Department*, p. 81.
41. Blanco, *American Army Hospitals*, pp. 358–9.
42. Gibson, *Bodo Otto and the Medical Background of the American Revolution*, p. 144.
43. Corner, *The Autobiography of Benjamin Rush*, p. 134.
44. Blanco, *American Army Hospitals*, p. 360.
45. Tilton, *Economical Observations on Military Hospitals*, pp. 29–30.
46. Duncan, *Medical Men in the American Revolution*, p. 224.
47. Duncan, *Medical Men in the American Revolution*, p. 217.
48. Corner, *The Autobiography of Benjamin Rush*, p. 133.
49. Duncan, *Medical Men in the American Revolution*, p. 239; Gillett, *The Army Medical Department*, p. 80.

50. Blanco, *American Army Hospitals*, p. 359.
51. Ferling, *Almost a Miracle*, p. 275.
52. Waldo, *Valley Forge 1777–78*, pp. 306–7.
53. Blanco, *American Army Hospitals*, pp. 362–3.
54. Gibson, *Bodo Otto and the Medical Background of the American Revolution*, p. 141.
55. Blanco, *American Army Hospitals*, pp. 359, 363.
56. Waldo, *Valley Forge 1777–78*, p. 312.
57. Waldo, *Valley Forge 1777–78*, p. 312.
58. Thacher, *Military Journal during the American Revolution*, p. 119.
59. Ferling, *Almost a Miracle*, p. 277.
60. Blanco, *Physician of the American Revolution*, p. 176; Gillett, *The Army Medical Department*, p. 84.
61. Saffron, *Surgeon to Washington*, p. 44; Gibson, *Bodo Otto and the Medical Background of the American Revolution*, p. 150.
62. Duncan, *Medical Men in the American Revolution*, p. 234; Blanco, *American Army Hospitals*, p. 362.
63. Fenn, *Pox Americana*, pp. 98–9.
64. Weedon, *Valley Forge Orderly Book*, pp. 254, 289.
65. Saffron, *Surgeon to Washington*, pp. 44–5.
66. Saffron, *Surgeon to Washington*, p. 220.

Chapter 10

1. Ferling, *Almost a Miracle*, p. 288.
2. Duncan, *Medical Men in the American Revolution*, p. 243.
3. Blanco, *Physician of the American Revolution*, p. 173.
4. Saffron, *Surgeon to Washington*, p. 50; Blanco, *Physician of the American Revolution*, p. 188.
5. Blanco, *Physician of the American Revolution*, p. 182.
6. Marshall, *Hygiene and Disease*, pp. 316–7; Marshall, *The Health of the British Soldier in America*, pp. 31–2.
7. Marshall, *The Health of the British Soldier in America*, p. 32.
8. Fortescue, *A History of the British Army*, vol. 3, pp. 253–4; Ferling, *Almost a Miracle*, pp. 288–303.
9. Fortescue, *A History of the British Army*, vol. 3, pp. 254–5; Ferling, *Almost a Miracle*, p. 306.
10. Ferling, *Almost a Miracle*, p. 306.

11. Peebles, *John Peebles' American War*, p. 194.
12. Cantlie, *A History of the Army Medical Department*, vol. 1, p. 149.
13. Duncan, *Medical Men in the American Revolution*, p. 267.
14. Schoepff, *The Climate and Diseases of America*, p. 13.
15. Greenman, *Diary of a Common Soldier in the American Revolution*, p. 122.
16. Gibbes, *Documentary History of the American Revolution*, pp. 255–9.
17. Peebles, *John Peebles' American War*, p. 195; Duncan, *Medical Men in the American Revolution*, p. 268.
18. Urban, *Fusiliers*, pp. 152–3.
19. Peebles, *John Peebles' American War*, p. 194.
20. Martin, *Private Yankee Doodle*, p. 131.
21. Saffron, *Surgeon to Washington*, p. 53; Founders Online, General Orders 29 June 1778.
22. Duncan, *Medical Men in the American Revolution*, p. 268; Blanco, *Physician of the American Revolution*, pp. 190–1; Gillett, *The Army Medical Department*, p. 99; Founders Online, General Orders 29 June 1778.
23. Ferling, *Almost a Miracle*, pp. 309–13; Symonds, *A Battlefield Atlas of the American Revolution*, p. 67.
24. Gillett, *The Army Medical Department*, p. 102.
25. Bouvet, *Le Service de Santé Français*, pp. 5–8.
26. Ferling, *Almost a Miracle*, pp. 323–5.
27. Cantlie, *A History of the Army Medical Department*, vol. 1, p. 150.
28. Ferling, *Almost a Miracle*, pp. 355–7; Symonds, *A Battlefield Atlas of the American Revolution*, p. 69.
29. Ferling, *Almost a Miracle*, pp. 380–2; Symonds, *A Battlefield Atlas of the American Revolution*, p. 71.
30. Symonds, *A Battlefield Atlas of the American Revolution*, pp. 72–3.
31. Gillett, *The Army Medical Department*, pp. 106–8.
32. Ferling, *Almost a Miracle*, pp. 388–90.
33. Bouvet, *Le Service de Santé Français*, pp. 16–21.
34. Thacher, *Military Journal during the American Revolution*, p. 149.
35. Saffron, *Surgeon to Washington*, p. 55.
36. Gibson, *Bodo Otto and the Medical Background of the American Revolution*, p. 181; Blanco, *Physician of the American Revolution*, pp. 194–5.

37. Gillett, *The Army Medical Department*, p. 103.
38. Thacher, *Military Journal during the American Revolution*, pp. 171, 176.
39. Saffron, *Surgeon to Washington*, pp. 51, 56; Blanco, *Physician of the American Revolution*, p. 173.
40. Gillett, *The Army Medical Department*, p. 112.
41. Gillett, *The Army Medical Department*, p. 115.
42. Saffron, *Surgeon to Washington*, pp. 56–7.
43. Gillett, *The Army Medical Department*, pp. 99, 103, 111.
44. Gibson, *Bodo Otto and the Medical Background of the American Revolution*, p. 180.
45. Tilton, *Economical Observations on Military Hospitals*, pp. 49–54.
46. Saffron, *Surgeon to Washington*, p. 58.
47. Gibson, *Bodo Otto and the Medical Background of the American Revolution*, pp. 259–60.
48. Gillett, *The Army Medical Department*, p. 108.
49. Gibson, *Bodo Otto and the Medical Background of the American Revolution*, p. 168.
50. Blanco, *Physician of the American Revolution*, p. 50.
51. Gillett, *The Army Medical Department*, pp. 102–3; Blanco, *Physician of the American Revolution*, pp. 191–2, 194–5.
52. Gillett, *The Army Medical Department*, p. 102.
53. Becker, *Smallpox in Washington's Army*, p. 429.
54. Gillett, *The Army Medical Department*, pp. 110–11.
55. Saffron, *Surgeon to Washington*, p. 136.
56. Cantlie, *A History of the Army Medical Department*, vol. 1, p. 151.
57. Marshall, *The Health of the British Soldier in America*, p. 34; Marshall, *Hygiene and Disease*, p. 317.
58. Jackson, *A Treatise on the Fevers of Jamaica*, pp. 293–5.
59. Marshall, *The Health of the British Soldier in America*, p. 34.
60. Schoepff, *The Climate and Diseases of America*, p. 17; Chadwick, *Dr Johann David Schoepff*, p. 159.
61. Peebles, *John Peebles' American War*, pp. 289, 291, 296.
62. Hagist, *Noble Volunteers*, p. 143.
63. Marshall, *Hygiene and Disease*, p. 318; Hayes Me C 29/28.
64. Marshall, *The Health of the British Soldier in America*, p. 37.
65. Marshall, *The Health of the British Soldier in America*, p. 37; Hagist, *Noble Volunteers*, pp. 142–3, 156.

66. Peebles, *John Peebles' American War*, pp. 290, 296.

67. Cantlie, *A History of the Army Medical Department*, vol. 1, p. 151.

68. Peebles, *John Peebles' American War*, p. 299.

69. Marshall, *Hygiene and Disease*, p. 318.

70. Marshall, *The Health of the British Soldier in America*, p. 36.

71. Jackson, *A Treatise on the Fevers of Jamaica*, pp. 295–8.

72. Cantlie, *A History of the Army Medical Department*, vol. 1, p. 150.

73. Kopperman, *The Medical Dimension in Cornwallis's Army*, p. 377.

Chapter 11

1. Symonds, *A Battlefield Atlas of the American Revolution*, pp. 79–89; Ferling, *Almost a Miracle*, pp. 409–67.

2. Kopperman, *The Medical Dimension in Cornwallis's Army*, pp. 378–89; Cantlie, *A History of the Army Medical Department*, vol. 1, pp. 151–3.

3. Duncan, *Medical Men in the American Revolution*, p. 310.

4. Blanco, *Medicine in the Continental Army*, p. 692.

5. Duncan, *Medical Men in the American Revolution*, p. 326; Gillett, *The Army Medical Department*, p. 117.

6. Blanco, *Medicine in the Continental Army*, pp. 692–3; Gillett, *The Army Medical Department*, pp. 115–18.

7. Ferling, *Almost a Miracle*, p. 427.

8. Kopperman, *The Medical Dimension in Cornwallis's Army*, pp. 369–70, 313; Urban, *Fusiliers*, p. 188.

9. McCandless, *Revolutionary Fever*, p. 227.

10. McCandless, *Revolutionary Fever*, p. 231.

11. Fenn, *Pox Americana*, pp. 116–18.

12. Kopperman, *The Medical Dimension in Cornwallis's Army*, p. 369; Marshall, *The Health of the British Soldier in America*, pp. 39–40.

13. Peebles, *John Peebles's American War*, p. 367.

14. Urban, *Fusiliers*, p. 188.

15. Kopperman, *The Cheapest Pay*, p. 467.

16. Marshall, *The Health of the British Soldier in America*, pp. 40–1.

17. Marshall, *The Health of the British Soldier in America*, p. 41; Kopperman, *The Medical Dimension in Cornwallis's Army*, p. 371.

18. Jackson, *A Treatise on the Fevers of Jamaica*, pp. 299–300.

19. Jackson, *A Treatise on the Fevers of Jamaica*, p. 299.

20. McCandless, *Revolutionary Fever*, pp. 232, 238–9.

21. Jackson, *A Treatise on the Fevers of Jamaica*, p. 247.

22. Duncan, *Medical Men in the American Revolution*, p. 313.

23. McCandless, *Revolutionary Fever*, p. 231.

24. Ferling, *Almost a Miracle*, pp. 435–7; Symonds, *A Battlefield Atlas of the American Revolution*, p. 85; Urban, *Fusiliers*, p. 96.

25. Tarleton, *A History of the Campaigns*, pp. 31–2.

26. Ferling, *Almost a Miracle*, pp. 441–2; Fortescue, *A History of the British Army*, vol. 3, p. 319.

27. Cantlie, *A History of the Army Medical Department*, vol. 1, p. 152.

28. Kopperman, *The Medical Dimension in Cornwallis's Army*, p. 385.

29. Tarleton, *A History of the Campaigns*, p. 110.

30. Hill, NA 30/11/64, pp. 93–4.

31. Blanco, *Medicine in the Continental Army*, p. 693.

32. Duncan, *Medical Men in the American Revolution*, p. 315.

33. Duncan, *Medical Men in the American Revolution*, p. 319.

34. Duncan, *Medical Men in the American Revolution*, pp. 319–20; Ferling, *Almost a Miracle*, p. 428.

35. Symonds, *A Battlefield Atlas of the American Revolution*, p. 89; Ferling, *Almost a Miracle*, pp. 402–3.

36. Cantlie, *A History of the Army Medical Department*, vol. 1, pp. 153, 168.

37. Johnson, *Uzal Johnson, Loyalist*, pp. 74–7, 82–3.

38. Gillett, *The Army Medical Department*, p. 118.

39. Marshall, *The Health of the British Soldier in America*, pp. 41–2.

40. Peebles, *John Peebles's American War*, p. 406.

41. Marshall, *The Health of the British Soldier in America*, p. 41.

42. Kopperman, *The Medical Dimension in Cornwallis's Army*, p. 372.

43. Kopperman, *The Medical Dimension in Cornwallis's Army*, p. 372.

44. Jackson, *A Treatise on the Fevers of Jamaica*, pp. 302–3.

45. McCandless, *Revolutionary Fever*, p. 237.

46. Kopperman, *The Medical Dimension in Cornwallis's Army*, p. 373.

47. Kopperman, *The Medical Dimension in Cornwallis's Army*, pp. 387–8.

48. Duncan, *Medical Men in the American Revolution*, p. 313.

49. McCandless, *Revolutionary Fever*, p. 227.

50. Duncan, *Medical Men in the American Revolution*, pp. 322–4.

51. Founders Online, Greene to Washington, 7 December 1780.

52. Founders Online, Greene to Washington, 28 December 1780.

53. Saffron, *Surgeon to Washington*, p. 64; Blanco, *Physician of the American Revolution*, p. 202; Duncan, *Medical Men in the American Revolution*, pp. 329–31.
54. Gillett, *The Army Medical Department*, p. 118; Duncan, *Medical Men in the American Revolution*, p. 322.
55. Duncan, *Medical Men in the American Revolution*, p. 323.
56. Kopperman, *The Medical Dimension in Cornwallis's Army*, p. 385.
57. Hayes, Me C 29/37.
58. Kopperman, *The Medical Dimension in Cornwallis's Army*, p. 384.

Chapter 12

1. Saffron, *Surgeon to Washington*, p. 66; Duncan, *Medical Men of the American Revolution*, pp. 331–2; Gillett, *The Army Medical Department*, p. 44.
2. Duncan, *Medical Men of the American Revolution*, pp. 335–9; Saffron, *Surgeon to Washington*, pp. 66–9.
3. Cochrane, *Medical Department of the Revolutionary Army*, p. 249.
4. Duncan, *Medical Men of the American Revolution*, p. 337.
5. Cochrane, *Medical Department of the Revolutionary Army*, p. 249.
6. Cochrane, *Medical Department of the Revolutionary Army*, pp. 252–3.
7. Gillett, *The Army Medical Department*, p. 46.
8. Duncan, *Medical Men of the American Revolution*, p. 343.
9. Duncan, *Medical Men of the American Revolution*, pp. 339–40.
10. Brown, *The Medical Department of the United States Army*, p. 61; Blanco, *Medicine in the Continental Army*, pp. 693–4; Gillett, *The Army Medical Department*, p. 118.
11. Brown, *The Medical Department of the United States Army*, p. 62.
12. Ferling, *Almost a Miracle*, pp. 465–79; Founders Online, Greene to Washington, 13 January 1781; Urban, *Fusiliers*, p. 227.
13. Hayes, Me C 29/38/1–2; Jackson, *A Treatise on the Fevers of Jamaica*, pp. 303–4.
14. Marshall, *The Health of the British Soldier in America*, p. 43.
15. Kopperman, *The Medical Dimension in Cornwallis's Army*, p. 374.
16. Kopperman, *The Medical Dimension in Cornwallis's Army*, pp. 377–8.
17. Marshall, *The Health of the British Soldier in America*, p. 43.
18. Schoepff, *The Climate and Diseases of America*, p. 23.

19. Thacher, *Military Journal during the American Revolution*, p. 249.
20. Fenn, *Pox Americana*, pp. 124–5.
21. Cochrane, *Medical Department of the Revolutionary Army*, p. 252.
22. Symonds, *A Battlefield Atlas of the American Revolution*, p. 91; Ferling, *Almost a Miracle*, pp. 485–7.
23. Howell, *Robert Jackson*, p. 124.
24. Howell, *Robert Jackson*, p. 124.
25. Myers, *Cowpens Papers*, p. 28.
26. Myers, *Cowpens Papers*, p. 29.
27. Kopperman, *The Medical Dimension in Cornwallis's Army*, p. 386.
28. Myers, *Cowpens Papers*, p. 30.
29. Myers, *Cowpens Papers*, p. 30.
30. Howell, *Robert Jackson*, p. 124.
31. Urban, *Fusiliers*, p. 232.
32. Ferling, *Almost a Miracle*, pp. 496–9; Kopperman, *The Medical Dimension in Cornwallis's Army*, p. 374.
33. Lamb, *An Original and Authentic Journal*, p. 357.
34. Tarleton, *A History of the Campaigns*, pp. 278–9.
35. Read, *Reminiscences of William Read*, p. 290.
36. Hill, TNA PRO 30/11/5, p. 127.
37. Hill, TNA PRO 30/11/5, pp. 117–18, 180.
38. Kopperman, *The Medical Dimension in Cornwallis's Army*, pp. 391–2.
39. Newsome, *A British Orderly Book*, pp. 388–9.
40. Hill, TNA PRO 30/11/5, p. 118.
41. Ferling, *Almost a Miracle*, pp. 518–19; Symonds, *A Battlefield Atlas of the American Revolution*, p. 95.
42. Dann, *Revolution Remembered*, p. 220.
43. Ferling, *Almost a Miracle*, pp. 500–30; Symonds, *A Battlefield Atlas of the American Revolution*, pp. 99–105.
44. Clinton, *Narrative*, p. 12.
45. Marshall, *The Health of the British Soldier in America*, p. 43.
46. Kopperman, *The Medical Dimension in Cornwallis's Army*, pp. 375–6.
47. Urban, *Fusiliers*, p. 262; Jackson, *A Treatise on the Fevers of Jamaica*, p. 304.
48. Kopperman, *The Medical Dimension in Cornwallis's Army*, p. 394.
49. Marshall, *The Health of the British Soldier in America*, p. 45.
50. Kopperman, *The Medical Dimension in Cornwallis's Army*, p. 390.
51. Ewald, *Diary of the American War*, p. 328.

52. Bender, *American Pharmacy*, p. 43.
53. Gillett, *The Army Medical Department*, pp. 105–6.
54. Saffron, *Surgeon to Washington*, p. 185.
55. Gillett, *The Army Medical Department*, pp. 118–19.
56. Cantlie, *A History of the Army Medical Department*, vol. 1, p. 153.
57. Gillett, *The Army Medical Department*, pp. 46, 121.
58. Duncan, *Medical Men of the American Revolution*, p. 348.
59. Saffron, *Surgeon to Washington*, pp. 155–6, 161–2; Gillett, *The Army Medical Department*, p. 48.
60. Dunkerly, *Eutaw Springs*, p. 86; Ferling, *Almost a Miracle*, pp. 512–20; Symonds, *A Battlefield Atlas of the American Revolution*, p. 86.
61. Dunkerly, *Eutaw Springs*, pp. 79–82; Saberton, *Cornwallis Papers*, vol. 6, pp. 171–2.

Chapter 13

1. Ferling, *Almost a Miracle*, pp. 523–53; Symonds, *A Battlefield Atlas of the American Revolution*, pp. 105–8.
2. Duncan, *Medical Men of the American Revolution*, p. 351; Blanco, *Physician of the American Revolution*, p. 70.
3. Duncan, *Medical Men of the American Revolution*, p. 351; Gillett, *The Army Medical Department*, p. 121.
4. Blanton, *Medicine in Virginia*, pp. 274–6; Gillett, *The Army Medical Department*, pp. 122–3.
5. Gillett, *The Army Medical Department*, p. 122.
6. Saberton, *The Cornwallis Papers*, vol. 6, pp. 95–6.
7. Lemaire, *Coste*, p. 91; Bouvet, *Le service de santé Français*, p. 30; Trénard, *Un défenseur des hôpitaux militaires*, p. 154; Wooden, *Dr Jean François Coste*, pp. 400–1.
8. Bouvet, *Le service de santé Français*, pp. 87–91.
9. Bouvet, *Le service de santé Français*, pp. 91, 94–6.
10. Blanton, *Medicine in Virginia*, pp. 277–8.
11. Saberton, *The Cornwallis Papers*, vol. 6, p. 51.
12. Drew, *Commissioned Officers in the Medical Services of the British Army*, p. 41; Blanton, *Medicine in Virginia*, p. 284.
13. Cantlie, *A History of the Army Medical Department*, vol. 1, p. 155; Duncan, *Medical Men of the American Revolution*, p. 353.
14. Thacher, *Military Journal during the American Revolution*, pp. 272–3.

15. Thacher, *Military Journal during the American Revolution*, p. 275.
16. Martin, *Private Yankee Doodle*, p. 239.
17. Bouvet, *Le service de santé Français*, p. 89.
18. Bouvet, *Le service de santé Français*, pp. 90–1.
19. Döhla, *A Hessian Diary of the American Revolution*, pp. 163–4, 167–9.
20. Saberton, *The Cornwallis Papers*, vol. 6, p. 31.
21. Kopperman, *The Medical Dimension in Cornwallis's Army*, p. 376; Marshall, *The Health of the British Soldier in America*, pp. 44–5.
22. Jackson, *A Treatise on the Fevers of Jamaica*, pp. 304–5.
23. Döhla, *A Hessian Diary of the American Revolution*, p. 162.
24. Ewald, *Diary of the American War*, pp. 328, 337.
25. Kopperman, *The Medical Dimension in Cornwallis's Army*, pp. 388–9.
26. Saffron, *Surgeon to Washington*, p. 187.
27. Gillett, *The Army Medical Department*, pp. 121–2; Thacher, *Military Journal during the American Revolution*, p. 277.
28. Martin, *Private Yankee Doodle*, p. 238.
29. Blanton, *Medicine in Virginia*, p. 277.
30. Gillett, *The Army Medical Department*, pp. 123–4.
31. Gillett, *The Army Medical Department*, p. 122.
32. Lemaire, *Coste*, pp. 93–4.
33. Fenn, *Biological Warfare in Eighteenth-Century North America*, p. 1572.
34. Thacher, *Military Journal during the American Revolution*, p. 272.
35. Bonsal, *The Cause of Liberty*, p. 144.
36. Fenn, *Biological Warfare in Eighteenth-Century North America*, pp. 1572–3.
37. Duncan, *Medical Men of the American Revolution*, p. 358; Blanco, *Medicine in the Continental Army*, p. 694.
38. Gillett, *The Army Medical Department*, p. 123; Blanton, *Medicine in Virginia*, p. 277.
39. Duncan, *Medical Men of the American Revolution*, pp. 356–7.
40. Blanton, *Medicine in Virginia*, p. 275.
41. Gillett, *The Army Medical Department*, p. 123.
42. Blanton, *Medicine in Virginia*, p. 280.
43. Blanton, *Medicine in Virginia*, p. 283.
44. Gillett, *The Army Medical Department*, pp. 125–7.
45. Blanton, *Medicine in Virginia*, p. 284.
46. Bouvet, *Le service de santé Français*, p. 95.

47. Tilton, *Economical Observations on Military Hospitals*, pp. 63–4.

48. Saberton, *The Cornwallis Papers*, vol. 6, p. 121.

49. Blanton, *Medicine in Virginia*, p. 284.

50. Blanton, *Medicine in Virginia*, p. 284.

51. Ewald, *Diary of the American War*, p. 342.

52. Lengel, *The 10 Key Campaigns of the American Revolution*, p. 214.

53. Duncan, *Medical Men of the American Revolution*, pp. 355–6; Bouvet, *Le service de santé Français*, p. 93.

54. Fenn, *Pox Americana*, pp. 130–33.

55. Cantlie, *A History of the Army Medical Department*, vol. 1, pp. 160–1.

56. Gillett, *The Army Medical Department*, p. 127.

57. Founders Online, General Orders, 18 May 1782.

58. Duncan, *Medical Men of the American Revolution*, p. 366.

59. Saffron, *Surgeon to Washington*, p. 246.

60. Brown, *The Medical Department of the United States Army*, p. 67.

61. Duncan, *Medical Men of the American Revolution*, p. 366.

Chapter 14

1. Duncan, *Medical Men of the American Revolution*, p. 70.

2. Saffron, *Surgeon to Washington*, p. 52.

3. Cox, *A Proper Sense of Honor*, p. 135.

4. Reide, *A View of the Diseases of the Army*, p. 97.

5. Marshall, *The Health of the British Soldier in America*, pp. 17–18.

6. Peckham, The Toll of Independence, pp. xi–xii, 132–3; Blanco, *Medicine in the Continental Army*, p. 695.

7. Dawson, *Les 2112 Français morts*.

8. Cantlie, *A History of the Army Medical Department*, vol. 1, p. 156; Kopperman, *The British Army in North America*, p. 75; Ferling, *Almost a Miracle*, p. 559.

9. Cantlie, *A History of the Army Medical Department*, vol. 1, p. 156.

10. Ferling, *Almost a Miracle*, p. 559.

11. Tilton, *Economical observations on Military Hospitals*, p. 34.

12. Hamilton, *The Duties of a Regimental Surgeon Considered*, vol. 2, p. 305.

13. Blanco, *Military Medicine in Northern New York*, p. 43.

14. Marshall, *Hygiene and Disease*, p. 321.

15. Cantlie, *A History of the Army Medical Department*, vol. 1, p. 156.
16. Kopperman, *The British Army in North America*, pp. 75–6.
17. Reide, *A View of the Diseases of the Army*, p. 164.
18. Hagist, *Noble Volunteers*, p. 145.
19. Marshall, *The Health of the British Soldier in America*, pp. 185–6.
20. Duncan, *Medical Men of the American Revolution*, p. 374; Schoepff, *The Climate and Diseases of America*, p. 10.
21. Marshall, *The Health of the British Soldier in America*, pp. 186–7; Duncan, *Medical Men of the American Revolution*, pp. 373–4.
22. Marshall, *The Health of the British Soldier in America*, pp. 15–17.
23. Urban, *Fusiliers*, p. 175.
24. Schoepff, *The Climate and Diseases of America*, p. 22.
25. Saberton, *The Cornwallis Papers*, vol. 6, pp. 203–5.
26. Cox, *A Proper Sense of Honor*, p. 146.
27. Urban, *Fusiliers*, p. 293.
28. Tilton, *Economical observations on Military Hospitals*, p. 64.
29. Saffron, *Surgeon to Washington*, p. 232.
30. Fenn, *Pox Americana*, pp. 264–9.
31. Duffy, *Epidemics in Colonial America*, pp. 222, 237–8.
32. Tilton, *Economical observations on Military Hospitals*, p. 61.
33. Marshall, *Hygiene and Disease*, pp. 313–14.
34. Peebles, *John Peebles' American War*, p. 94.
35. Kopperman, *The British High Command and Soldiers' Wives in America*, p. 31.
36. Fenn, *Pox Americana*, pp. 107–8.
37. Jones, *Medicine in Virginia*, p. 258.
38. Ramsay, *A History of South Carolina*, vol. 2, pp. 92–4.
39. Duffy, *Epidemics in Colonial America*, p. 245.
40. Fenn, *Pox Americana*, p. 131.
41. Rees, *They Were Good Soldiers*, p. 16.
42. Rees, *They Were Good Soldiers*, pp. 16, 79–80.
43. Fenn, *Pox Americana*, p. 131.
44. Rush, *Medical Inquiries and Observations*, p. 211.
45. Rees, *They Were Good Soldiers*, p. 80.
46. Covey, *African American Slave Medicine*, p. 5.
47. Vogel, *American Indian Medicine*, pp. 62–3.

48. Rush, *Medical Inquiries and Observations*, p. 209.
49. Calloway, *The American Revolution in Indian country*, pp. 4–5.
50. Calloway, *The American Revolution in Indian country*, pp. 58–9.
51. Fenn, *Pox Americana*, p. 23.
52. Duffy, *Epidemics in Colonial America*, p. 244.
53. Fenn, *Pox Americana*, pp. 24–6.
54. Vogel, *American Indian Medicine*, pp. 262–3.
55. Furtado, *Plague, Pestilence and Pandemic*, pp. 202–3.
56. Spring, *With Zeal and with Bayonets Only*, pp. 31–2.
57. Blanco, *Military Medicine in Northern New York*, p. 52.
58. Becker, *Smallpox in Washington's Army*, p. 421.
59. McCandless, *Revolutionary Fever*, p. 243.
60. Fenn, *Pox Americana*, p. 88.
61. Becker, *Smallpox in Washington's Army*, pp. 420–1; Gibson, *Bodo Otto and the Medical Background of the American Revolution*, pp. 101–2.
62. Becker, *Smallpox in Washington's Army*, pp. 410, 414.
63. Cash, *The Canadian Military Campaign*, p. 55.
64. Becker, *Smallpox in Washington's Army*, p. 412.
65. Becker, *Smallpox in Washington's Army*, p. 412.
66. Gibson, *Bodo Otto and the Medical Background of the American Revolution*, p. 95; Reiss, *Medicine and the American Revolution*, p. 98.
67. Atkinson, *The British are Coming*, p. 294.
68. Fenn, *Pox Americana*, p. 82.
69. McCandless, *Revolutionary Fever*, p. 235.
70. McCandless, *Revolutionary Fever*, pp. 237–8; Dorney, *An Imprudent and Unnecessary Measure*, p. 157.
71. Kopperman, *The Medical Dimension in Cornwallis's Army*, p. 398.
72. McCandless, *Revolutionary Fever*, p. 242; Saberton, *The Cornwallis Papers*, vol. 6, p. 11.
73. Kopperman, *The Medical Dimension in Cornwallis's Army*, p. 392.
74. Marshall, *Hygiene and Disease*, p. 320.
75. McCandless, *Revolutionary Fever*, pp. 229–30, 238–42; Kopperman, *The Medical Dimension in Cornwallis's Army*, pp. 396–7.
76. Dorney, *An Imprudent and Unnecessary Measure*, p. 157.
77. McCandless, *Revolutionary Fever*, pp. 225–7; Kopperman, *The Medical Dimension in Cornwallis's Army*, pp. 397–8.

Chapter 15

1. Chaplin, *Medicine in England during the Reign of George III*, pp. 6–7.
2. Garrison, *Notes on the History of Military Medicine*, p. 137.
3. Tröhler, *To Improve the Evidence of Medicine*, p. 4.
4. Charters, *Disease, War, and the Imperial State*, p. 118.
5. Kopperman, *Medical Services in the British Army*, p. 455.
6. Marshall, *The Health of the British Soldier in America*, pp. 190–2.
7. Cantlie, *A History of the Army Medical Department*, vol. 1, p. 171.
8. Gibson, *Bodo Otto and the Medical Background of the American Revolution*, pp. 49–50; Shyrock, *Medicine and Society in America*, pp. 20–1, 33; Duncan, *Medical Men in the American Revolution*, pp. 7–8.
9. Blanco, *Medicine in the Continental Army*, pp. 695–6, 699; Applegate, *The American Revolutionary War Hospital Department*, pp. 303–4; Tilton, *Economical Observations on Military Hospitals*, p. vi.
10. Gillett, *The Army Medical Department*, p. 128.
11. Gillett, *The Army Medical Department*, p. 129.
12. Ranby, *Nature and Treatment of Gunshot Wounds*, pp. 31–3.
13. Howard, *Wellington's Doctors*, p. 68.
14. Gillett, *The Army Medical Department*, pp. 166–7.
15. Kopperman, *Medical Services in the British Army*, p. 453.
16. Marshall, *The Health of the British Soldier in America*, p. 84.
17. Howard, *Wellington's Doctors*, pp. 93–4.
18. Tilton, *Economical Observations on Military Hospitals*, p. vi.
19. Gillett, *The Army Medical Department*, pp. 163, 167.
20. Blanco, *Physician of the American Revolution*, p. 207.
21. Chaplin, *Medicine in England during the Reign of George III*, pp. 20–1.
22. Blanco, *Medicine in the Continental Army*, p. 697.
23. Blanco, *Wellington's Surgeon General*, p. 14.
24. Tröhler, *To Improve the Evidence of Medicine*, pp. 95–9; Billroth, *Historical Studies on the Nature and Treatment of Gunshot Wounds*, pp. 227–8; Kaufman, *Surgeons at War*, p. 15.
25. Blanco, *Physician of the American Revolution*, p. 208.
26. Tilton, *Economical Observations on Military Hospitals*, p. 62.
27. Warren, *The Life of John Warren M.D.*, pp. 243–4.
28. Binney, *A Remarkable Case of Gunshot-Wound*, pp. 574–5.

29. Jones, *Plain Concise Practical Remarks*, pp. 3–4; Ravitch, *Surgery in 1776*, p. 292; Shyrock, *Medicine and Society in America*, p. 59.

30. Griffenhagen, *Drug Supplies in the American Revolution*, pp. 130–4.

31. Reide, *A View of the Diseases of the Army*, pp. 361–96; Van Swieten, *The Diseases Incident to Armies*, pp. 104–12.

32. Griffenhagen, *Drug Supplies in the American Revolution*, pp. 126–7.

33. Blanco, *Medicine in the Continental Army*, p. 698.

34. Bender, *American Pharmacy in the Colonial and Revolutionary Periods*, pp. 35–6.

35. Abrams, *Revolutionary Medicine*, p. 58.

36. Blanton, *Medicine in Virginia*, p. 267.

37. Applegate, *Preventative Medicine in the American Revolutionary Army*, p. 381; Blanco, *Medicine in the Continental Army*, p. 697.

38. Marshall, *Hygiene and Disease*, pp. 328–31.

39. Tröhler, *To Improve the Evidence of Medicine*, p. 115.

40. Reide, *A View of the Diseases of the Army*, p. xii.

41. Charters, *Disease, War, and the Imperial State*, pp. 130–5.

42. McCausland, *Facts and Observations*, pp. 247–64; Maehle, *Four Early Clinical Studies*, pp. 151–3; Tröhler, *To Improve the Evidence of Medicine*, p. 53.

43. Robertson, *Observations on the Jail, Hospital or Ship Fever*, pp. 227–9; Maehle, *Four Early Clinical Studies*, pp. 153; Tröhler, *To Improve the Evidence of Medicine*, pp. 39–41.

44. Blanco, *Physician of the American Revolution*, pp. 209–10.

45. Shyrock, *Medicine and Society in America*, p. 60.

46. Duncan, *Medical Men in the American Revolution*, p. 6; Toner, *The Medical Men of the Revolution*, pp. 96–7.

47. Duncan, *Medical Men in the American Revolution*, p. 368.

48. Heaton, *Medicine in New York*, p. 37.

49. Gibson, *Bodo Otto and the Medical Background of the American Revolution*, p. 321.

50. Blanton, *Medicine in Virginia*, p. 268.

51. Applegate, *The Effect of the American Revolution*, pp. 551–3; Blanco, *Physician of the American Revolution*, p. 211.

52. Shyrock, *Medicine and Society in America*, p. 119; Abrams, *Revolutionary Medicine*, pp. 31–2.

53. Jones, *Medicine in Virginia*, p. 270.

54. Abrams, *Revolutionary Medicine*, pp. 236–7.

55. Fenn, *Pox Americana*, p. 30.

56. Fenn, *Pox Americana*, pp. 36, 38.

57. Becker, *Smallpox in Washington's Army*, pp. 390–1.

58. Hasselgren, *The Smallpox Epidemics in America*, p. 2838.

59. Blanco, *Medicine in the Continental Army*, p. 684; Becker, *Smallpox in Washington's Army*, p. 430.

60. Howe, *General Sir William Howe's Orderly Book*, pp. 148, 156; Becker, *Smallpox in Washington's Army*, p. 395; Fenn, *Pox Americana*, p. 49.

Bibliography

Abrams, JE, *Revolutionary Medicine : The Founding Fathers and Mothers in Sickness and in Health* (New York, 2013).

Advice to the Officers of the British Army (London, 1782).

Agnew, D, 'A Biographical Sketch of Governor Richard Howell of New Jersey', *The Pennsylvania Magazine of History and Biography*, vol. 22, no. 2, 1898, pp. 221–30.

An account of men lost and disabled in his Majesty's Land Service in North America and the West Indies from 1 November 1774, British Museum, Add. Mss. 38, 378.

Anburey, T, (ed. Jackman, S), *With Burgoyne from Quebec* (Toronto, 1963).

Applegate, HL, 'Preventive Medicine in the American Revolutionary Army', *Military Medicine*, vol. 126, 1961, pp. 379–82.

Applegate, HL, 'The American Revolutionary War Hospital Department', *Military Medicine*, vol. 126, 1961, pp. 296–306.

Applegate, HL, 'The Effect of the American Revolution on American Medicine', *Military Medicine*, vol. 126, 1961, pp. 551–3.

Applegate, HL, 'The Medical Administrators of the American Revolutionary Army', *Military Affairs*, vol. 25, 1961, pp. 1–10.

Atkinson, CT, 'Some Evidence for Burgoyne's Expedition'. *Journal of the Society for Army Historical Research*, vol. 26, no. 108, 1948, pp. 132–142.

Atkinson, R, *The British are Coming: The War for America 1775–1777* (London, 2019).

Balderston, M, Syrett, D, *The Lost War: Letters from British Officers during the American Revolution* (New York, 1975).

Bangs, I, *Journal of Lieutenant Isaac Bangs April 1 to July 29 1776* (Cambridge, 1890).

Barker, J, *The British in Boston* (Cambridge, 1924).

Beardsley, Ebenezer, 'History of a Dysentery in the 22nd Regiment of the late Continental Army', *The American Museum*, vol. 5, 1789, pp. 249–50.

Beck, J, *Medicine in the American Colonies* (New Mexico, 1966).

Becker, AM, 'Smallpox in Washington's Army', *The Journal of Military History*, vol. 68, no. 2, 2004, pp. 381–430.

Bell, WJ, *John Morgan Continental Doctor* (Philadelphia, 1965).

Bender GA, and Parascandola, J, *American Pharmacy in the Colonial and Revolutionary Periods* (Madison, 1977).

Billroth, T, *Historical Studies on the Nature and Treatment of Gunshot Wounds from the Fifteenth Century to the Present Time* (Connecticut, 1933).

Binney, B, 'A Remarkable Case of Gunshot-Wound', *The New York Medical and Physical Journal*, vol. 7, 1828, pp. 574–5.

Bird, H, *Attack on Quebec* (New York, 1968).

Blake, JB, Medicine and the Revolution, *Military Medicine*, vol. 149, no. 4, 1984, pp. 189–95.

Blanco, RL, 'American Army Hospitals in Pennsylvania during the Revolutionary War', *Pennsylvania History: A Journal of Mid-Atlantic Studies*, vol. 48, no. 4, 1981, pp. 347–368.

Blanco, RL, 'Henry Marshall (1775–1851) and the Health of the British Army', *Medical History*, vol. 14, no. 3, 1970, pp. 260–76.

Blanco, RL, 'Medicine in the Continental Army 1775–81', *Bulletin of the New York Academy of Medicine*, vol. 57, no. 8, 1981, pp. 677–701.

Blanco, RL, 'Military Medicine in Northern New York 1776–1777', *New York History*, vol. 63, no. 1, 1982, pp. 39–58.

Blanco, RL, *Physician of the American Revolution Jonathan Potts* (New York, 1979).

Blanco, RL, 'The Prestige of British Army Surgeons', *Societas: Review of Social History*. vol. 2, 1972, pp. 333–51.

Blanco, RL, 'The Soldier's Friend: Sir Jeremiah Fitzpatrick, Inspector of Health for Land Forces', *Medical History*, vol. 20, no. 4, 1976, pp. 402–21.

Blanco, RL, *Wellington's Surgeon General, Sir James McGrigor* (Durham, 1974).

Blanton, W, *Medicine in Virginia in the Eighteenth Century* (Richmond, 1931).

Bloch, H, 'Medical Conditions at Valley Forge', *New York State Medical Journal*, vol. 70, 1970, pp. 3010–3012.

Bloomfield, A, (ed. Lender, ME and Martin, JK), *Citizen Soldier: The Revolutionary War Journal of Joseph Bloomfield* (Yardley, 2018).

Bonsal, S, *The Cause of Liberty* (London, 1947).

Bouvet, M, *Le service de santé Français pendant la guerre d'indépendance des États-Unis* (Paris, 1933).

Brocklesby, R, *Oeconomical and Medical Observations* (London, 1764).

Brown, HE, *The Medical Department of the United States Army from 1775 to 1873* (Washington, 1873).

Brown, M (ed.), *Baroness Von Riedesel and the American Revolution. Journal of Tour of Duty* (Chapel Hill, 1965).

Brownlee, J, 'The Health of London in the Eighteenth Century', *Royal Society of Medicine Proceedings*, vol. 18, no. 2, 1925, pp. 73–85.

Butterfield, LH, *Letters of Benjamin Rush: Memoirs of the American Philosophical Society*, 2 vols. (Princeton, 1951).

Calloway, CG, *The American Revolution in Indian Country* (Cambridge, 1995).

Cantlie, N, *A History of the Army Medical Department*, Vol. I (Edinburgh, 1974).

Cash, P, *Medical Men at the Siege of Boston* (Philadelphia, 1973).

Cash, P, 'The Canadian Military Campaign of 1775–1776: Medical Problems and Effects of Disease', *Journal of the American Medical Association*, vol. 236, no. 1, 1976, pp.52–56.

Chadwick, JR, 'Dr Johann David Schoepf Surgeon of the Anspach-Bayreuth Troops in America 1777–1784', *Medical Library and Historical Journal*, vol. 3, 1905, pp. 157–165.

Chaplin, A, *Medicine in England during the Reign of George III* (London, 1919).

Charters, E, *Disease, War, and the Imperial State* (Chicago, 2014).

Chase, E, *The Beginnings of the American Revolution*, Vol. III (London, 1911).

Clarke, J, *An Impartial and Authentic Narrative of the Battle of Bunker Hill* (London, 1775).

Clinton, H, *Narrative relative to his conduct during part on his command of the King's Troops in North America* (London, 1783).

Cochrane, J, 'Medical Department of the Revolutionary Army', *Magazine of American History*, vol. 12, 1884, pp. 241–60.

Cohn, A, 'An Incident not Known to History: Squire Ferris and Benedict Arnold at Ferris Bay, October 13, 1776', *The Proceedings of the Vermont Historical Society*, vol. 55, no. 2, 1978, pp. 96–112.

Collins, VL, *A Brief Narrative of the Ravages of the British and Hessians at Princeton in 1776–1777* (Princeton, 1906).

Colombier, J, *Preceptes sur la Santé des gens de guerre ou Hygiene Militaire* (Paris, 1775).

Considerations upon the different modes of finding recruits for the Army (London, 1775).

Conway, S, *The British Isles and the War of American Independence* (Oxford, 2000).

Corner, GW, *The Autobiography of Benjamin Rush* (Princeton, 1948).

Corsar, KC, 'Letters from America, 1780 and 1781', *Journal for the Society of Army Historical Research*, vol. 20, no. 79, 1941, pp. 130–5.

Covey, HC, *African American Slave Medicine* (Lanham, 2008).

Cowen, DC, *Medicine in Revolutionary New Jersey* (Trenton, 1975).

Cox, C, *A Proper Sense of Honor: Service and Sacrifice in George Washington's Army* (Chapel Hill, 2004).

Curtis, EE, *The Organization of the British Army in the American Revolution* (New Haven, 1926).

Cutbush, E, *Observations on the Means of Preserving the Health of Soldiers and Sailors* (Philadelphia, 1808).

Cuthbertson, B, *A System for the Compleat Interior Management and Oeconomy of a Battalion of Infantry* (Bristol, 1776).

Dann, JC, *Revolution Remembered* (Chicago, 1986).

Davis, DB, 'Medicine in the Canadian Campaign of the Revolutionary War: The Journal of Doctor Samuel Fisk Merrick', *Bulletin of the History of Medicine*, vol. 44, no. 5, 1970.

Dawson, HB, 'Bunker's Hill', *The Historical Magazine*, vol. 3, 1868, pp. 321–442.

Dawson, W, 'Les 2112 Français morts au États-Unis de 1777 à 1783 en combattant pour l'indépendance américaine', *Journal de la Société des Américanistes*, vol. 28, 1935, pp. 1–154.

Digby, Lieutenant William, *Journal 1776–1777*. In Baxter, JP, *The British Invasion from the North, the Campaigns of Generals Carleton and Burgoyne from Canada 1776–1777* (Albany 1887).

Doblin, H, Lynn, MC, *An Eyewitness Account of the American Revolution and New England life: The Journal of JF Wasmus German Company Surgeon 1776–83* (Westport, 1990).

Döhla, JC, *A Hessian Diary of the American Revolution* (Oklahoma, 1983).

Dorney, DR, 'An Imprudent and Unnecessary Measure: Major Problems in the First Invasion of North Carolina, September–October 1780', *Journal of the Society for Army Historical Research*, vol. 99, 2021, pp. 152–69.

Drew, R, *Commissioned Officers in the Medical Services of the British Army 1660–1960*, Vol. I (London, 1968).

Drew, R, 'John Hunter and the Army', *Journal Royal Army Medical Corps*, vol. 113, 1967, pp. 5–17.

Drowne, HR, 'Dr Solomon Drowne, A Surgeon of the Revolution', *The Bulletin of the Fort Ticonderoga Museum*, vol. 8, no. 3, 1949, pp. 110–12.

Duffy, J, *Epidemics in Colonial America* (Baton Rouge, 1953).

Duffy, J, 'Public Health in New York City in the Revolutionary Period', *Journal of the American Medical Association*, vol. 236, no. 1, 1976, pp. 47–51.

Duncan, LC, *Medical Men in the American Revolution* [1775–1783] (Pennsylvania, 1931).

Dunkerly, RM, Boland, IB, *Eutaw Springs: The Final Battle of the American Revolution's Southern Campaign* (Columbia, 2017).

Elmer, E, 'Extracts from the Journal of Surgeon Ebenezer Elmer of the New Jersey Continental Line September 11–19, 1777', *The Pennsylvania Magazine of History and Biography*, vol. 35, no. 1, 1911, pp. 103–7.

Elmer, E, 'Journal of Ebenezer Elmer', *New Jersey Historical Society*, vol. 2, 1847, pp. 95–146, 150–4; vol. 3, 1848–1849, pp. 21–56, 90–102.

Essame, H, 'A Redcoat Surgeon's Account of 1776', *Military Review*, vol. 42, 1962, pp. 66–78.

Estes, JW, 'A Disagreeable and Dangerous Employment: Medical letters from the Siege of Boston 1775', *Journal of the History of Medicine and Allied Sciences*, vol. 31, no. 3, 1976, pp. 271–91.

Evelyn, WG, *Memoirs and Letters of Captain W Glanville Evelyn* (ed. Scull, GD) (Oxford, 1879).

Ewald, Captain J, *Diary of the American War: A Hessian Journal* (Yale, 1979).

Farnsworth, A, 'Amos Farnsworth's Diary', *Proceedings of the Massachusetts Historical Society*, vol. 12, 1898, pp. 74–107.

Fenn, EA, 'Biological Warfare in Eighteenth-Century North America: Beyond Jeffrey Amherst', *Journal of American History*, vol. 86, no. 4, 2000, pp. 1552–1580.

Fenn, EA, *Pox Americana* (New York, 2002).

Ferling, J, *Almost a Miracle: The American Victory in the War of Independence* (Oxford, 2007).

Fifth Report of the Commissioners of Military Enquiry: Army Medical Department (London, 1808).

Fitzpatrick, JC, *The Writings of George Washington* (Washington, 1931–44).

Forster, T, Diary of Thompson Forster. Staff Surgeon to His Majesty's Detached Hospital in North America. October 19th 1775 to October 23rd 1777. Transcribed in 1938 from the original in the possession of Robert Ethelstone Thompson Forster (in author's possession).

Fortescue, J, *A History of the British Army*, Vol. III. (London, 1902).

Founders Online, US National Archives and Records Administration, Washington (https://founders. archives. gov).

Frey, SR, *The British Soldier in America* (Austin, 1981).

Fried, S, *Rush: Revolution, Madness and the Visionary Doctor who became a Founding Father* (New York, 2018).

Frothingham, R, *History of the Siege of Boston* (Boston, 1849).

Furtado, P, *Plague, Pestilence and Pandemic* (London, 2021).

Garrison, FH, *Notes on the History of Military Medicine* (Hildesheim, 1970).

Gates, D, *The British Light Infantry Arm c. 1790–1815* (London, 1987).

General Hospital Department, TNA WO 28/6 (1778–1783).

General Orders re Hospitals, TNA WO 36/1.

Gibbes, RW, *Documentary History of the American Revolution* (Columbia, 1853).

Gibson, J, 'The Role of Diseases in the 70,000 Casualties in the American Revolutionary Army', *College of Physicians of Philadelphia Transactions and Studies*, vol. 17, 1949, pp. 121–7.

Gibson, JE, *Bodo Otto and the Medical Background of the American Revolution* (Springfield, 1937).

Gibson, JE, 'Captured Medical Men and Army Hospitals of the American Revolution', *Annals of Medical History*, vol. 10, 1938, pp. 382–9.

Gillett, MC, *The Army Medical Department 1775–1818* (Washington, 1981).

Gillman, CMB, 'Military Surgery in the American Revolution', *Journal of the Medical Society of New Jersey*, vol. 57, 1960, pp. 491–96.

Gooch, B, *A Practical Treatise on Wounds and other Chirurgical Subjects* (Norwich, 1767).

Gordon, MB, *Naval and Maritime Medicine during the American Revolution* (Ventnor, 1978).

Grant, A, *Observations on the Use of Opium in removing symptoms supposed to be owing to Morbid Irritability* (London, 1785).

Greenman, J, (ed. Bray, RC and Bushnell, PE), *Diary of a Common Soldier in the American Revolution 1775–1783* (DeKalb, 1978).

Griesemer, AD, 'John Jones M.D.: pioneer, patriot and founder of American surgery', *World Journal of Surgery*, vol. 34, no. 4, 2010, pp. 605–9.

Griffenhagen, GB, 'Drug Supplies in the American Revolution', *Bulletin of the United States National Museum*, vol. 225, 1961, pp. 110–134.

Guerra, F, *American Medical Bibliography 1639–1783* (New York, 1962).

Hagist, DH, *British Soldiers American War* (Yardley, 2014).

Hagist, DH, *Noble Volunteers: The British Soldiers who Fought the American Revolution* (Yardley, 2020).

Hagist, DH, 'Unpublished Writings of Roger Lamb Soldier in the American War of Independence', (Part 1), *Journal of the Society for Army Historical Research*, vol. 89, 2011, pp. 280–290.

Hamilton, R, *The duties of a regimental surgeon considered* (London, 1787).

Hasselgren, P-O, *Revolutionary Surgeons* (New York, 2021).

Hasselgren, P-O, 'The Smallpox Epidemics in America in the 1700s', *World Journal of Surgery*, vol. 44, 2020, pp. 2837–41.

Hayes, JM, Letters to Charles Mellish, University of Nottingham Library, Me C 29/1–60.

Headquarters Records America, TNA PRO WO 28/2–10.

Heaton, CE, 'Medicine in New York during the English Colonial Period 1664–1775', *Bulletin of the History of Medicine*, vol. 17, 1945, pp. 9–37.

Heighes, GL, 'Letters Relating to the Continental Military Hospitals in Lancaster County', *Lancaster County Historical Society Papers*, vol. 52, 1948, pp. 73–96.

Hill, Surgeon Hill's Report, TNA PRO 30/11/5.

Hill, Surgeon, to Cornwallis, TNA PRO 30/11/64.

Hope, R, Letters 1770–1782, TNA PRO 30/39/1.

Howard, MR, *Napoleon's Doctors: The Medical Services of the Grande Armée* (Stroud, 2006).

Howard, MR, *Walcheren 1809: The Scandalous Destruction of a British Army* (Barnsley, 2012).

Howard, MR, *Wellington's Doctors: The British Army Medical Services in the Napoleonic Wars* (Staplehurst, 2002).

Howe, W, General Orders by Major General The Honourable William Howe, *Collections of the New-York Historical Society*, 1883, pp. 251–585.

Howe, W, *General Sir William Howe's Orderly Book* (London, 1890).

Howell, HAL, 'Robert Jackson MD Inspector of Hospitals', *Journal Royal Army Medical Corps*, vol. 16, 1911, pp. 121–139.

Howell, HAL, 'The Story of the Army Surgeon and the Care of the Sick and Wounded in the British Army from 1715 to 1748', *Journal Royal Army Medical Corps*, vol. 22, 1914, pp. 320–4, 455–71.

Hudson, GL (ed.), *British Military and Naval Medicine 1600–1830* (Amsterdam, 2007).

Hughes, BP, *Firepower: Weapons Effectiveness on the Battlefield 1630–1850* (London, 1974).

Hume, IN, *1775: Another Part of the Field* (London, 1966).

Hunter, J, *A Treatise on the Blood, Inflammation and Gun-shot Wounds* (London, 1794).

Hunter, J, *Hunterian Reminiscences* (London, 1833).

Inman, G, 'George Inman's Narrative of the American Revolution', *The Pennsylvania Magazine of History and Biography*, vol. 7, no. 3, 1883, pp. 237–48.

Instructions for the Direction of the Hospital (September 1775), TNA PRO 30/55.

Jackson, R, *A System of Arrangement and Discipline for the Medical Department of Armies* (London, 1805).

Jackson, R, *A Systematic View of the Formation, Discipline and Economy of Armies* (London, 1804).

Jackson, R, *A Treatise on the Fevers of Jamaica* (London, 1791).

Jelenko, C, 'Emergency Medicine in Colonial America, Revolutionary War Casualties', *Annals of Emergency Medicine*, vol. 11, no. 1, 1982, pp. 40–43.

Johnson, U, (ed. Moss BG), *Uzal Johnson, Loyalist: Revolutionary War Diary of Surgeon to Ferguson's Command* (Blacksburg, 2000).

Jones, GW, 'Medicine in Virginia in Revolutionary Times', *Journal of the History of Medicine and Allied Sciences*, vol. 31, 1976, pp. 250–270.

Jones, J, *Plain Concise Practical Remarks on the Treatment of Wounds and Fractures* (Philadelphia, 1776).

Jordan JW, *The Military Hospitals at Bethlehem and Lititz during the Revolution* (Philadelphia, 1896).

Kaufman, MH, *Surgeons at War* (Westport, 2001).

Kemble, S, *Journal of Lieut. Col. Stephen Kemble 1773–1780* (Boston, 1972).

Kemensky, J and Gray, EG, *The Oxford Handbook of the American Revolution* (Oxford, 2012).

Kennedy, S, 'Letters of Dr Samuel Kennedy to his Wife in 1776', *Pennsylvania Magazine of History and Biography*, vol. 8, 1885, pp. 111–116.

Kennett, L, *The French Forces in America 1780-1783* (Westport, 1977).

Ketchum, RM, *Saratoga: Turning Point of America's Revolutionary War* (New York, 1997).

Ketchum, RM, *The Battle for Bunker Hill* (London, 1963).

Ketchum. RM, *The Winter Soldiers: The Battles for Trenton and Princeton* (London, 1973).

King, LS, *The Medical World of the Eighteenth Century* (Chicago, 1958).

Kirkland, FR, 'Journal of a Physician Lewis Beebe', *The Philadelphia Magazine*, vol. 59, no. 4, 1935, pp. 321–61.

Knox, R, 'Dr Robert Knox's Account of the Battle of Valcour October 11–13 1776', *Vermont History*, vol. 46, 1978, p. 141.

Kopperman, PE, 'Medical Services in the British Army 1742–1783', *Journal of the History of Medicine and Allied Sciences*, vol. 34, 1979, pp. 428–55.

Kopperman, PE, 'The British Army in North America and the West Indies 1755–83: A Medical Perspective', in Hudson, GL (ed.), *British Military and Naval Medicine 1600–1830* (Amsterdam, 2007).

Kopperman, PE, 'The British High Command and Soldiers' Wives in America 1755–1783', *Journal of the Society for Army Historical Research*, vol. 60, no. 24, 1982, pp. 14–34.

Kopperman, PE, 'The Cheapest Pay: Alcohol Abuse in the Eighteenth-Century British Army', *The Journal of Military History*, vol. 60, no. 3, 1996, pp. 445–70.

Kopperman, PE, 'The Medical Dimension in Cornwallis's Army 1780-1781', *North Carolina Historical Review*, vol. 89, 2012, pp. 367–398.

Kopperman, PE, 'The Numbers Game: Health Issues in the Army that Burgoyne Led to Saratoga', *New York History*, vol. 88, no. 3, 2007, pp. 256–85.

Lamb, R, *An Original and Authentic Journal of Occurrences during the Late American War* (Dublin, 1809).

Lamb, R, *Memoir of his Own Life* (Dublin, 1811).

Lemaire, J-F, *Coste: Premier Médecin des Armées de Napoléon* (Paris, 1997).

Lengel, EG, *The 10 Key Campaigns of the American Revolution* (Washington, 2020).

Lenihan, P, *Fluxes, Fevers, and Fighting Men* (Warwick, 2019).

Lesser, CH, *The Sinews of Independence; Monthly strength reports of the Continental Army* (Chicago, 1976).

Lind, J, *A Treatise on the Scurvy* (Edinburgh, 1753).

Lind, J, *An Essay on Diseases* (London, 1768).

Lister, J, *The Concord Fight: Being so Much of the Narrative of Jeremy Lister of the 10th Regiment of Foot* (Cambridge, 1931).

Lloyd, C and Coulter, JS, *Medicine and the Navy 1200–1900*, Vol. 3 (Edinburgh, 1961).

Lushington, SR, *The Life and Services of General Lord Harris, G.C.B.* (London, 1840).

Mackenzie, F, *A British Fusilier in Revolutionary Boston* (New York, 1969).

Mackesy, P, *The War for America 1775–1783* (Lincoln, 1992).

Maehle, A-H, 'Four Early Clinical Studies to assess the effects of Peruvian bark', *Journal of the Royal Society of Medicine*, vol. 106, 2013, pp. 150–55.

Marshall, T, 'Hygiene and Disease: The British Army in North America 1775–81', *Journal of the Society for Army Historical Research*, vol. 88, 2010, pp. 311–331.

Marshall, T, 'Surgeons Reconsidered: Military Medical Men of the American Revolution', *Canadian Bulletin of Medical History*, vol. 27, no. 2, 2010, pp. 299–319.

Marshall, T, 'The Health of the British Soldier in America 1775–1781', PhD Thesis (McMaster, 2006).

Marston, D, *The American Revolution 1774–1783* (Oxford, 2002).

Martin, H, *A Narrative of a Discovery of a Sovereign Specific for the Cure of Cancers* (Philadelphia, 1782).

Martin, JP (ed. GE Scheer), *Private Yankee Doodle* (Boston, 1962).

McCandless, P, 'Revolutionary Fever: Disease and War in the Lower South 1776–1783', *Transactions of the American Clinical and Climatological Association*, vol. 118, 2007, pp. 225–49.

McCausland, RM (Surgeon to the King's or 8th Regiment of Foot), 'Facts and Observations on Different Medical Subjects', *Medical Commentaries*, 1781, pp. 247–96.

Medical Department Letters 1766–1775, PRO, Adm. 97/86–87 Admiralty Office.

Medical Department 1781–1789, PRO, WO 7/96 War Office.

Middleton, WS, 'Medicine at Valley Forge', *Annals of Medical History*, vol. 3, no. 6, 1941, pp. 461–86.

Monro, D, *An Account of the Diseases which were Most Frequent in the British Military Hospitals in Germany* (London, 1764).

Monro, D, *Observations on the Means of Preserving the Health of Soldiers* (London, 1780).

Morgan, J, *A Vindication of his Public Character in the Station of Director-General* (Boston, 1777).

Myers, TB, *Cowpens Papers being Correspondence of General Morgan and the Prominent Actors* (Charleston, 1881).

Nadeau, G, 'A German Military Surgeon in Rutland Massachusetts during the Revolution', *Bulletin History of Medicine*, vol. 18, 1945, pp. 243–300.

Neimeyer, CP, *America Goes to War: A Social History of the Continental Army* (New York, 1996).

Newsome, AR, 'A British Orderly Book 1780-1781', *North Carolina Historical Review*, vol. 9, 1932, pp. 57–78, 163–86, 273–98, 366–9.

Nooth, JM, Letters written by John Mervyn Nooth, Physician with the Army in North America 1778–1782, NAM 1992-10-43.

Norwood, WMF, 'Deborah Sampson alias Robert Shirtliff Fighting Female of the Continental Line', *Bulletin of the History of Medicine*, vol. 31, no. 2, 1957, pp. 147–61.

O'Callaghan, EB, *Orderly Book of Lieut. Gen. John Burgoyne* (Albany, 1860).

Owen, M, *Medical Department of the United States Army during the Revolution* (New York, 1920).

Peckham, HH, *The Toll of Independence* (Chicago, 1974).

Peebles, J, (ed. Gruber, ID), *John Peebles' American War 1776–1782* (Stroud, 1998).

Perron, Joachim du, Comte de Revel, *Journal Particuliere d'une Campagne aux Indies Occidentales (1781–1782)* (Paris, 1898).

Pfister, A, *The Voyage of the First Hessian Army from Portsmouth to New York 1776* (New York, 1915).

Philbrick, N, *Bunker Hill: A City, a Siege, a Revolution* (London, 2014).

Pindell, R, 'A Militant Surgeon of the Revolution: Some Letters of Richard Pindell', *Maryland Historical Magazine*, vol. 18, 1923, pp. 309–23.

Pringle, J, *Observations on the Diseases of the Army* (London, 1775).

Ramsay, D, *A History of South Carolina* (Charleston, 1809).

Ranby, J, *Nature and Treatment of Gunshot Wounds* (Philadelphia, 1776).

Ravitch, MM, 'Surgery in 1776', *Annals of Surgery*, vol. 186, no. 3, 1977, pp. 291–300.

Read, W, Reminiscences of William Read, in Gibbes, RW, *Documentary History of the American Revolution* (New York, 1857), pp. 248–293.

Records of Military Headquarters, America, General Hospital Department, TNA WO 28/6

Rees, JU, *They Were Good Soldiers: African-Americans Serving in the Continental Army, 1775–1783* (Warwick, 2019).

Reide, TD, *A View of the Diseases of the Army in Great Britain, America, The West Indies and on Board of King's Ships and Transports* (London, 1793).

Reiss, O, *Medicine and the American Revolution: How Diseases and their Treatments Affected the Colonial Army* (Jefferson, 1998).

Rhodehamel, J, *George Washington: The Wonder of the Age* (New Haven, 2017).

Riedesel, Baroness F, *Letters and Journals* (New York, 1968).

Roberts, A, *George III* (London, 2021).

Roberts, RK, *March to Quebec* (Garden City, 1953).

Robertson, J, 'Remarks on the Management of the Scalped-Head', *The Philadelphia Medical and Physical Journal*, vol. 2, part 2, 1806, pp. 27–30.

Robertson, R, *Observations on the Jail, Hospital or Ship Fever* (London, 1783).

Rogers, BO, 'Surgery in the Revolutionary War: Contributions of John Jones MD (1729–1791)', *Plastic Reconstructive Surgery*, vol. 49, no. 1, 1972, pp. 1–13.

Rowley, W, *Medical Advice for the use of the army and navy in the present American expedition* (London, 1776).

Rush, B, *Directions for Preserving the Health of Soldiers* (Philadelphia, 1777).

Rush, B, *Medical Inquiries and Observations* (Philadelphia, 1789).

Saberton, I, *The Cornwallis Papers: The Campaigns of 1780 and 1781*, vol. VI (Uckfield, 2010).

Sabourin, VM, 'The War of Independence: a surgical algorithm for treatment of head injury in the continental army', *Journal of Neurosurgery*, vol. 124, no. 1, 2016, pp. 234–43.

Saffron, M, 'Rebels and Disease. The New York Campaign 1776'. *Academy of Medicine New York Bulletin*, vol. 13, 1967, pp. 104–18.

Saffron, M, *Surgeon to Washington, Dr John Cochrane (New York, 1977)*.

Schmitz, R, *The Medical and Pharmaceutical Care of the Hessian Troops in the American Revolution*, in Bender GA, and Parascandola, J, *American Pharmacy in the Colonial and Revolutionary Periods* (Madison, 1977).

Schoepff, JD, *The Climate and Diseases of America* (Boston, 1875).

Secretary-at-War, Out-Letters, America, TNA WO 4/275.

Selevan, IC, 'Nurses in American History: The Revolution', *American Journal of Nursing*, vol. 75, no. 4, 1975, pp. 592–4.

Senter, I, *The Journal of Isaac Senter* (Tarrytown, 1915).

Shippen, W, 'Text of William Shippen's First Draft of a Plan for the Organization of the Military Hospital During the Revolution', *Annals of Medical History*, vol. 1, 1917–18, pp. 174–6.

Shryock, RH, *Medicine and Society in America: 1660–1860* (Ithaca, 1960).

Shute, D, 'The Journal of Dr Daniel Shute, Surgeon in the Revolution 1781–1782', *New England Genealogical Register*, vol. 84, 1930, pp. 383–9.

Simes, T, *The Military Guide for Young Officers* (London, 1781).

Spiegel, AD, 'James McHenry, M.D.: Physician, Patriot, Politician and Poet', *Journal of Community Health*, vol. 24, no. 4, 2003, pp. 281–302.

Spring, MH, *With Zeal and with Bayonets Only: The British Army on Campaign in North America 1775–1783* (Norman, 2008).

Stacy, KR, 'Venereal Disease in the 84th Regiment of Foot during the American Revolution', *Journal of the Society for Army Historical Research*, vol. 77, no. 312, 1999, pp. 237–9.

Starbuck, DR, 'Military Hospitals on the Frontier of Colonial America', *Expedition*, vol. 39, no. 1, 1997, pp. 33–45.

State of the Troops which arrived in the Fleet from England 1779, TNA CO 5/98.

Stedman, C, *The History of the American War* (Dublin, 1794).

Steuben, Baron FW von, *Regulations for the Order and Discipline of the Troops of the United States* (Boston, 1807).

Stewart, J, (ed. Wickman, D), 'A Most Unsettled Time on Lake Champlain: The October 1776 Journal of Jahiel Stewart', *The Proceedings of the Vermont Historical Society*, vol. 64, no. 2, 1996, pp. 89–98.

Sullivan, T, (Boyle, JL, ed.), *From Redcoat to Rebel; The Thomas Sullivan Journal* (2019).

Symonds, CL, Clipson, WJ, *A Battlefield Atlas of the American Revolution* (1986).

Syrett, D, 'Living Conditions on the Navy Board's Transports during the American War 1775–1783', *Mariner's Mirror*, vol. 55, 1969, pp. 87–94.

Tarleton, Lt-Col, *A History of the Campaigns of 1780 and 1781 in the Southern Provinces of North America* (London, 1787).

Thacher, J, *Military Journal during the American Revolution from 1775 to 1783* (Mineola, 2019).

1776: The British Story of the American Revolution (Greenwich, 1976).

Thursfield, H, 'Smallpox in the American War of Independence', *Annals of Medical History.* vol. 2, 1940, pp. 312–18.

Tilton, J, *Economical Observations on Military Hospitals* (Wilmington, 1803).

Toner, JM, *The Medical Men of the Revolution* (Philadelphia, 1876).

Torres-Reyos, R, *Morristown National Historical Park: 1779–1780 Encampment. A Study of Medical Services* (Washington, 1971).

Townsend, J, *Some Account of the British army under the command of General Howe and of the Battle of Brandywine* (Philadelphia, 1846).

Trénard, L, 'Un défenseur des hôpitaux militaires: Jean-François Coste', *Revue du Nord*, vol. 75, 1993, pp. 149–180.

Tröhler, U, *To Improve the Evidence of Medicine: The 18th Century British origins of a critical approach* (London, 2000).

Urban, M, *Fusiliers: How the British Army Lost America but Learnt to Fight* (London, 2008).

Van Swieten, G, *The Diseases Incident to Armies* (Philadelphia, 1776).

Vernon, HA, 'Medical Crisis at Fort Niagara 1779–80', *Niagara Frontier*, vol. 24, 1977, pp. 92–3.

Vess, DH, *Medical Revolution in France 1789–1796* (Gainesville, 1975).

Vogel, VJ, *American Indian Medicine* (Norman, 1990).

Waldo, A, 'Valley Forge 1777-78. Diary of Surgeon Albigence Waldo of the Connecticut Line', *Pennsylvania Magazine of History and Biography*, vol. 21, 1897, pp. 199–323.

Wangensteen, OH and SD, *The Rise of Surgery: From Empiric Craft to Scientific Discipline* (Minneapolis, 1978).

Ward, HM, *The War for Independence and the Transformation of American Society* (London, 1999).

Waring, JI, 'Medicine in Charleston at the Time of the Revolution', *Journal of the American Medical Association*, vol. 236, no. 1, 1976, pp. 31–34.

Warren, E, *The Life of John Warren M.D.* (Boston, 1874).

Weedon, G, *Valley Forge Orderly Book* (New York, 1902).

Wilbur, CK, *Revolutionary Medicine 1700–1800* (Chester, 1980).

Willard, MW, *Letters on the American Revolution 1774–1776* (Port Washington, 1968).

Williams, WH, 'Independence and Early American Hospitals 1751-1812', *Journal of the American Medical Association*, vol. 236, no. 1, 1976, pp. 35–39.

Wooden, AC, 'Dr Jean François Coste and the American Army in the American Revolution', *Delaware Medical Journal*, vol. 48, no. 7, 1976, pp. 397–404.

Wooden, AC, 'The Wounds and Weapons of the Revolutionary War 1775–1783', *Delaware Medical Journal*, vol. 44, no. 3, 1972, pp. 59–65.

Wurtele, FC, *Blockade of Quebec in 1775–1776 by the American Revolutionists* (Quebec, 1905).

Young, W, 'Journal of Sergeant William Young', *Pennsylvania Magazine of History and Biography*, vol. 8, no. 3, 1884, pp. 255–278.

Index